CLOSED RHINOPLASTY

ILLUSTRATED TECHNICAL MANUAL

ACTA MEDICA

If you wish to consult the entire catalogue of Acta Medica, go to the website www.griffineditore.it in the plastic surgery section, or scan the QR Code

CLOSED RHINOPLASTY
ILLUSTRATED TECHNICAL MANUAL

Editorial coordination: Giuseppe Roccucci
Writing and editing: Lucia Oggianu
Graphic design and layout: Marco Redaelli

Printing: Starprint srl
Printed in Italy: march 2022

With the collaboration of
Paolo Gasperoni
Vania Moro Packo
Paolo Messercola for anaesthesia in rhinoplasty
Valentina Pino for the revision and for the chapter on instrumental tests

English translation by Valentina Pino and Caterina Alberti

PUBLISHER
Griffin srl unipersonale
Via Cavalluccio 2/B 22060 Carimate (Como)
Tel. 031.789085
customerservice@griffineditore.it
www.griffineditore.it

ISBN 978-88-97438-71-7

To my wife Cristiana and to my daughters Sandy and Giorgia

You can do better, but the worst is in ambush

If there are two ways to do one thing, the simplest one is the one that will give the least problems (Eugenio Farallo)

Rhinoplasty is a relatively simple procedure with which it is difficult to have constant results (Gustav Aufricht)

This work is dedicated to my past, present and future family members and to those who have been close to me with affection and competence in my profession.

This book is intended to be a practical guide to closed rhinoplasty and is aimed at those who have not yet fully understood it's philosophy and therefore think it is a very difficult operation. I tried to give a clear view of the nose in its anatomical, functional and surgical aspects, so as not to lease areas of shadow that could be a source of doubts.
Having carried out my practice as a plastic surgeon in a predominantly european context, I am unfamiliar with ethnic rhinoplasty and therefore I refer to other publications the in-depth information necessary to perform it. Secondary rhinoplasty, on the other hand, is the practical application of a whole wealth of experience that has been made over the years and therefore it is almost impossible to bring back to a single algorithm the decisions to be made. With the regain of old techniques, the so-called open rhinoplasty have been proposed again. In open rhinoplasty the subversion of the normal human anatomy of the nose make it impossible for those called to correct noses in which this technique was applied to be reasonably sure not to cause further damage or to perform the correction successfully.
At the moment that I'm writing, Cottle's rhinoplasty proposed in 1954 is back in vogue and it is called "preservation rhinoplasty". Repurposing this technique constitutes a backtrack on the part of the major popularizers of "open rhinoplasty". With time and experience everyone will come to decide which one work best in his hands.

In my hands, closed rhinoplasty gives excellent results and I think that repurposing it will bring many colleagues back to choosing this approach which is reliable and satisfying.
Rhinoplasty, even if well performed, may not give the desired result. It is therefore necessary to know that further adjustments are possible, even if not frequent. The rhinoplasty according to Joseph, from which the one performed by me derives, which limits itself to changing the morphology of the various anatomical components, can be further retouched, even by those who have not performed primary rhinoplasty. Those who undertake this task will not find themselves facing a new entity, which happens in the "open" case, where there is an unknown anatomy, with cicatricial stratifications and grafts that turn the product of this technique a surprise. Instead, it may refer to an anatomy that has not been much altered and which therefore constitutes a new reliable starting point, which allows further modifications without fear of taking risks.
You need a good knowledge of nasal anatomy and physiology to perform a rhinoplasty. Texts that explore these topics are available, and it is advisable to have a broad knowledge of them, since the correction of the nose will recur countless times in the life of a plastic surgeon. In his book we will not dwell on the anatomical description of the nose, which can be found in any basic book, but will explain the key elements to perform a rhinoplasty or a rhinoseptoplasty that does not give functional problems. Rhinoplasty is a logical operation, not an imaginative one. The steps to follow with the relative useful comments to understand what are the reasons of what is done are explained In this book.

by Doctor Giuseppe Leopizzi
Specialist in Plastic Surgery and Otolaryngology

For me it is a particular source of pride to write the presentation of this work by my friend Carlo Gasperoni, to whom I am linked by an old friendship. We met in the distant past in residency school in Parma with Prof. Alberto Azzolini. Since then we always stayed in close contact, so I was able to experience Carlo's professional technical evolution first hand, which led him to be, in a short time, one of the most appreciated plastic surgeons in Italy and abroad. It is from this wide experience that the idea of writing this text on rhinoplasty arose, being it a much discussed topic and, in my opinion, the most fascinating one in aesthetic surgery. It is not sufficient to simply learn the surgical technique to make a good nose, but it is necessary to get inside the physiognomy of our patient, understand it in order to preserve it. Only by achieving a respectful result of this principle, a true aesthetic gesture is made and this text leads us precisely on this complex path. The so-called close rhinoplasty appears at first sight out of fashion, in a world where the open way reigns. But it is precisely through the closed path and only through it, that maximum naturalness can be obtained, thanks to the fact that the structures that make up the soft triangle, the interdomal and medial intercrural ligaments, usually interrupted with the open path, are respected. None of us knows the answers to the several problems about rhinoplasty, but certainly all of those who are interested about this topic, independently from their beliefs about the technique to be used, are interested about the expansion of their notions in order to expand their surgical horizons. This book constitutes an unpublished and excellent guide for those who do not settle for only making a nose, but want to make the right nose for that face.

Introduction

Acknowledgements

Preface

CHAPTER 1 Medical history pag. 10

CHAPTER 2 Nose inspection pag. 12

CHAPTER 3 Photographic documentation pag. 21

CHAPTER 4 Nasal cavity inspection and functional considerations pag. 23

CHAPTER 5 Instrumental tests pag. 32

CHAPTER 6 Anatomical considerations pag. 34

CHAPTER 7 Execution pag. 52

CHAPTER 8 Septoplasty pag. 125

CHAPTER 9 Turbinates treatment pag. 140

CHAPTER 10 Osteotomies pag. 145

CHAPTER 11 Shaping the base of the nostrils pag. 158

CHAPTER 12 Dressing pag. 162

CHAPTER 13 Nasal packing pag. 169

CHAPTER 14 Postoperative period pag. 171

CHAPTER 15 Synechiae pag. 173

CHAPTER 16 Post-rhinoplasty breathing problems pag. 174

CHAPTER 17 Spreader grafts pag. 176

CHAPTER 18 Use of cartilage grafts. How and why pag. 183

CHAPTER 19 Alloplastic materials pag. 194

CHAPTER 20 The humpless or saddle nose pag. 203

CHAPTER 21 Cases pag. 206

CHAPTER 1

Medical history

A medical history is the first essential step and should cover any trauma, breathing, allergies and any episodes of nosebleeds.

Usually, a nose that is always blocked on one side suggests a mechanical obstruction. However, breathing difficulties may be subjectively important, even if the anatomical situation does not appear objectively abnormal. Worsening in the breathing at bedtime indicates excessive swelling of the turbinates, which does not necessarily occur during the day. If the nose closes up in certain environments, the cause may be an allergy or very delicate mucous membranes that suffer from irritation caused by a wide variety of substances.

Difficulty in breathing given by allergens usually occurs over periods. Certain allergies, such as the one linked to the widespread presence of mites, tend to be always present with more or less accentuated recrudescence in dusty environments or at times when the heating of the rooms moves the air with its convective movements, putting into circulation the allergens that were deposited on the floor surface. In these cases it is advisable to have an allergist examination to make the patient understand that it is possible that the intervention does not completely solve the breathing problems, because in reality they are due to other causes, not just related to an abnormal conformation of the nose. The restoration of a normal anatomical situation contributes in any case to an improvement of symptoms due to concomitant allergic factors.

The nasal bleeding (epistaxis) that the patient sometimes reports in the anamnesis may be occasional or repeated, unilateral or bilateral. In both cases it may be due to varices, but environmental factors such as being in places that are too dry or where irritants are present, may be also taken into account. Hypertensive crises can also cause nosebleeds. Rhinoscopy will be decisive in determining whether irritated mucous membranes or varicose veins are involved. The presence of angiomas is very rare, and particularly dangerous are those of the skull base, because they can be responsible for profuse bleedings that are difficult to stop. They are usually not diagnosed before surgery, but if in doubt, a CT scan will be decisive for the diagnosis.

CHAPTER 2

Nose inspection

The nose should be observed in order to evaluate the thickness and quality of the skin, and whether asymmetries are present.

Thick skin will take much longer to settle than thin skin. The skin is normally thicker in the lower half of the nose because it is richer in sebaceous glands and will therefore take longer to settle after rhinoplasty.

Asymmetries can be acquired through recent trauma, or they can be due to growth under the influence of a deviated septum. Acquired asymmetries are easier to correct, while those caused by asymmetrical growth are more difficult because in these cases the bones, and especially the cartilages, have grown asymmetrically and with different curvatures between right and left. When the differences are caused by asymmetrical cartilage curvatures, it is difficult and sometimes impossible to achieve perfect symmetry.

The width must be assessed. If excessive, suggests a malformation or bone cyst, the diagnosis of which can be made by a CT scan. It should be borne in mind that when a hump is reduced, the nasal pyramid is transformed into a truncated pyramid, and it will therefore be necessary to carry out osteotomies to return to a pyramid shape. The nose will therefore be narrower than at the start, but since a new harmony will be created with rhinoplasty, the narrowing of the pyramid will not be evident, except on careful examination of the pre-operative photos.

The dorsum may have a hump, a normal or very low profile.

A hump should be reduced, while a low back should be increased instead.

The position of the nasion (the root of the nose) should also be observed: it may be normal (fig. 1), more posterior (fig. 2a) or more anterior (fig. 2b).

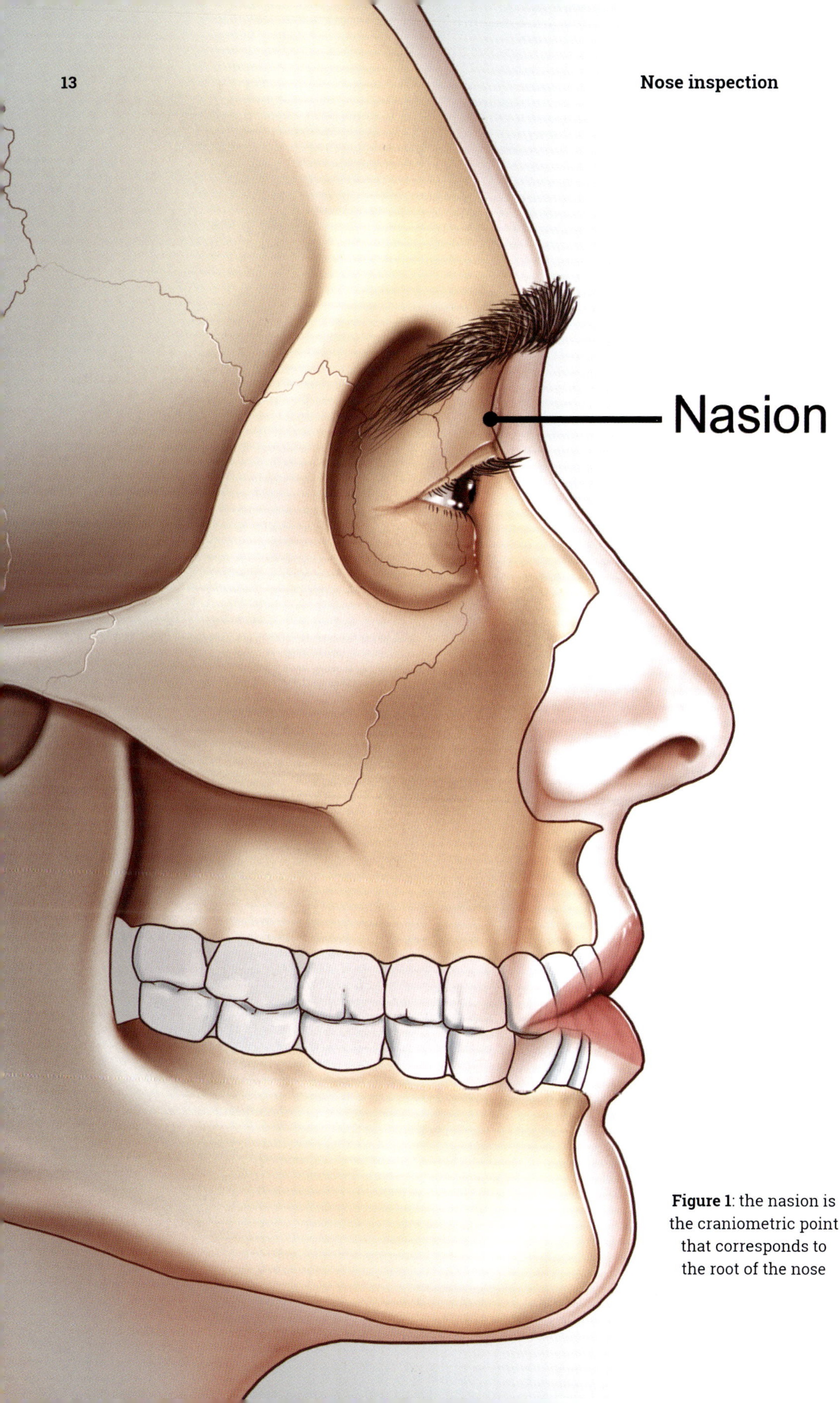

Figure 1: the nasion is the craniometric point that corresponds to the root of the nose

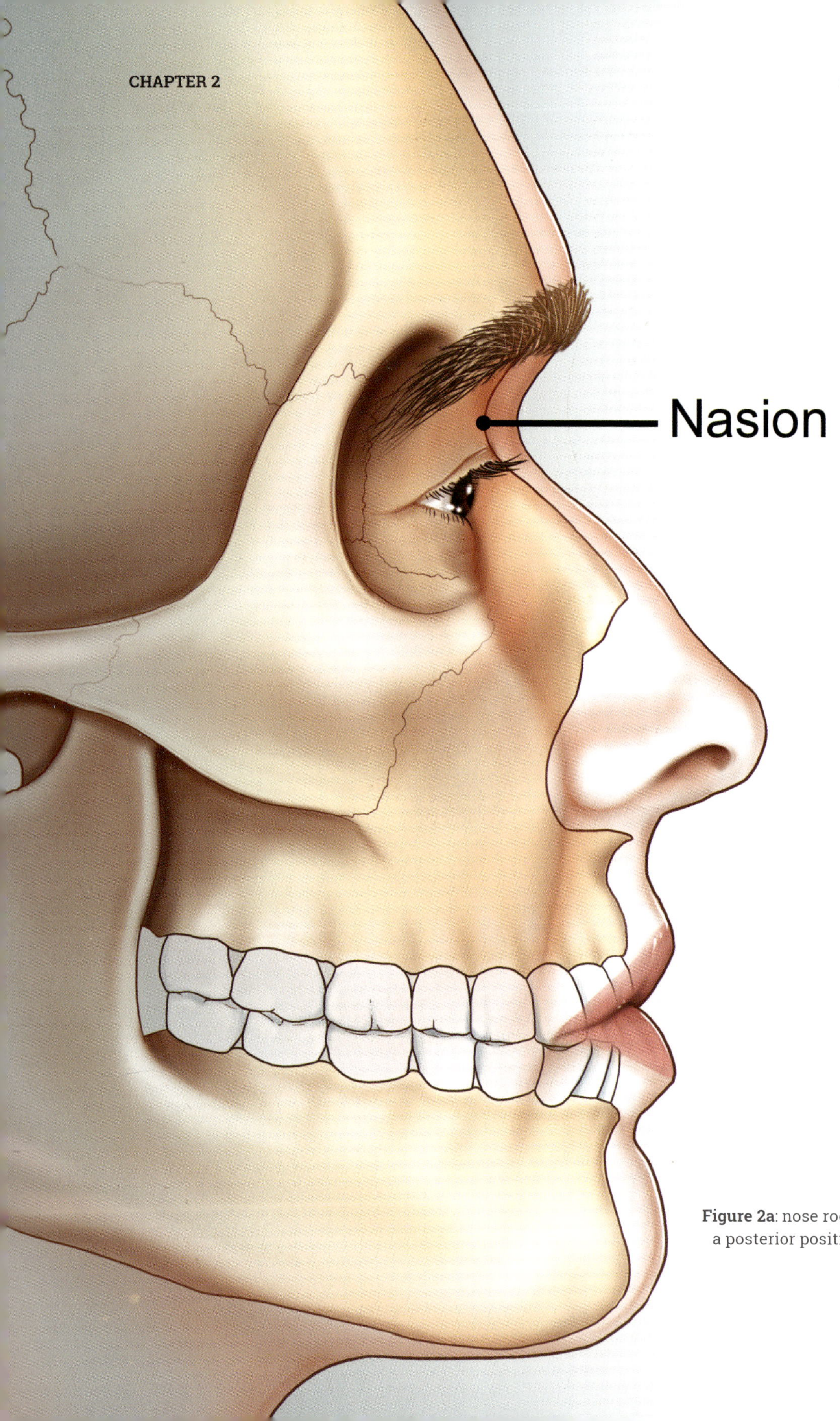

Figure 2a: nose root in a posterior position

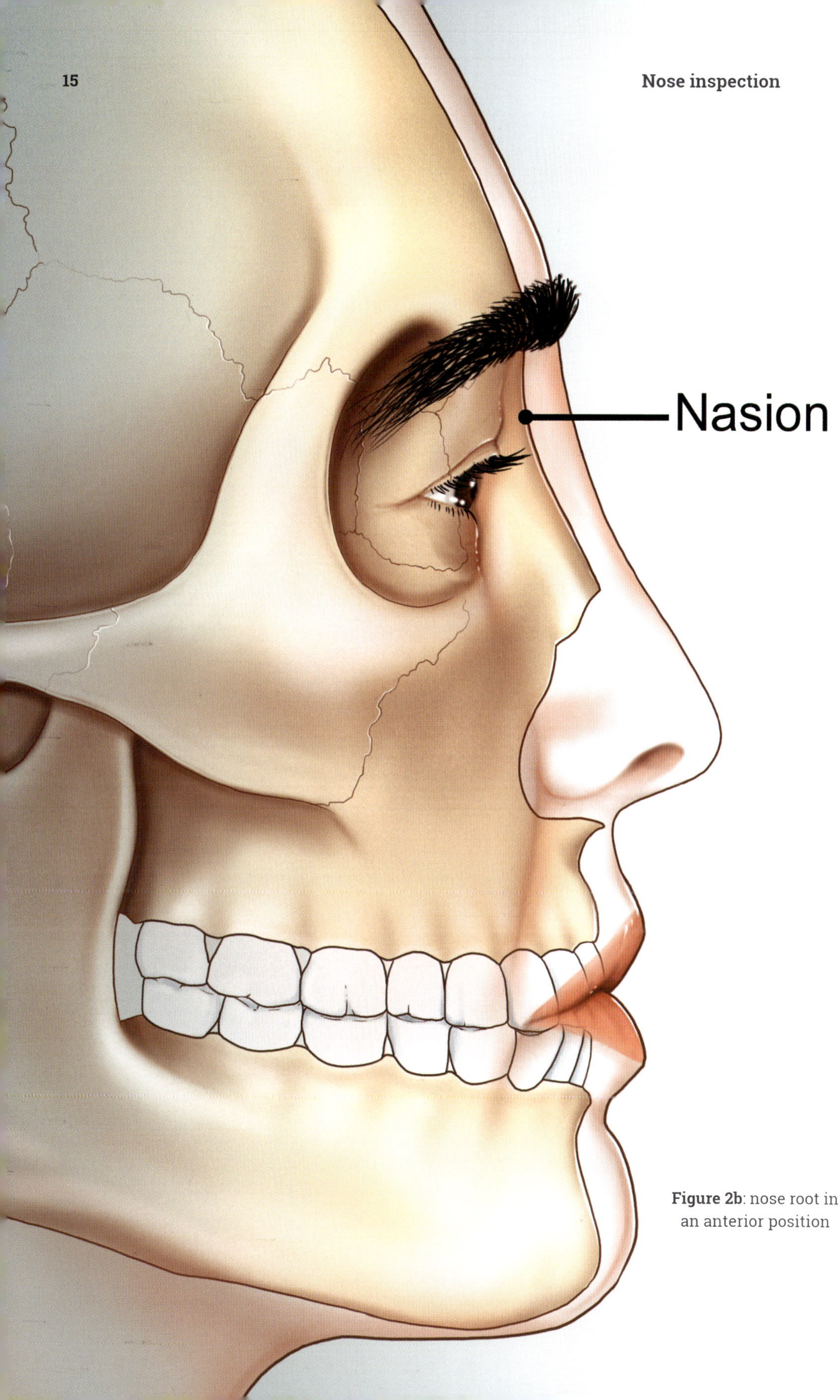

Figure 2b: nose root in an anterior position

The nasion is the root from which it is possible to design the new nasal profile. In the vast majority of cases it should not be modified because it is normal.

An anterior position of the nasion is responsible for a greek profile and, except in cases where this is not preferable, should be hollowed out.

If the nasion is in a posterior position, it may be convenient to proceed with the rhinoplasty without trying to keep it more anterior, because it would be necessary to place grafts which over time can be a source of problems and dissatisfaction due to their possible displacement or visibility. These defects, even if not immediately evident, can appear over the years, because the movements of the glabella tend to dislocate grafts over time. The nose should therefore be planned in such a way that it appears natural, even if perhaps in abstract terms it will not adhere to the theoretical canons of beauty. However, it is often possible to achieve a pleasing and normal shape even without bringing the nasion in a more anterior position (figs. 2c, d, e, f).

The nasolabial angle should be observed and should be slightly open, of around 100-105 degrees. Protrusion of the anterior nasal spine supports an open nasolabial angle. Its back-position results in a closed nasolabial angle. In the first case the anterior nasal spine should be reduced with the help of a bone rongeur, while in the second case, if tilting of the septum (figs. 3a, b) is not sufficient, a cartilage graft must be inserted to fill it. The anterior nasal spine may also be displaced to a side, in which case it must be fractured to be repositioned on the midline (fig. 4a). A lateral position of the anterior nasal spine may be evident on observation but should be better assessed by feeling with the fingers whether or not the nasal spine is in axis.

A lateral position of the anterior nasal spine will displace the anterior septum, and therefore should always be corrected.

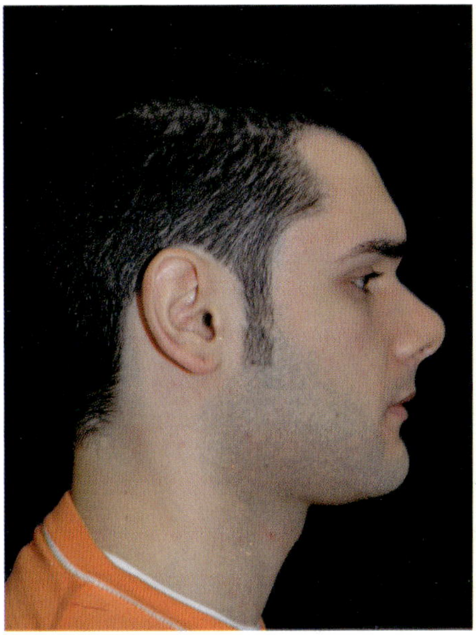

Figure 2c: nasion in a posterior position

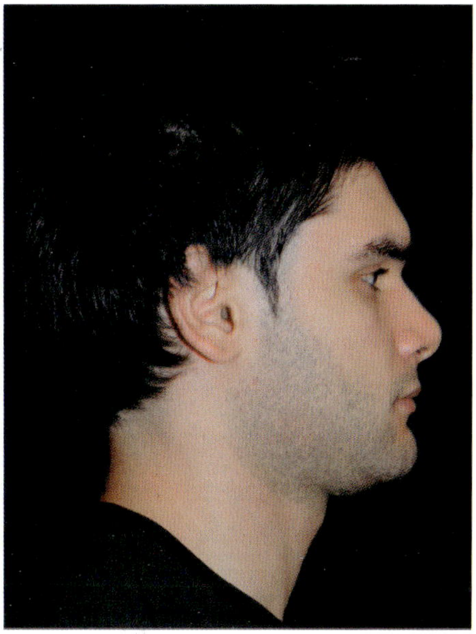

Figure 2d: post-op image of a good result achieved without bringing the Nasion anteriorly

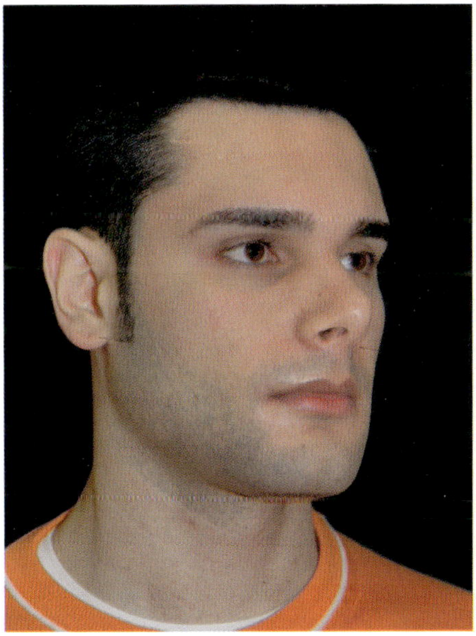

Figure 2e: three-quarters preoperative photo

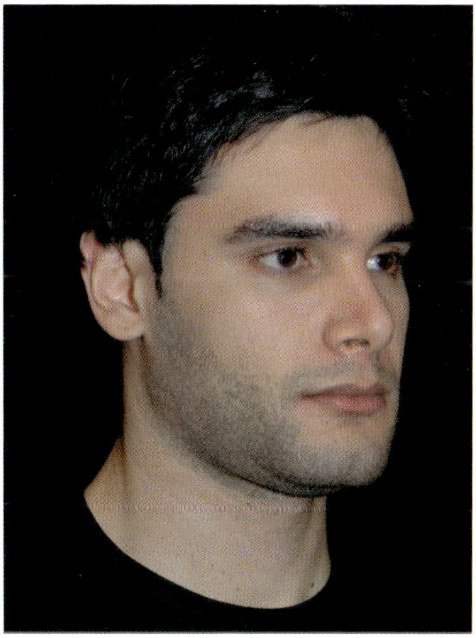

Figure 2f: post-op image. In the three-quarters view it is possible to appreciate the harmony of the transition between the eyebrows and the nose profile

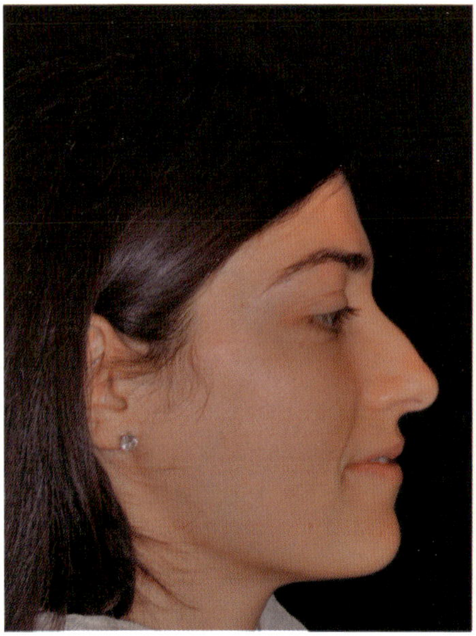

Figure 3a: patient with the nasolabial angle not sufficiently open

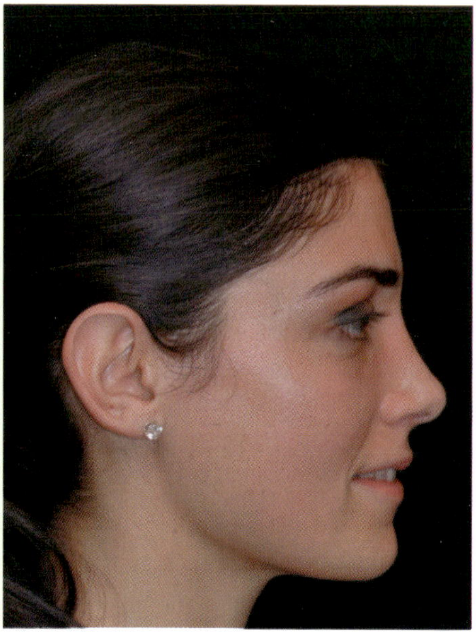

Figure 3b: correction of the nasolabial angle brought to approximately 110°

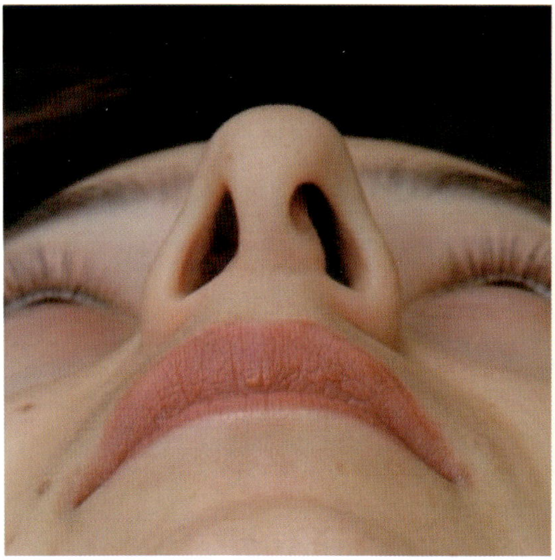

Figure 4a: the nasolabial spine protrudes into the left nasal cavity and needs to be fractured with a chisel to allow the caudal portion of the septum to get into axis

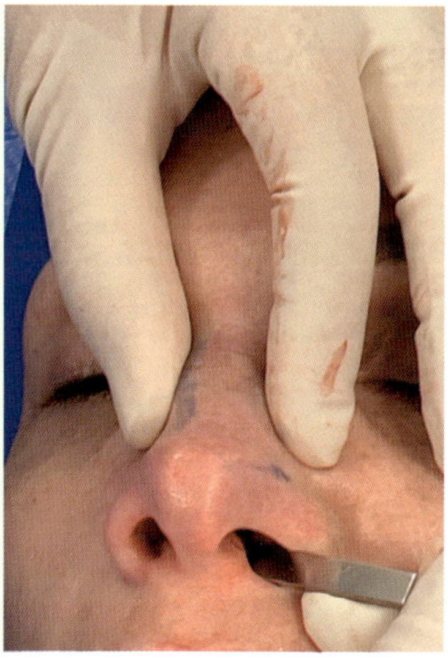

Figure 4b: anterior nasal spine is fractured with a chisel

The correction of the lateral position of anterior nasal spine is accomplished fracturing it with a chisel (fig. 2.5b) and guiding its healing on axis with stitches placed to stabilize the anterior part of the septum.
The nasolabial angle conditions the entry of air flow into the nasal cavities. For an optimal breathing, this airflow must be directed towards the lower portion of the nasal cavity, i.e. the one that is close to the palate. An acute angle will force the air to travel along its nasal tract with non-physiological vorticity. The correct air flow into the nasal cavity allows adequate air warming and filtering. When the nasolabial angle has a correct inclination (around 100/105°), the air is channeled towards the floor of the nasal fossa without abnormal whirling. If the angle is too open or too closed, the air is forced into tortuous paths, causing a difficult breathing (figs. 5a, b, c).

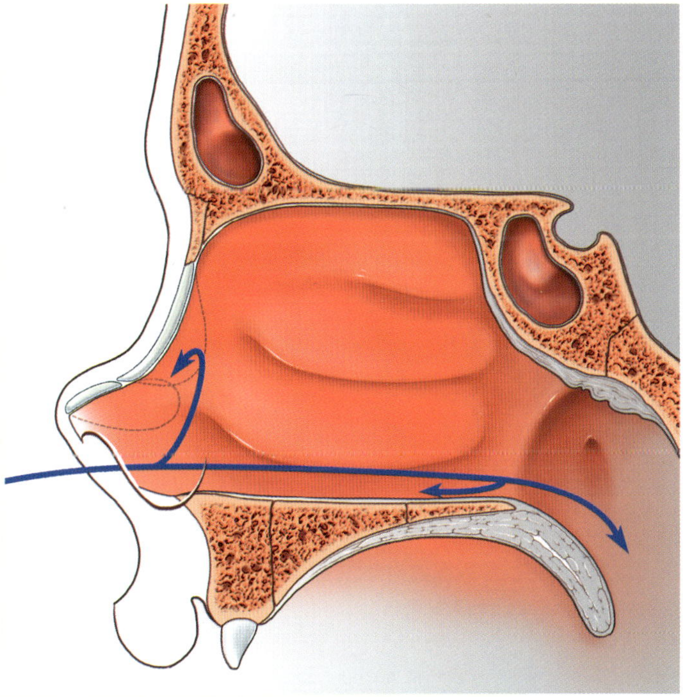

Figure 5a: air flows in the nose with an open nasolabial angle

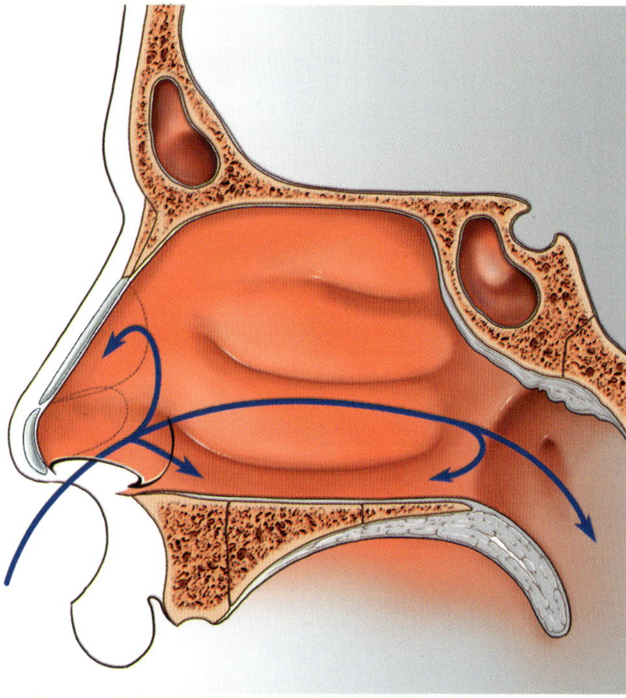

Figure 5b: air flows in the nose with a normal nasolabial angle

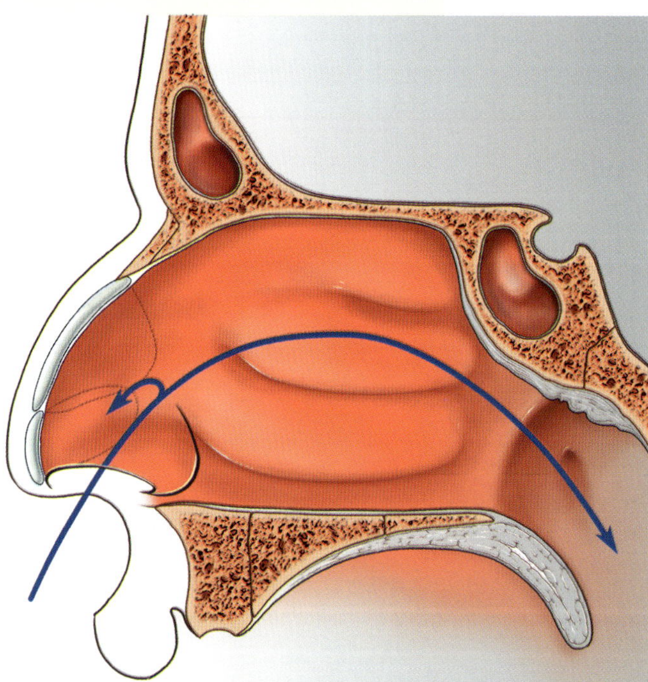

Figure 5c: air flows in the nose with a closed nasolabial angle

CHAPTER 3

Photographic documentation

- Photos should be taken from the front, at three-quarters, from below and the two profiles. The black background does not highlight the shadows of the flash and it is therefore preferable, unless you have a photo studio where a professional can do better.
- Three-quarters shots should include the tip of the nose within the contour of the face. It is advisable to have a camera with a lens without zoom and to always photograph at the same distance in order not to have image deformations induced by different optics. The flash in the profile and

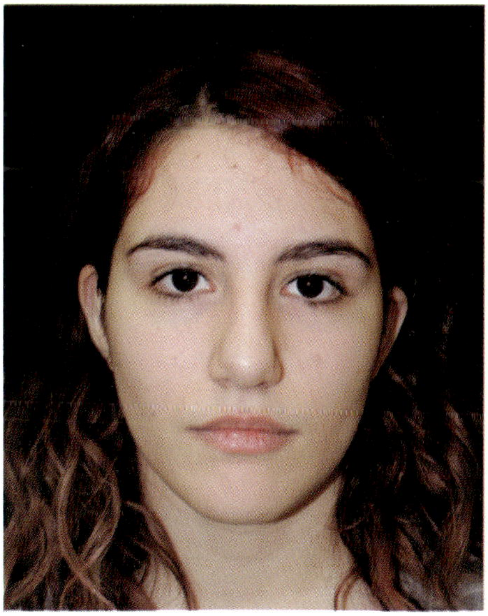

Figure 1: front view

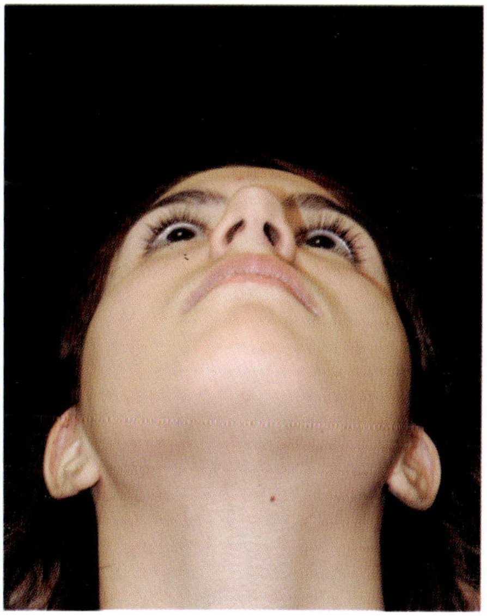

Figure 2: photo from below

three-quarters photos should be rotated on the same side as the tip of the nose to avoid casting shadows of the face.

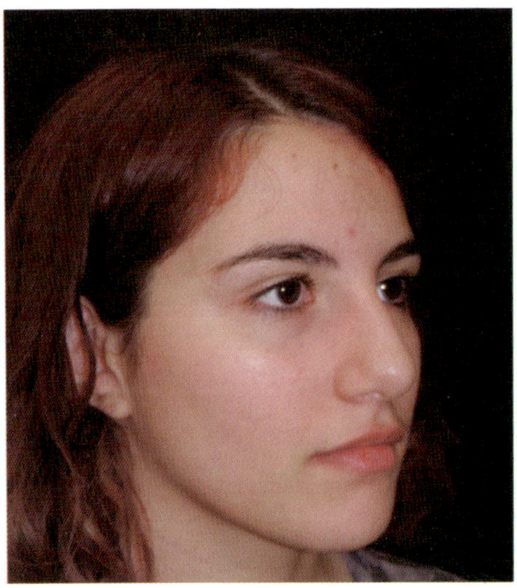

Figure 3: three-quarters photo of the right side including tip of nose within cheekbone features

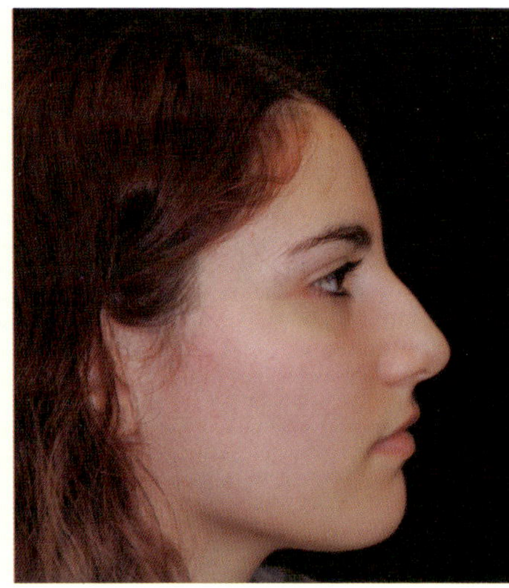

Figure 4: right profile photo

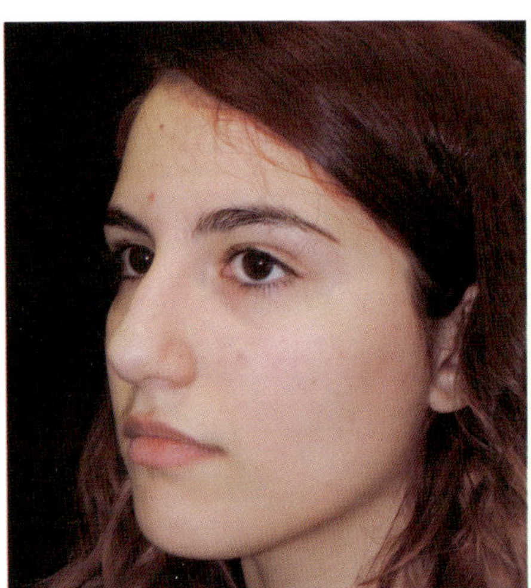

Figure 5: three-quarters photo of the left side including tip of nose within cheekbone features

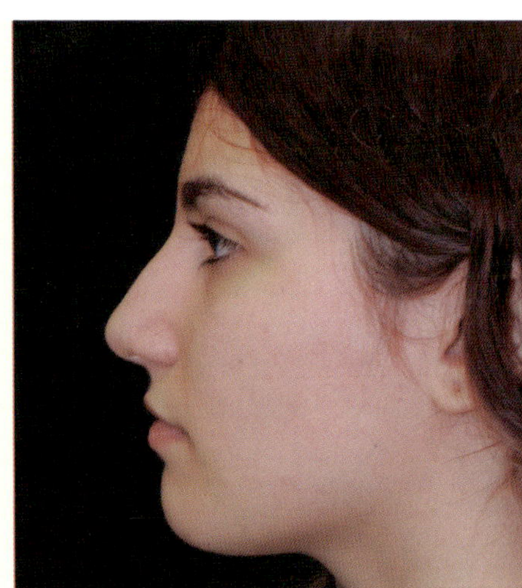

Figure 6: left profile photo

CHAPTER 4

Nasal cavities inspection and functional considerations

The nostrils may be symmetrical or asymmetrical. Their fibrous lateral portion may be more or less developed, and the alar cartilages may also be symmetrical or asymmetrical. The conformation of the alar cartilages must be evaluated: their lower margin may be close or far from the margin of the nostrils; the curvatures may be different between right and left alar cartilages.

Cartilages with different curvatures are difficult to treat in order to achieve perfect symmetry, so never promise it, especially in these cases. If the lower margin of the lateral crus of the alar cartilage diverges two much upwards from the margin of the nostrils, it may be advisable to bring them down to achieve pleasing results (figs. 1a, b).

Rhinoscopy is normally performed with the aid of the Nasal Speculum and can be completed with a nasal fibroscope. Rhinoscopy is used to observe the nasal septum and the turbinates (fig. 2)

The nasal septum can be on axis or have deviations that can be cartilaginous, bony or both. Normally the deviations are left-convex due to dislocation of the septum that occurs during birth due to the passage through the birth canal. The septum may not return to axis so its growth nuclei cause ossification and growth of the septal cartilage shifted to the left.

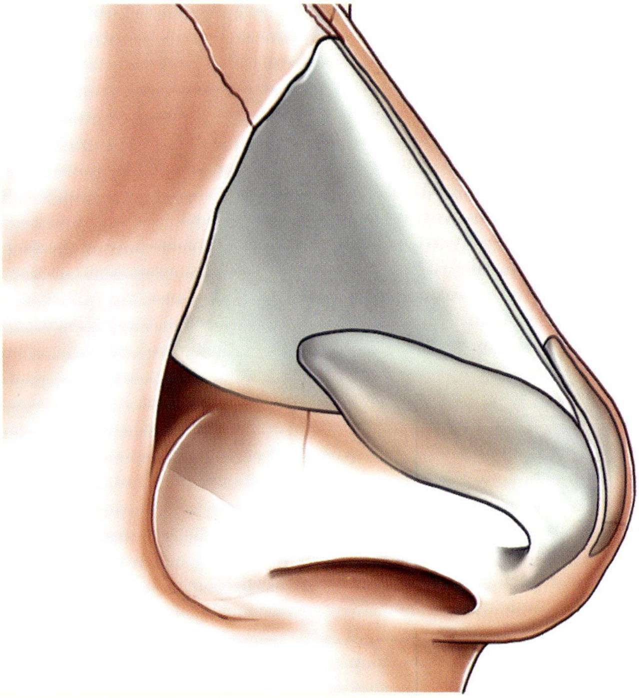

Figure 1a: if the lateral crus of the alar cartilages is oriented upwards, its orientation must be changed by bringing it closer to the margin of the nostril. Otherwise, once its cephalic margin has been resected, there would not be a sufficient strip of cartilage (measuring at least 2mm) left along the nostril to prevent the nasal ala from collapsing

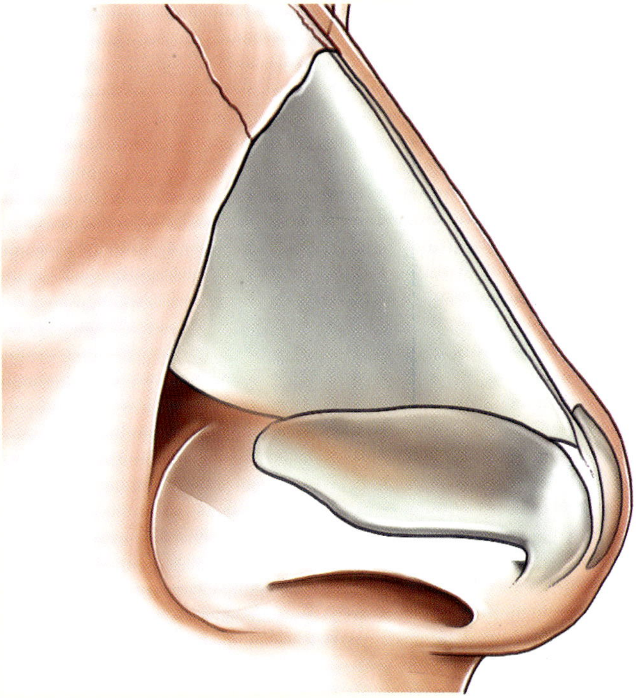

Figure 1b: normal orientation of the lateral crus fairly close to the edge of the nostril

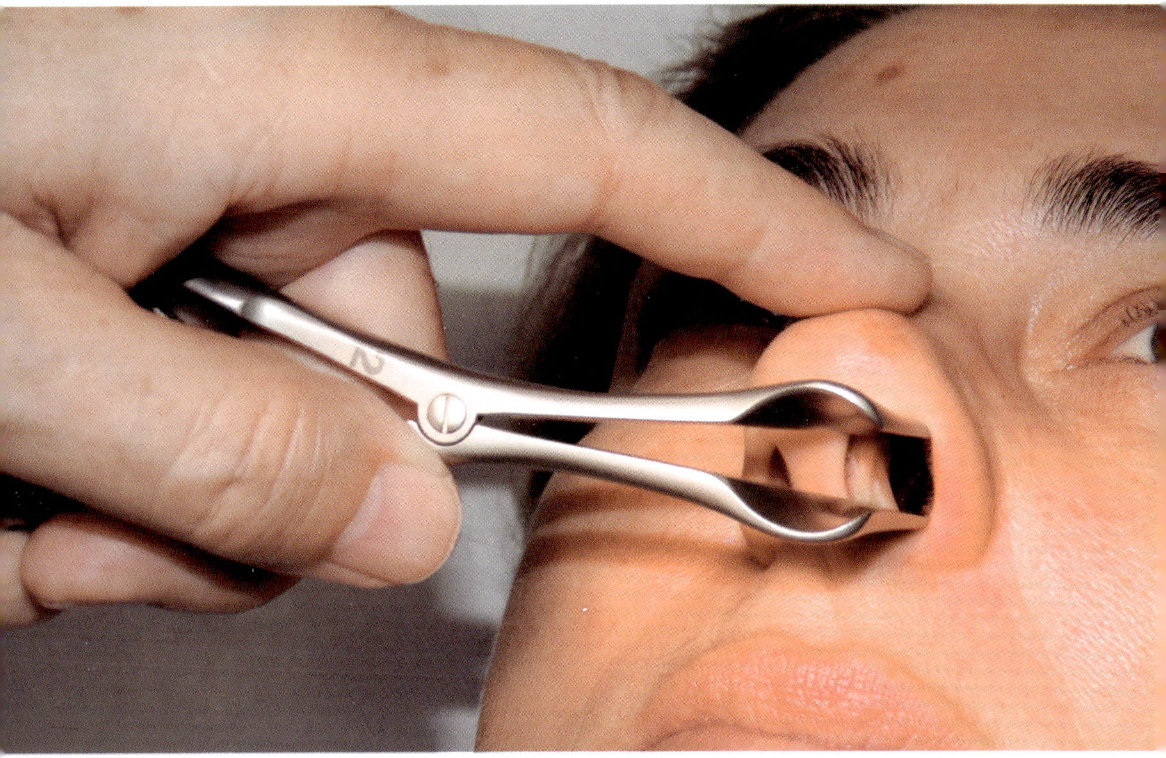

Figure 2: to perform a rhinoscopy, a Killian speculum is introduced and the index finger is used to stabilize its position

It is called left deviation because the base of the septum occupies the left nasal fossa, but almost invariably the upper part of the septum is tilted to the opposite side and thus the nose is visually tilted to the right! It should be better described as right-convex or left-convex deviation, indicating which side is the obstacle given by the deviation.

The deviation areas were described by Cottle and were divided into 5 areas: area 1 - vestibular area; area 2 - valve area; area 3 - attic area; area 4 - anterior area of turbinates and area 5 - posterior area of turbinates (figs. 3a, b, c, d, e).

Right-convex deviations are of traumatic nature. Particular attention should be paid to deviations in the valve area and the attic area. These are the

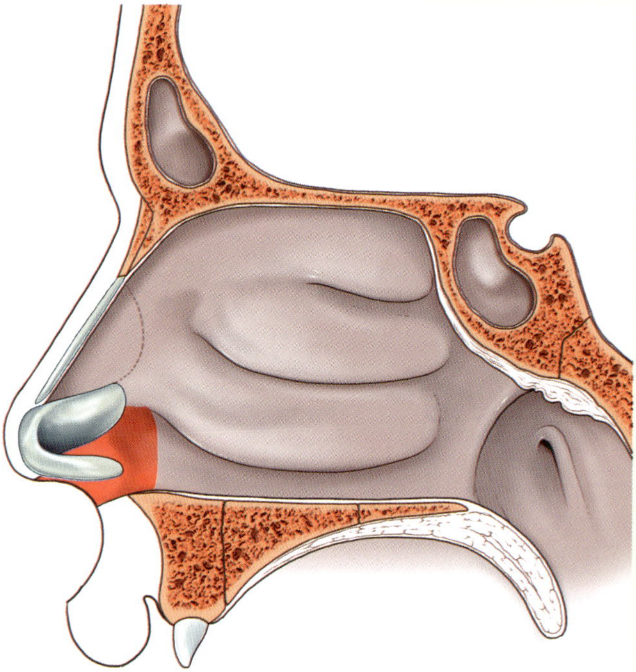

Figure 3a: Cottle area 1. Deviation in area 1 give moderate breathing problems. It usually causes a distortion of the nostrils

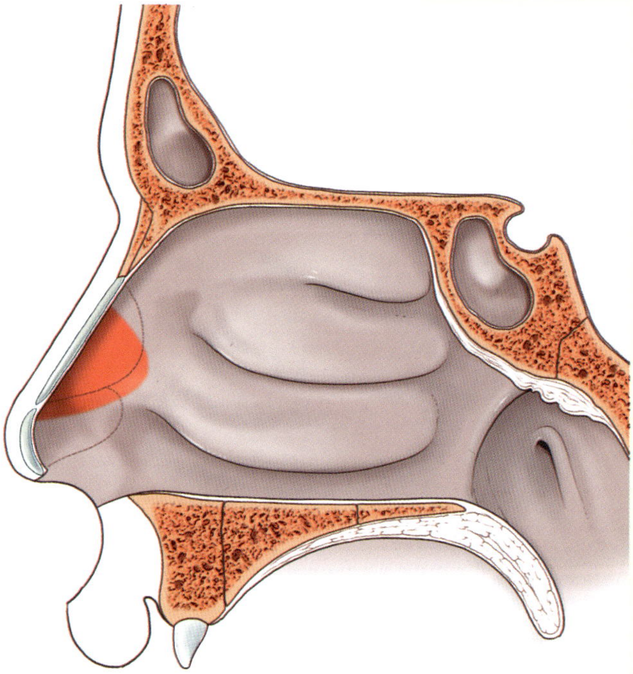

Figure 3b: Cottle area 2. Deviation in area 2 prevents the Mink Valve from functioning properly and cause breathing problems

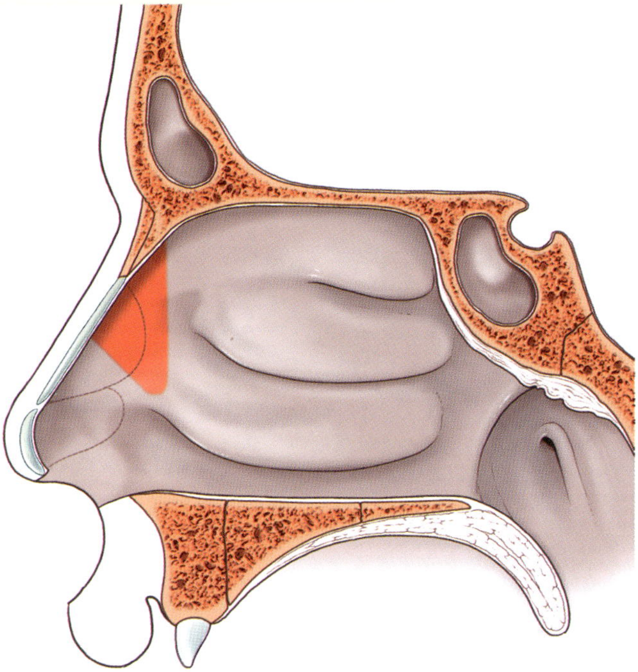

Figure 3c: Cottle area 3. Deviation in area 3 do not cause evident breathing disorders but can support a nasal deviation that is difficult to correct and is most often masked by placing grafts in the depressed areas to give an optical impression of a straight nose

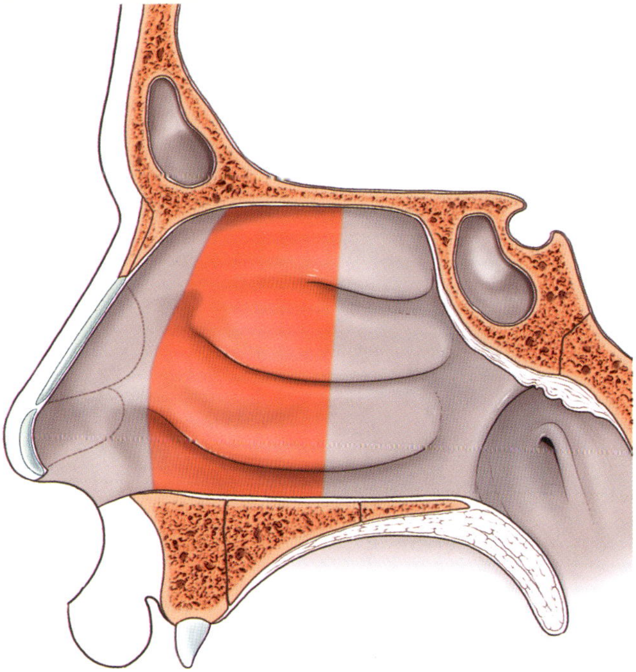

Figure 3d: Cottle area 4. Deviation in area 4 cause breathing difficulties, frontal headache, cough, rhinitis and sinusitis

injecting, as is done with any other injection, makes sure you are not inside a blood vessel (fig. 4).

When a deviation of the septum is to be corrected, the turbinate which is located in the widest nasal fossa is hypertrophic because it has to arrive to touch the septum in order to perform its function correctly (as explained earlier). It

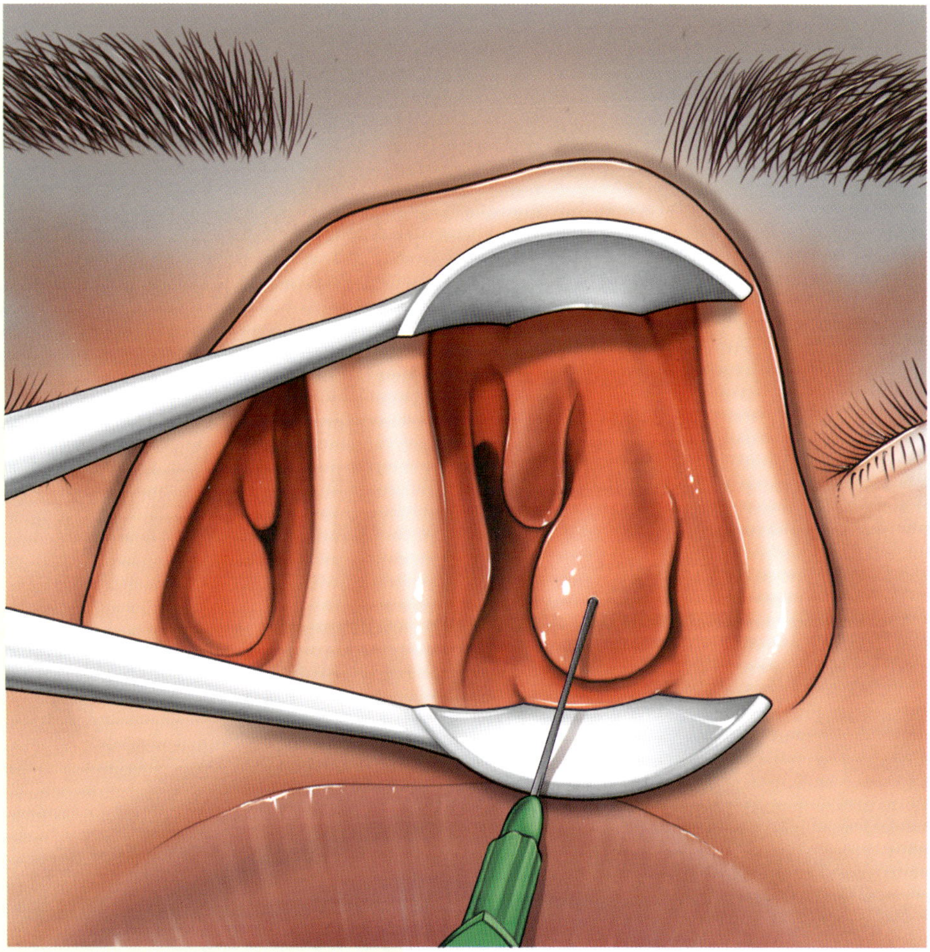

Figure 4: infiltration of triamcinolone in the head of the turbinate. This is effective when the allergic component is predominant, but dangerous because the substance injected can cause blindness via the bloodstream. If you decide to proceed, you must remain very superficial, aspirating before injecting, to be sure that you have not penetrated a blood vessel

is therefore advisable to reduce the hypertrophy with diathermocoagulations or even better with devices that produce a plasma such as the coblator (Smith&Nephew) or the Meghan (meghan-europe.com). With the plasma that these devices produce, the tissues inside the turbinate, where the tip of the device is inserted, dissolve at a molecular level with a minimal thermal effect on the surrounding tissues. These devices use radiofrequency to create a focused plasma field that breaks up tissue molecules between 40° and 70° C, causing a volumetric reduction with minimal thermal effect (see chapter 9) (fig. 5).
Diathermocoagulation leads to the formation of a healing process on the surface of the turbinate. Its proximity to the septum may result in synechiae formation (see chapter 15). Plasma is preferred because it acts within the turbinate and therefore if synechiae formation occurs, it is not attributable to this technique of turbinate reduction.

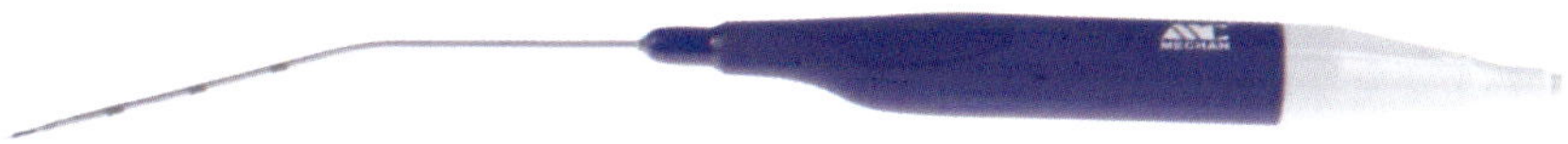

Figure 5: tip of a plasma-producing device. It is introduced from the head of the turbinate along its length. It has three black marks help that help to judge the depth of the tip. Once the tip is inserted, the plasma is generated with the control of a foot-switch

References

1 Kayser R Die exacte messun der luftdurgängigkeit der nase. Arch Laryngol Rhinology, Berlin 3:101, 1895.

2 Meyer R Secondary and Functional Rhinoplasty-The difficult Nose. Grune & Stratton inc, p 22, 1988.

3 Rees T.D, Aethetic Plastic Surgery, Vol 1. p 92-93 ; W.B.Saunders 1980.

CHAPTER 5

Instrumental tests

author Valentina Pino

There are no indispensable instrumental tests before performing a rhinoplasty, however in some selected cases it is advisable to perform instrumental exams. Among them there are fiber-optic endoscopy, rhinomanometry and CT scan.

Fiber-optic endoscopy

Can be performed with both a flexible or a rigid endoscope. Subluxation of the quadrangular cartilage, the antero-inferior part of which can protrude into the nasal vestibule or the presence of thickenings, spurs or bone ridges may be observed. In the preoperative phase, fiber-optic endoscopy allows to highlight undetected morphological or pathological alterations. So it is possible to evaluate preoperatively the characteristics of the lower and middle turbinates (structure, hypertrophy, malposition) and of the nasal septum (deviations), inflammatory or allergic diseases, vascular abnormalities or tumors.

Rhinomanometry

Rhinomanometry measures nasal permeability using the principles of fluid dynamics making it possible to evaluate the patency of the nasal cavities through measurements of the air flow and the pressure gradient between the nostrils, anterior nasal pressure and choana (posterior nasal pressure).

The detection of these parameters, both inspiratory and expiratory, is carried out through a mask applied to the face during the spontaneous breathing. The rhinomanometric flux and pressure data can be expressed graphically through a “sigmoid” graph or through the Cottle rhinogram. The numerical expression of rhinomanometric data is linked to nasal resistance which makes use of Poiseouille’s law: R= D P/V. The comparison between basal rhinomanometric measurements and those after the topical application of vasoconstrictors, after the insufflation of allergen extracts and after position changes, allows the differentiation between anatomical and functional cause of nasal patency alterations. However, the rhinomanometric examination in aesthetic rhinoplasty has an almost exclusively a medico-legal interest to document pre-existing breathing problems.

CT scan

CT scan is required in selected cases, not routinely. The purpose is to highlight the internal nasal morphology.
CT scan is usually made without contrast medium in the axial and coronal projections. The main information that can be deducted from the CT concerns anatomy of the nasal cavity, especially as regards the morphology of the nasal septum, the turbinates and the presence of space-occupying lesions (polyps, neoplasms) which could be responsible for bone erosions.

CHAPTER 6

Anatomical considerations

The anatomy we need to know

The nose is roughly shaped like a pyramid. The actual pyramid is its upper portion, made up of the nasal processes of the maxilla, the nasal bones and their cartilaginous extension, the upper lateral cartilages also named triangular cartilages. The tip of the nose is a unit separated from the pyramid. The tip consists of nostrils, which are supported by the alar cartilages, that give the tip different shapes, depending on how they are shaped. These two structures, pyramid and tip, are connected trough a fibrous system that allows the mobility of the tip and of the upper lateral cartilages. The membranous septum connects the tip to the cartilaginous septum, and a mucosal cul-de-sac between the upper lateral and lateral crus of the alar cartilages called by Rees "intercartilagineous groove" (1) to the terminal part of the pyramid, the upper lateral cartilages. These soft connective structures allow the mobility of the tip, while the pyramid itself has some mobility only in its cartilaginous part. This mobility of the cartilaginous part of the pyramid permits the movement of the Mink valve and i.e. of the upper lateral cartilages in relation to the septum (2).

Mobility is indispensable for the function of the upper lateral cartilages, which are also, in addition to the turbinates, the main regulators of inspiratory and expiratory airflows. The nose must allow an air flow that varies according to the needs. If physical activity is increased, as during a run, the nose must allow a greater air flow; if it is minimal, as during sleep, the air flow must also be minimal. Obviously between these two extremes there is a normal condition of activity, to which a relative air flow corresponds.

In chapter 9 the function of the turbinates has been analyzed, now let's analyze the function of the upper cartilages as air flow regulators. The upper lateral cartilages articulate with the lower margin of the nasal bones. Straatma and Straatma in 1951 described this relationship and showed that the nasal bones overlap with the upper lateral cartilages for 2 to 11 mm (3) (fig. 1).

Care must be taken not to cause the detachment of these cartilages when reducing the hump (fig. 2) If the upper lateral cartilage is detached, a characteristic step and depression occurs just below the nasal bone due to cartilage displacement toward the septum, and its ability to perform its valve function is lost, causing respiratory problems (fig. 3). In fact, the nose also has the important function of providing resistance to air inlet, which is mainly carried out by the upper lateral cartilages. The limited air flow entering the lungs when the muscles of respiration dilate the thoracic cage produce a negative pressure which is an important factor in pulmonary blood circulation. The triangular shape of the upper lateral cartilages must be maintained to enable them to perform their function properly (figs. 4a, b).

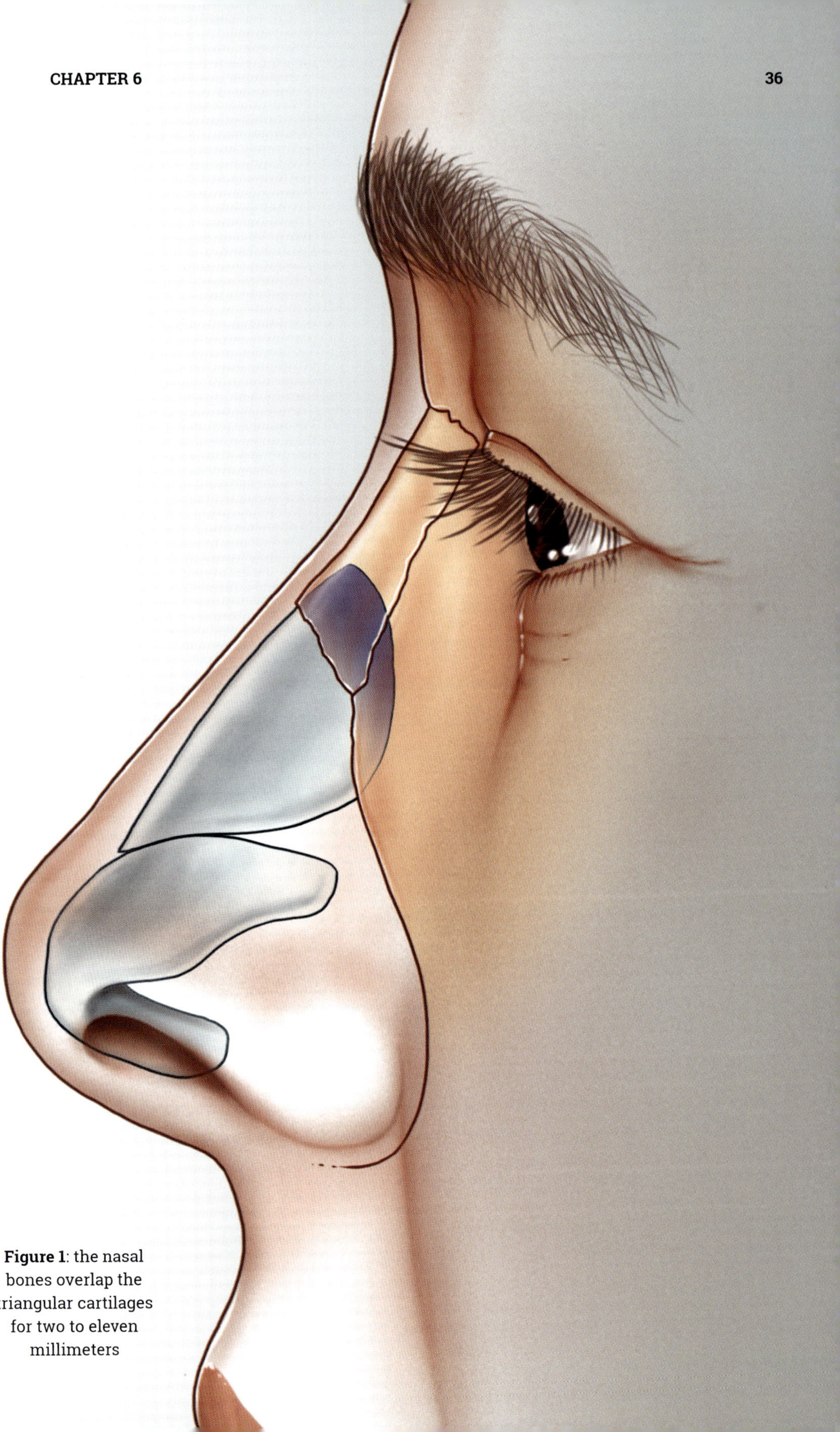

Figure 1: the nasal bones overlap the triangular cartilages for two to eleven millimeters

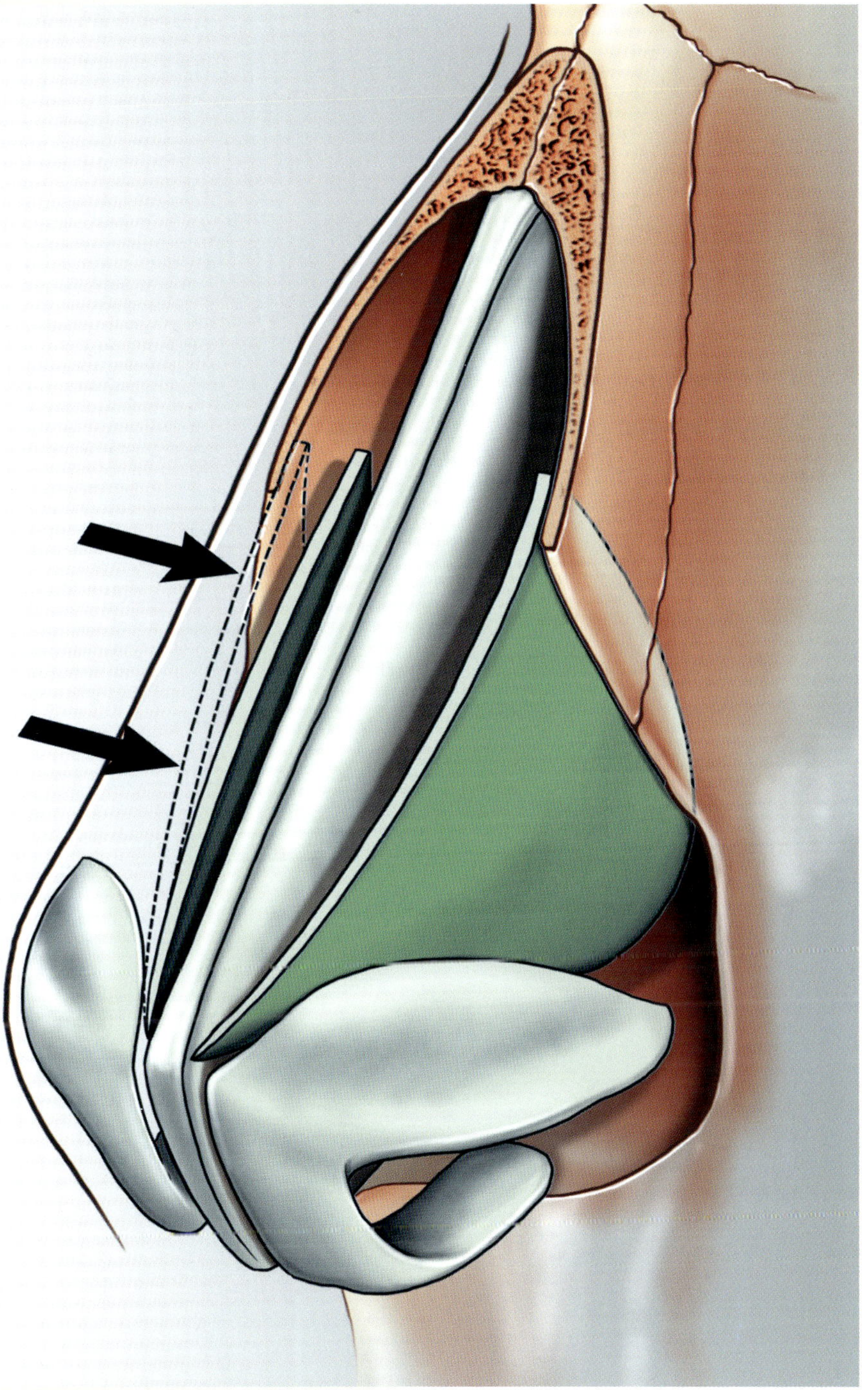

Figure 2: detachment of the triangular cartilage caused by incorrect maneuvers, usually by the use of rasps that hook it exerting a traction instead of consuming it

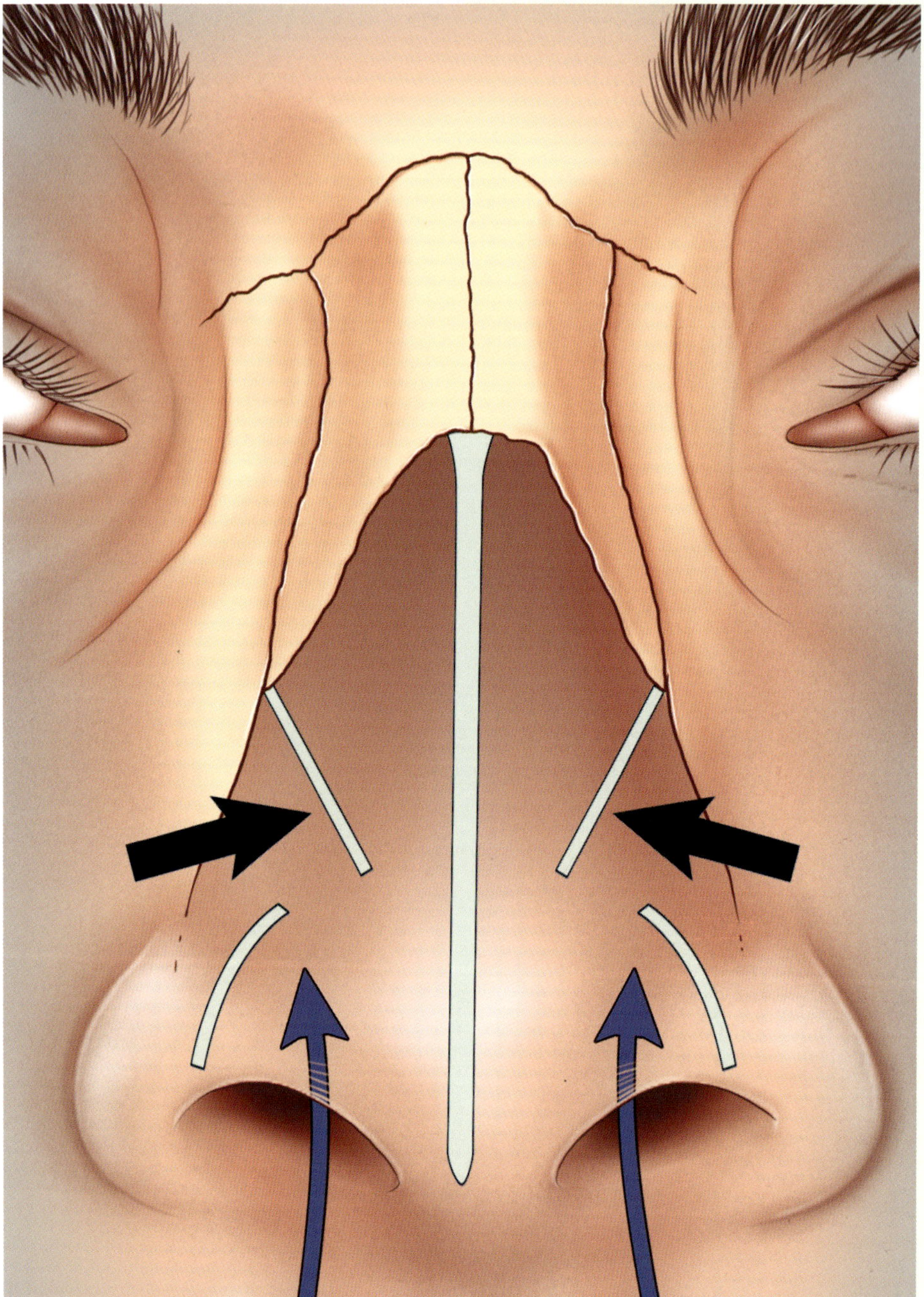

Figure 3: during inhalation the airflow exerts a negative pressure on the walls of the nasal cavities and therefore the free edge of the triangular cartilages approaches the septum

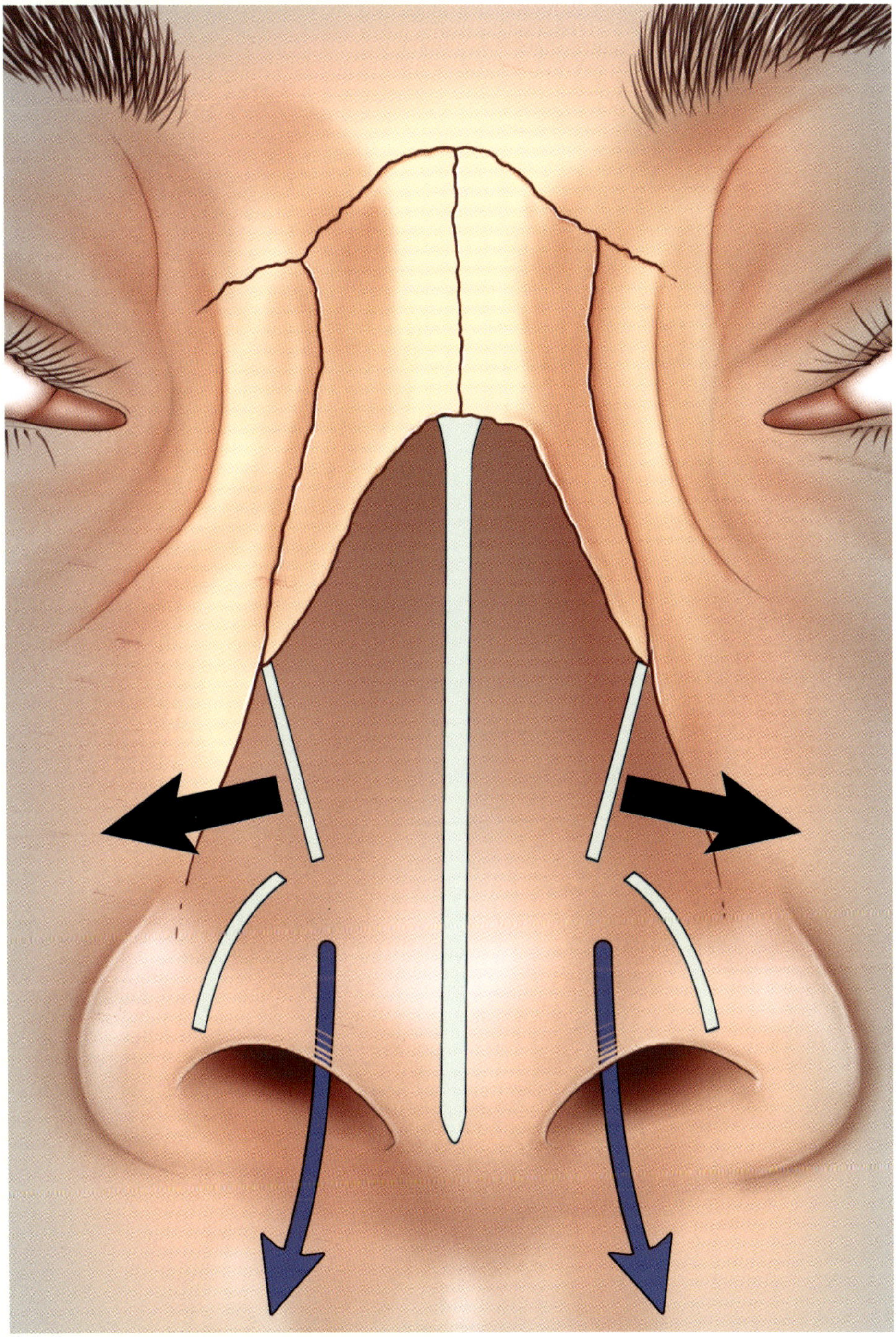

Figure 4: during exhalation the airflow exerts a positive pressure so the triangular cartilages move away from the nasal septum

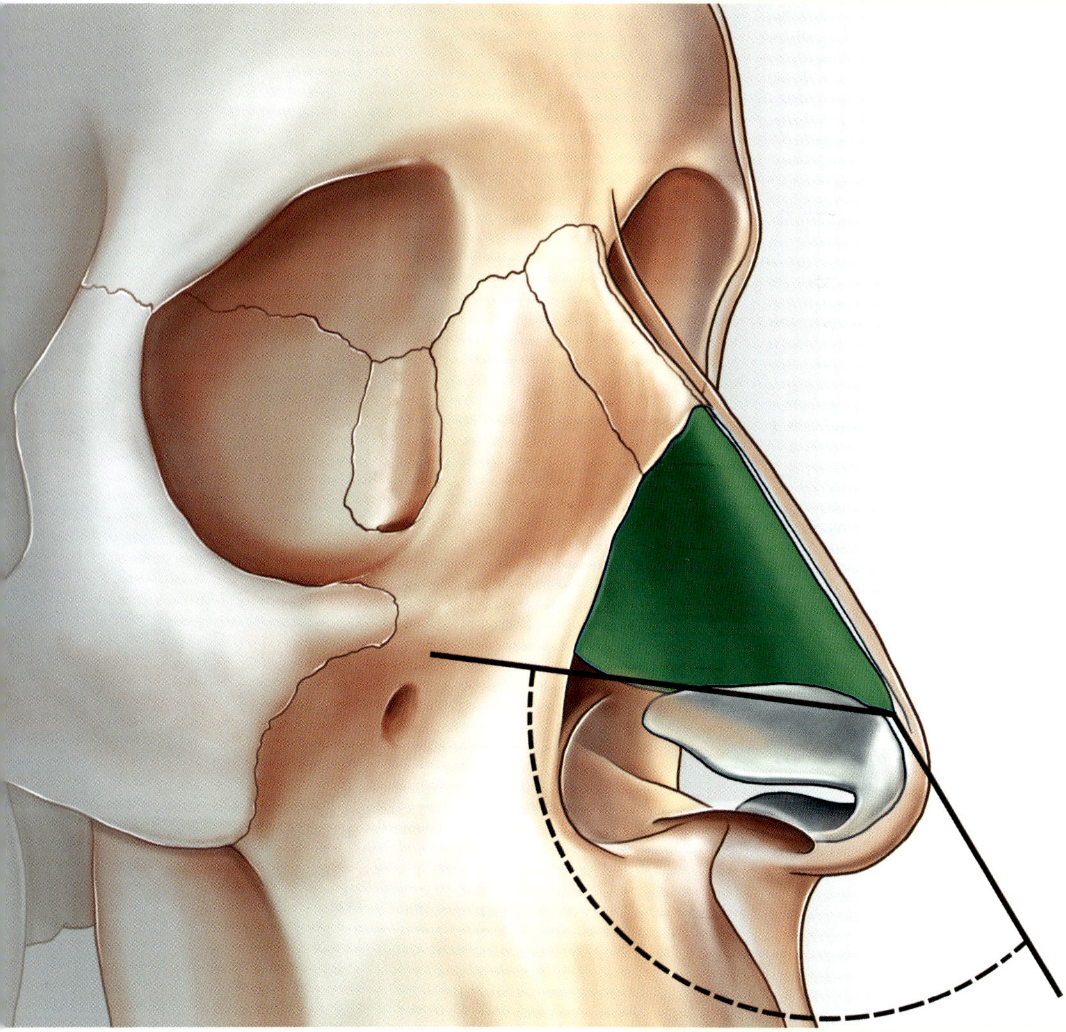

Figure 5: the angle that the free edge of the triangular cartilage makes with the septum should be approximately 120°

Mechanism of valve operation and how the upper lateral cartilages act in the inspiratory phase

The faster the inspiratory flow, the greater the valve effect. In fact, according to Bernoulli's equation, a decrease in the section of the cavity where a fluid flows, in this case air, corresponds to an increase in the velocity of the latter, which causes a decrease in the internal pressure at that point. As a consequence, the external pressure will be greater than the internal one and will tend to push the upper lateral cartilage towards the septum reducing the section of the nasal cavity.

Therefore the relationship between the nasal septum and the triangular cartilage must have parameters within which no disturbances occur. We have already said that the triangular (upper lateral) cartilage must keep its shape, and if the nose is shortened, it must also be shortened maintaining an acute angle with the nasal dorsum. This angle must be about 120°, according to Sheen (4) (fig. 5).

The dihedral angle that the lower part of the cartilage forms with the septum must not be too small, i.e. not less than 10/15° (tension according to Cottle) nor too large, i.e. more than 15° (ballooning according to Cottle). If it is too small, the closing function of the valve is excessive and restricts the air flow too easily. If it is too large, the valve effect is not carried out, with negative consequences on breathing and pulmonary circulation caused by the reduced negative inspiratory pressure (5) (figs. 6a, b).

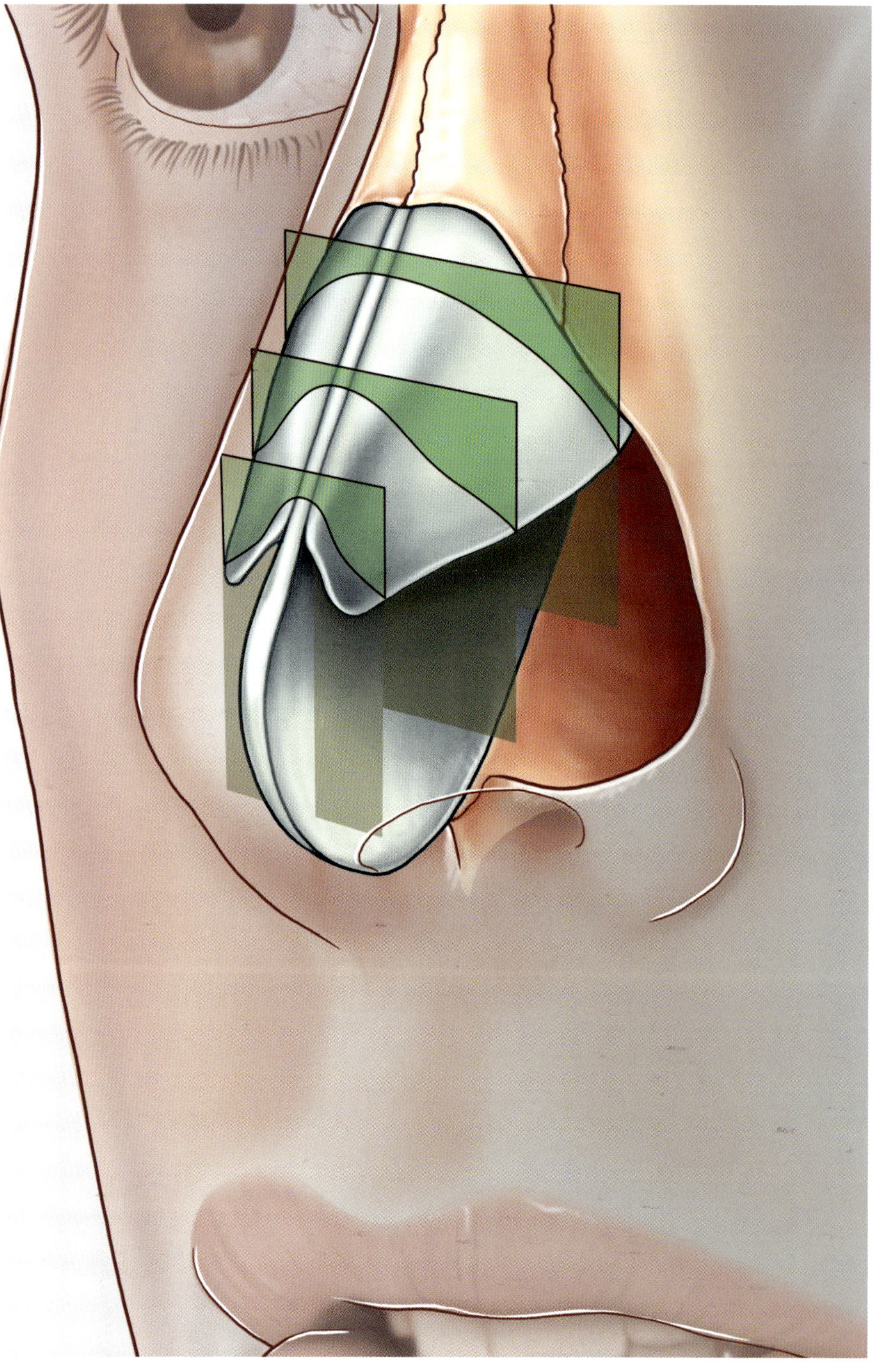

Figure 6a: the dihedral angle that the triangular cartilages make with the septum is narrower at the bottom and wider at the top. At the bottom, a large angle allows too much air to pass through, adversely affecting the pulmonary blood circulation

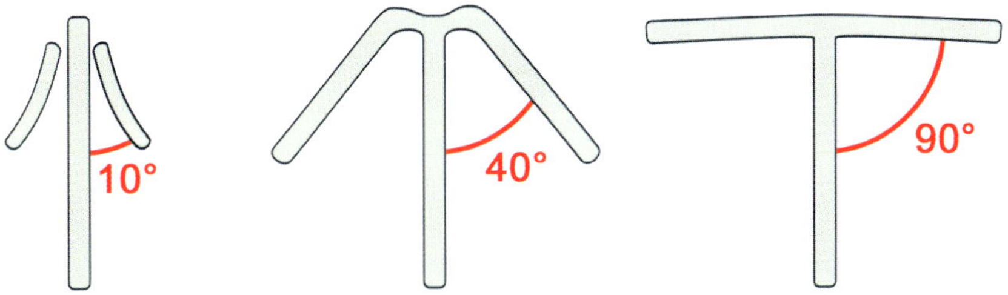

Figure 6b: the angle that the caudal portion of the triangular cartilage does with the septum should measure 10 degrees, but it can also measure up to 90 degrees in the negroid nose

The Tip

The nasal tip is a separate entity, connected to the pyramid by soft fibrous tissues that allow its mobility. Its cavity is called the nasal vestibule and its function is to direct the air flow into the nasal cavities (6). The nasal tip is supported by the alar cartilages. These cartilages have a medial part, the medial crus and a lateral part or lateral crus. Some authors describe a middle crus between these two. The shape of the alar cartilages is of great importance for both aesthetics and functionality of the nose (fig. 7).

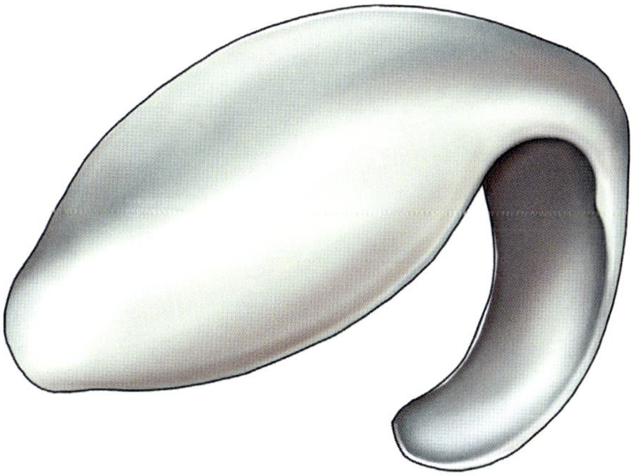

Figure 7: right ala cartilage. The medial crus goes down and the lateral crus goes laterally. At the top of the anterior margin of the medial crus there is a small point which I have named Deneb and which forms a landmark when applying the cartilage delivery technique

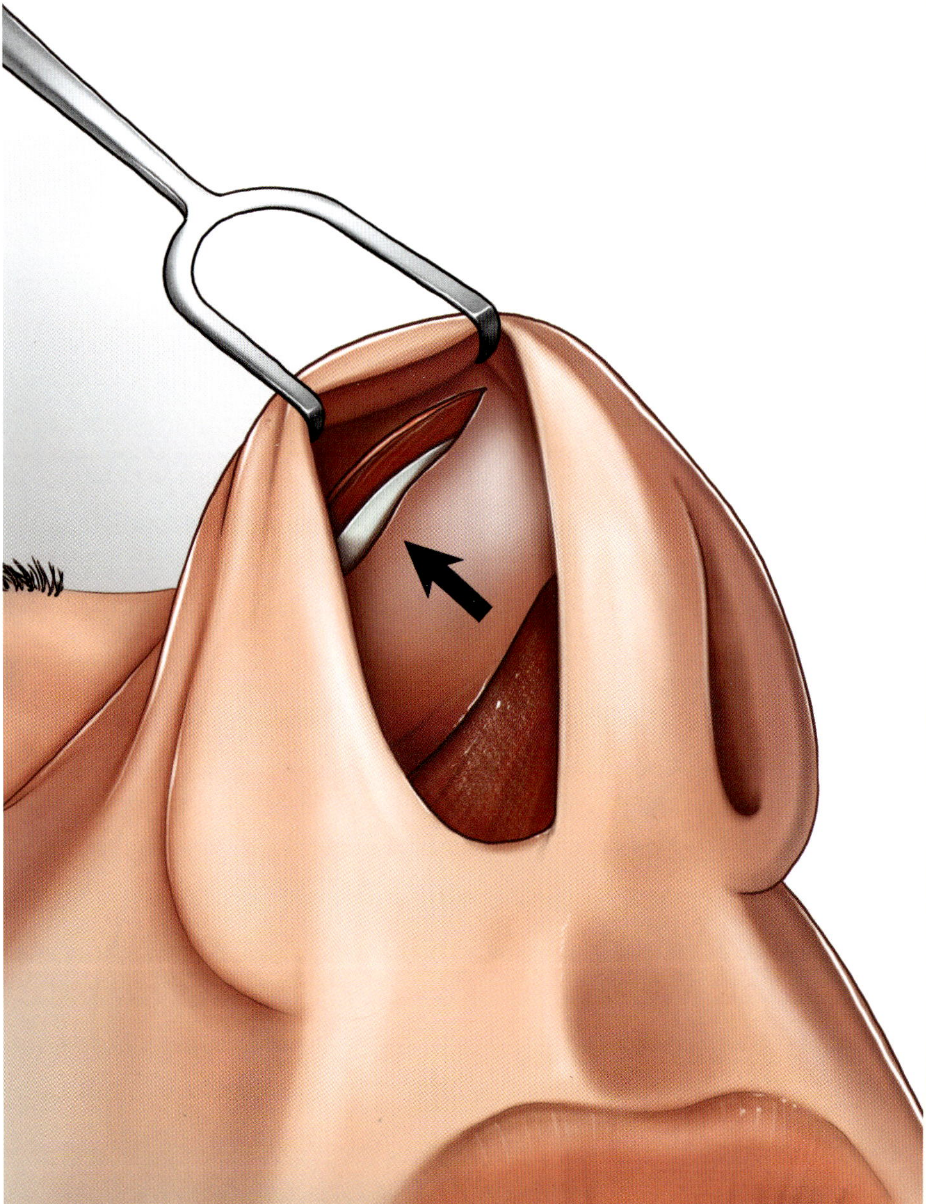

Figure 8b: removal of a lozenge of vestibular skin caudal to the lower margin of the lateral crus corresponding to how much you want to lower it

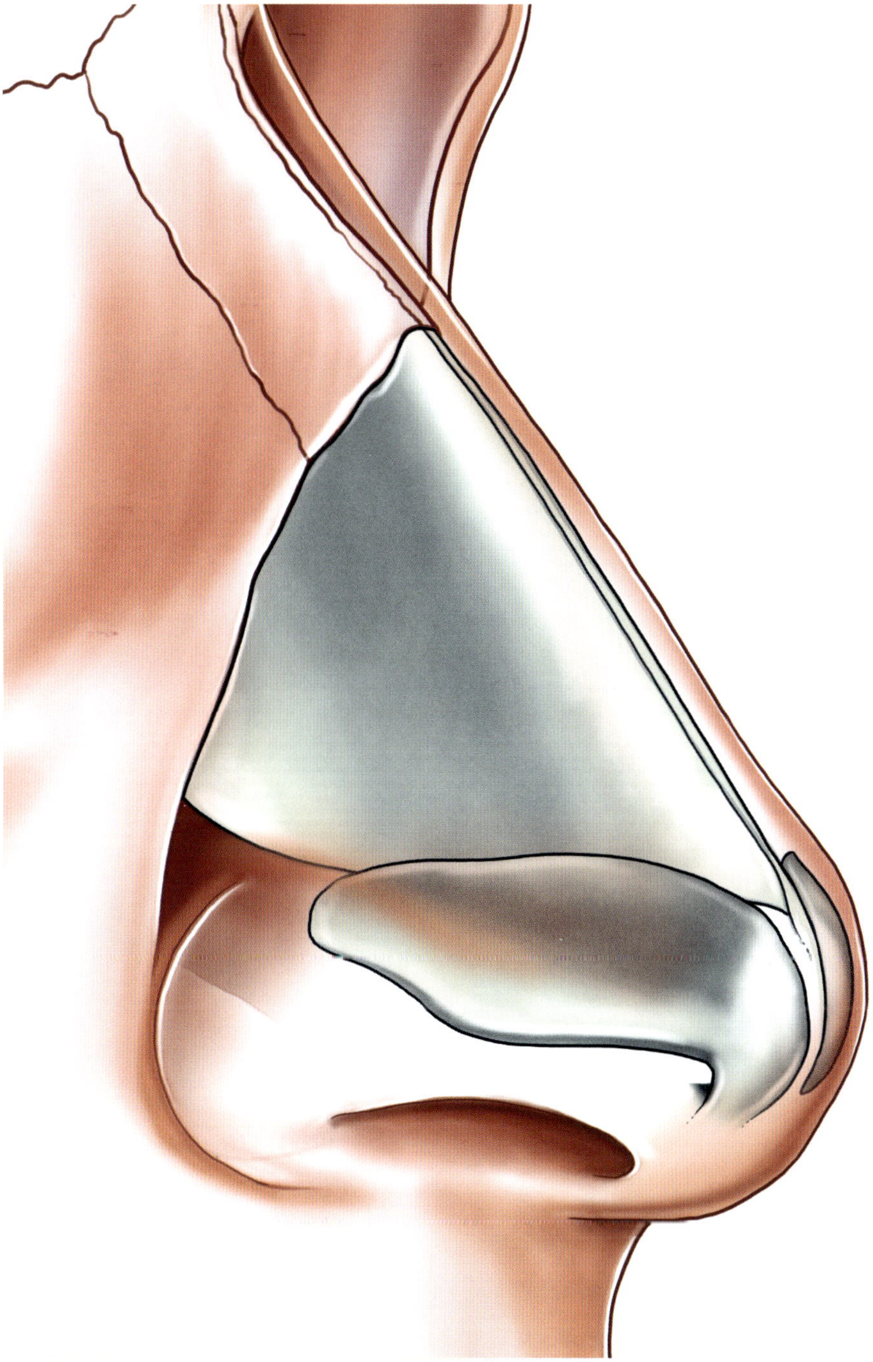

Figure 8c: once the cartilage has been brought closer to the edge of the nostril, resection of its cephalic margin can be planned without fear of not leaving a sufficient strip of cartilage to support the nasal ala

At the junction between the middle crus and medial crus, along the lower margin, there is a very small cartilage tip, not described in anatomy texts, that has been shown to me by the great surgeon Lionello Ponti. This tip (fig. 7), that I named Deneb, like the star of the swan constellation, is present in some drawings of the alar cartilages and is a fundamental landmark to maintain the symmetries when delivering the alar cartilages is necessary to correct the tip of the nose.
When the alar cartilages are delivered, the presence of a landmark makes it possible to shape the nasal tip maintaining, or rather allowing to reach, its symmetry even if both cartilages are exposed from only one nostril. The exposition of the tip through a rim incision and the delivery of the alar cartilages do not allow the certainty of symmetry if Deneb is not known and therefore used as a landmark (see chapter 7). The lack of knowledge of the existence of Deneb as a landmark has pushed many to dust off the technique of Rethi of 1934 (9) giving new life to the open rhinoplasty that perhaps would have as advantage, compared to the closed rhinoplasty, the direct vision of the alar cartilages and therefore a better achievement of the symmetry (figs. 9a, b). Since the knowing of the existence of the Deneb tip, open rhinoplasty becomes needless in the majority of cases because the alar cartilages can be modelled under direct vision with reasonable certainty of obtaining a symmetrical tip. When necessary, grafts can also be placed, and can be fixed under direct vision as easily as in open rhinoplasty.
The lower part of the medial crus has a curvature called the cartilage foot (10), which gives the air a vorticity that is important in respiratory physiology. In fact, the air is humidified and filtered by the turbinates in an effective manner because it enters the nostrils not only with the right inclination, but also with the right vorticity.

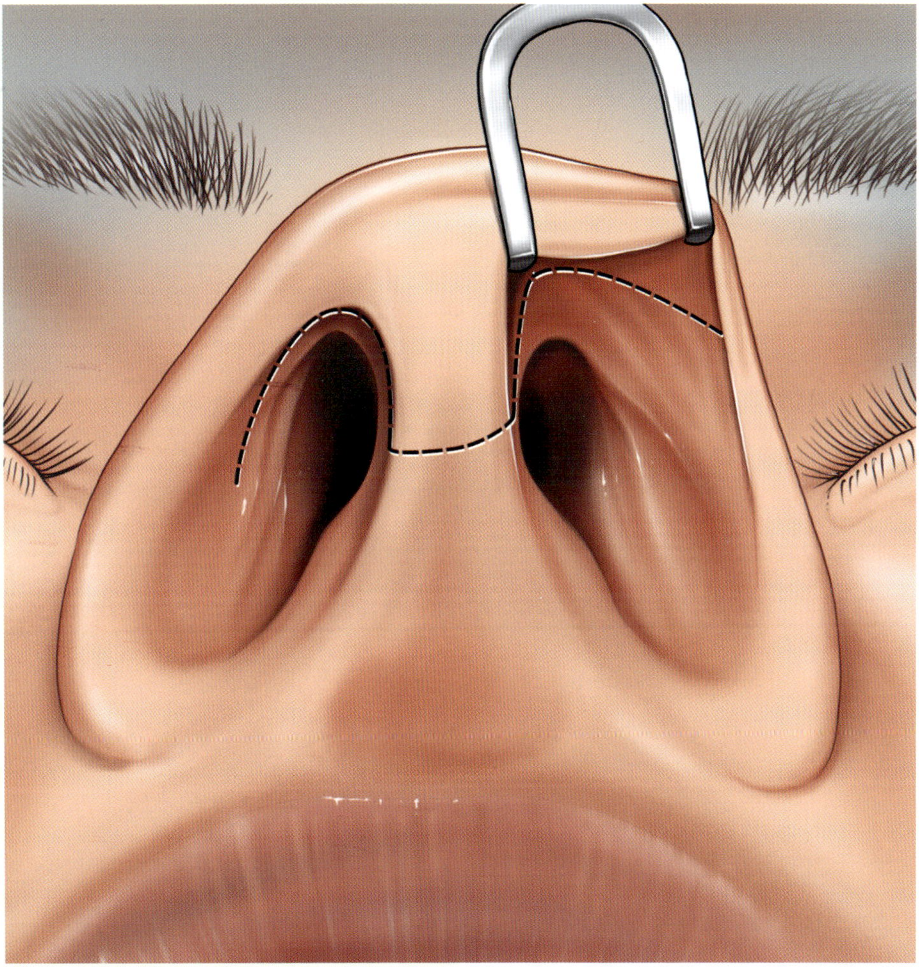

Figure 9a: Rethi incision, the first author to propose ‚open' rhinoplasty in 1934

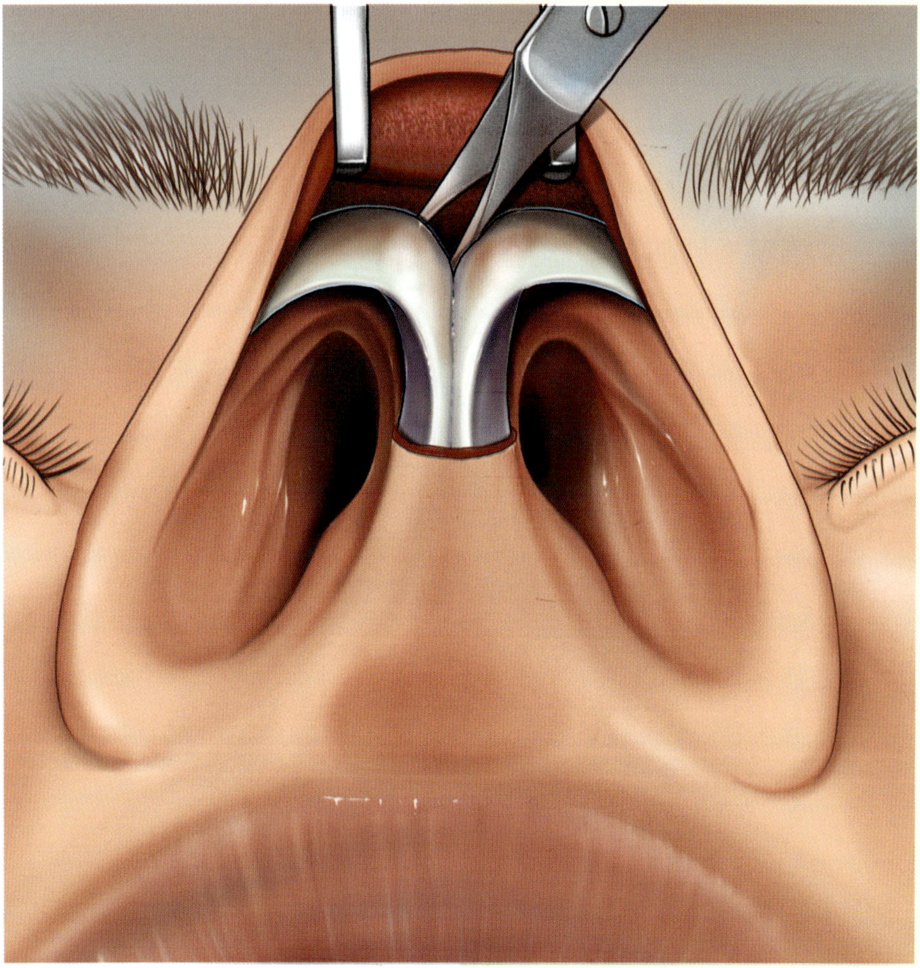

Figure 9b: open rhinoplasty approach

References

1. Rees T.D Aesthetic Plastic Surgery. W. B. Saunders Philadelphia London Toronto, 1980; p. 117.

2. Mink P.J. The nose as a means of breathing. Presse Otolaryngol. Belge, 1903; 21, 481-496.

3. Gonzales -Ulloa M. Aesthetic Plastic Surgery Vol 3, Piccin 1988; p. 29.

4. Sheen J H. Aethetic Rhinoplasty. C.V. Mosby Company 1978; p. 26.

5. Sulsenti G. Chirurgia Funzionale ed Estetica del Naso. Officine Grafiche Arsitalia di Ozzano Emilia, 1972; p. 33.

6. Sulsenti G. Lezioni di Chirurgia Funzionale del Setto e della Piramide Nasale. Poligrafici Luigi Parma S.P.A. Bologna, 1978; p. 40.

7. Converse Reconstructive Plastic Surgery vol. 2. W.B. Saunders Company, 1977; p. 1047.

8. Converse Reconstructive Plastic Surgery vol. 2. W.B. Saunders Company 1977, p. 1049.

9. Rethi A. Raccourcissement du nez trop long. Rev.Chir.Plast, 1934; 2:85.

10. Converse Reconstructive Plastic Surgery vol. 2. W.B. Saunders Company 1977; p. 1048.

CHAPTER 7

Execution

Anaesthesiological introduction

edited by Paolo Messercola anaesthesiologist

Anesthesia for rhinoplasty has the particular purpose to restrict intraoperative bleeding. Over the years, different techniques have been proposed, also in relation to technological and pharmacological evolution: general anesthesia with orotracheal intubation and local anesthesia with or without sedation.

Different techniques have different advantages and disadvantages, but have the common goal to reduce bleeding, and permit a good surgical result with patient and operator satisfaction.

The anesthesiologist, the surgeon and, of course, the patient work together towards the same goal.

Local anesthesia with or without sedation has been the most widely used technique for many years.

The disadvantages of this technique are: patient mobility; difficult management of adverse events; lack of pressure control with increased risk of bleeding; risk of inhalation ab ingestis in case of deep sedation with loss of cough and swallowing reflexes; the difficult rapid access to the upper airways due to the location of the surgical site; not suitable for anxious or unmotivated patients. These disadvantages make, in our opinion, general anesthesia the technique of first choice.

The objectives of general anesthesia are: obtaining hypnosis, i.e. the loss of awareness of the events related to the operation; akinesia, i.e. the possibility of positioning the patient as desired; muscle relaxation to facilitate

surgical access; control of the autonomic nervous system and analgesia to control pain reflexes. In addition, in Rhinoplasty surgery, the use of systemic pressure control allows for optimal bleeding reduction.
General anesthesia, which is currently well-tolerated and has few side effects, promotes total control of the procedure, permits continuous monitoring and facilitates emergency intervention on a motionless patient, in the desired position, without time restrictions.

Peculiarities of general anesthesia in rhinoplasty

Anesthesia in rhinoplasty is characterized by a number of factors including the potential problems with effective airway control, the mixing of skills between surgeon and anesthesiologist, which requires a good working relationship between the specialists involved. Careful control of bleeding is also necessary because it may increase the possibility of complications such as hypovolemia and blood inhalation, as well as adversely affecting surgery and its outcome.
Pressure control thus arises from the need to meet several requirements: to ensure the reduction of blood loss, to improve the working conditions of the surgeon, but at the same time it must be compatible with a satisfactory preservation of perfusion flow to the tissues, especially in the brain, coronaries and kidney.
Anesthesia in nose surgery must be sufficiently deep to avoid hypertensive episodes and coughing containing bleeding.

Anesthesia techniques

The introduction of short-acting drugs such as propofol and remifentanil has enabled a more precise control and better intraoperative conditions for rhinoplasty than in the past.
The most effective techniques confirmed by numerous randomized and controlled trials, focus on the use of total intravenous anesthesia (TIVA) with propofol and remifentanil.
The use of combined techniques of local anesthesia by infiltration obtained through the use of 2% lidocaine with adrenaline 1:50.000 produces only transient hemodynamic effects, characterized by variation in arterial pressure, without significant alterations in tissue perfusion, and it is accompanied by a better control of intraoperative bleeding. This results in reduction of the surgical procedure duration and improvement of the post-operative course.

Surgical technique

What to do first

The upper lip should be observed: often when the nose is thin and has a very prominent hump, the nasal tip in growth has been pushed up by the septum and therefore the upper lip remains raised uncovering the incisors, the lip looks thin and voluntary movement may be required to close the buccal rim (fig. 1a). Typically in these cases, even if only to speak, there is a noticeable and unsightly movement of the nasal tip when moving the lips. However, this movement can also be present if the anatomical conformation is different from that described above. Since with rhinoplasty, in most cases, the aim is to reduce the hump, the septum will not support anymore the tip, which will therefore move backwards, reducing the nasal projection. This movement cannot take place completely if the connections between

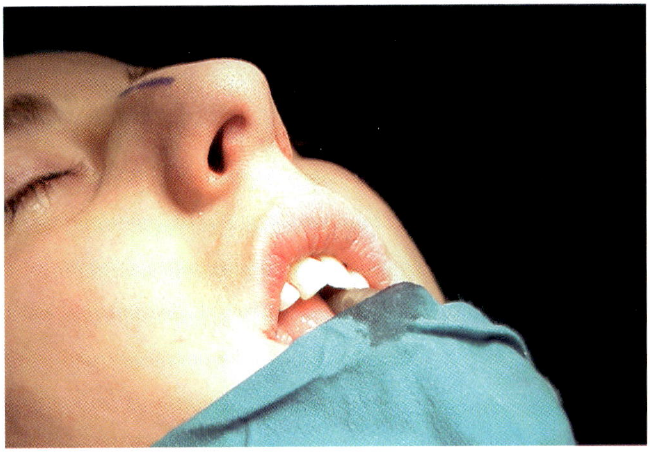

Figure 1: the lip remains elevated in the central part due to excessive projection of the tip of the nose

the lip and the anterior nasal spine are not interrupted, in order to allow the soft tissues to slide in relation to the underlying bone structure.

The procedure to perform this is: an incision is made along the labial frenulum, a Joseph's elevator is introduced, and the soft tissues are elevated from the anterior nasal spine and the lower part of the upper maxilla, just below the piriform aperture. The depressor septi nasi muscle, disengaged with this maneuver, will no longer exert its nasal tip depressing action when speaking or smiling. In profile lowering rhinoplasties the tension on the tip decreases as a result of the reduction of its projection, and after the above-described detachment has been performed, the soft tissues under the nose will eventually settle down. This will result in a better harmonization of the nose-upper lip ratio, and the lip will also appear visually fuller.

The labial frenulum is not normally modified but only used as a natural point to make the incision through which it is possible to introduce Joseph's elevator (figs. 2a, b). However, if deemed necessary it can also be lengthened and not only incised. In this case the lengthening can be done cutting it with scissors or with a simple Z-plastic.

The root of the nose (nasion is the name of the craniometric point that

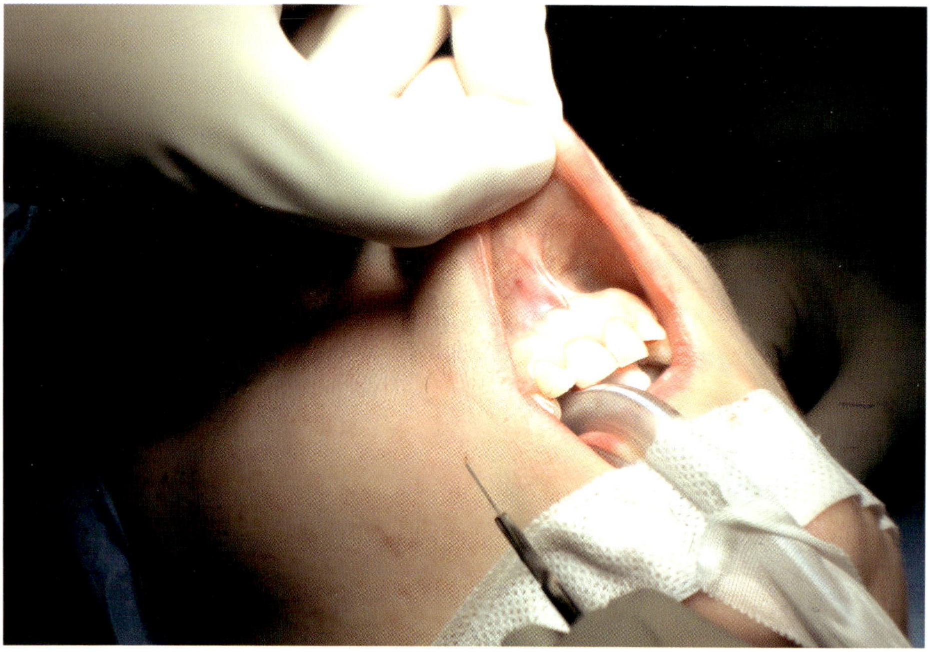

Figure 2a: longitudinal incision of the labial frenulum

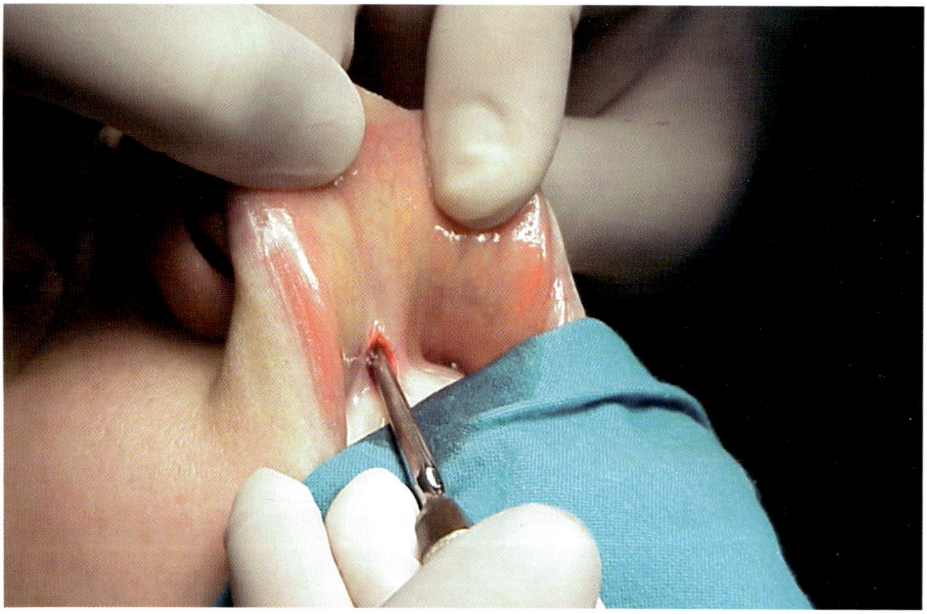

Figure 2b: septal depressor muscle detachment with Joseph's elevator

corresponds to the root of the nose) is then assessed (fig. 3). In the vast majority of cases the nasion doesn't need to be changed and is the point from which the ideal line of the new dorsum originates (fig. 4a). In some cases the nasion needs to be brought further back excavating the root of the nose using a curved rasp (fig. 5).
To bring anteriorly the nasion bone, cartilage or alloplastic grafts may be used. The use of grafts must be well thought out and carried out only if indispensable, because due to the typical motility of the glabella it is difficult to stabilize such grafts. For this reason, if it is not really indispensable to advance the nasion, it is advisable to change the drawing of the nose and to find an aesthetically different solution that does not involve its advancement.
In some cases the profile has to be augmented. In this case, various materials can be used: e.g. bone, cartilage, muscle fascia and also alloplastic products. Each of these have advantages and disadvantages. As an alloplastic material it is preferable to use polytetrafluoroethylene (PTFE or goretex) because of its broad tolerable qualities, because it is durable and virtually free of complications. Bone is indicated for augmentation with rigidity, that is advisable for example to restore rigidity and support in the noses of former boxers. Cartilage is easier to find. Cartilage from the nose is the most suitable. Once removed from a context in which they exerted and were subjected to the action of forces, due to the fact that these forces are lacking, cartilages tend to bend. The alar cartilages need to be weakened with Rubin's morselizer (fig. 6), or crushed with Cottle's cartilage crusher (fig. 7) to make them lose the memory of their shape.
The cartilages can also be diced and wrapped in a muscular fascia or in absorbable surgicel polyanhydroglucuronic acid or tabotamp made of oxidized and regenerated cellulose tissue (fig. 8) to be placed on the dorsum, but this is a second-best solution because it will never be possible to be sure to

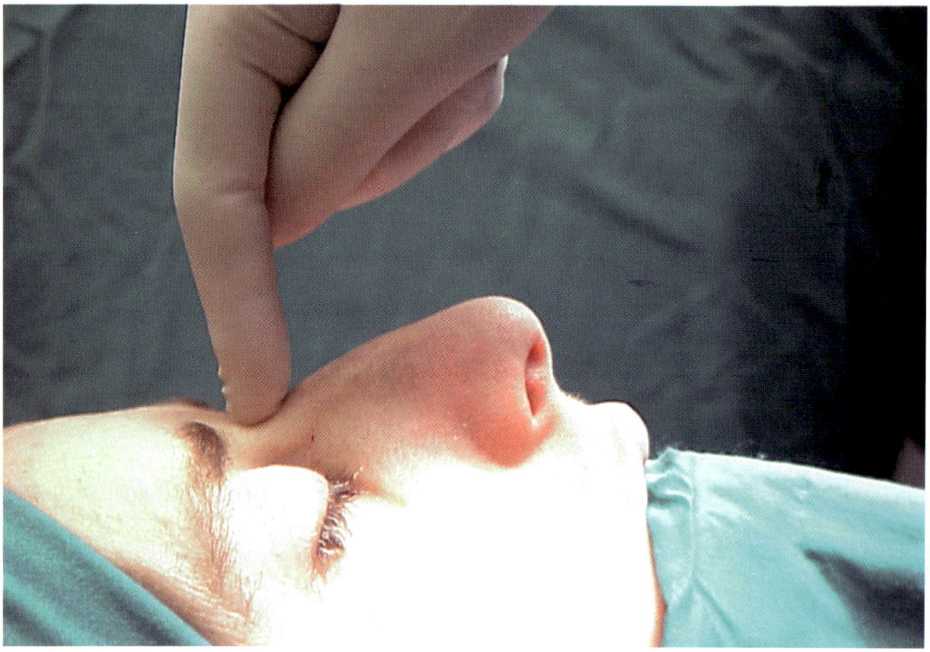

Figure 3: assessment of the root of the nose, pressing the soft tissues with a finger

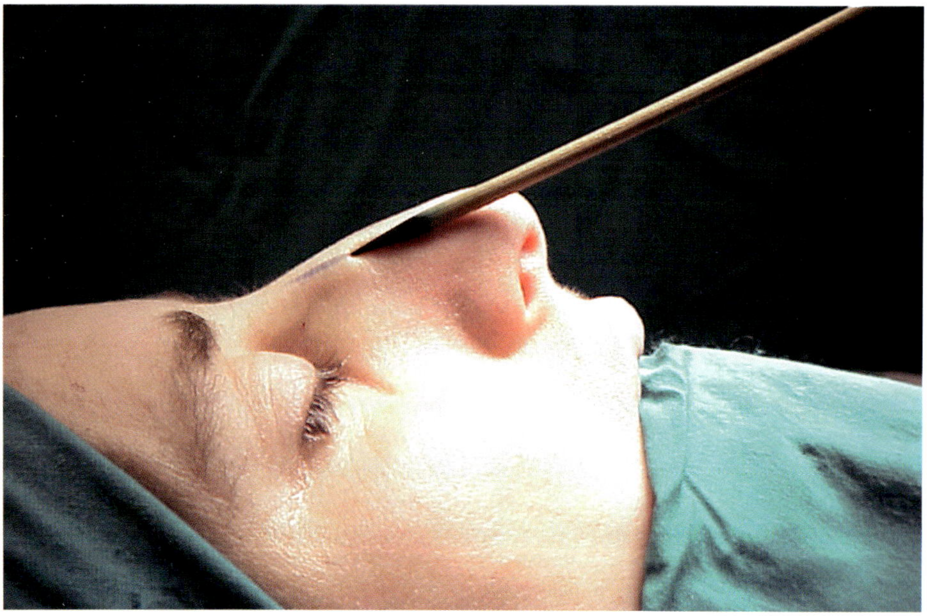

Figure 4: the new line of the dorsum is drawn

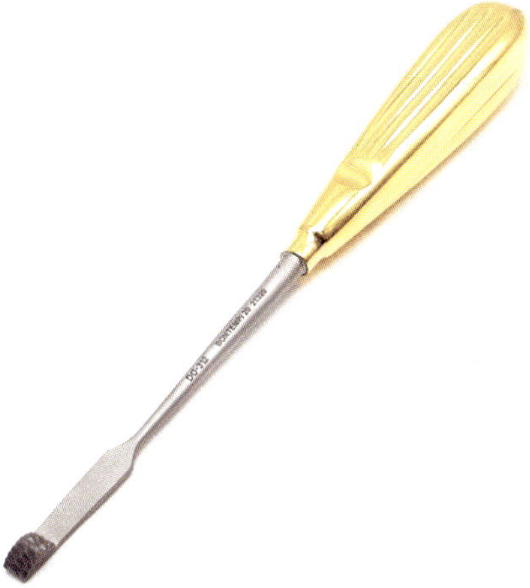

Figure 5: rasps for digging the glabella

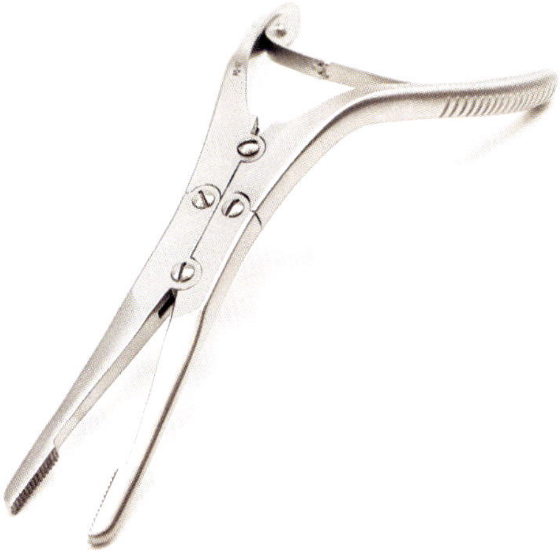

Figure 6: Rubin's morselizer, used to weaken the cartilage and make it loose its memory in order to prevent subsequent curling

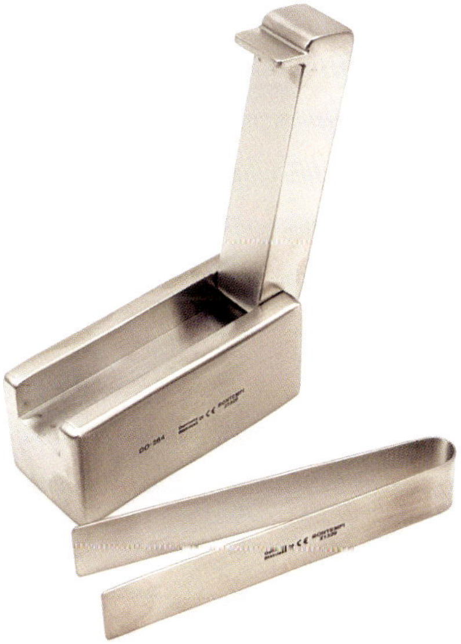

Figure 7: Cottle's cartilage crusher, which serves the same purpose as Rubin's morselizer, but crushes a lot the fragment to be used

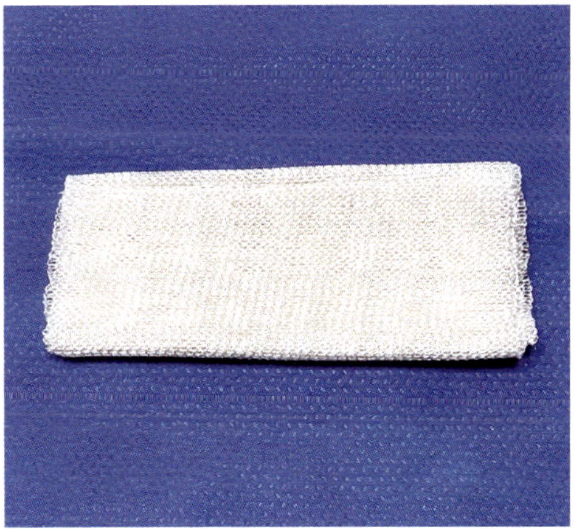

Figure 8: surgicel polyanhydroglucuronic. Similar to tabotamp, consisting of oxidized and regenerated cellulose

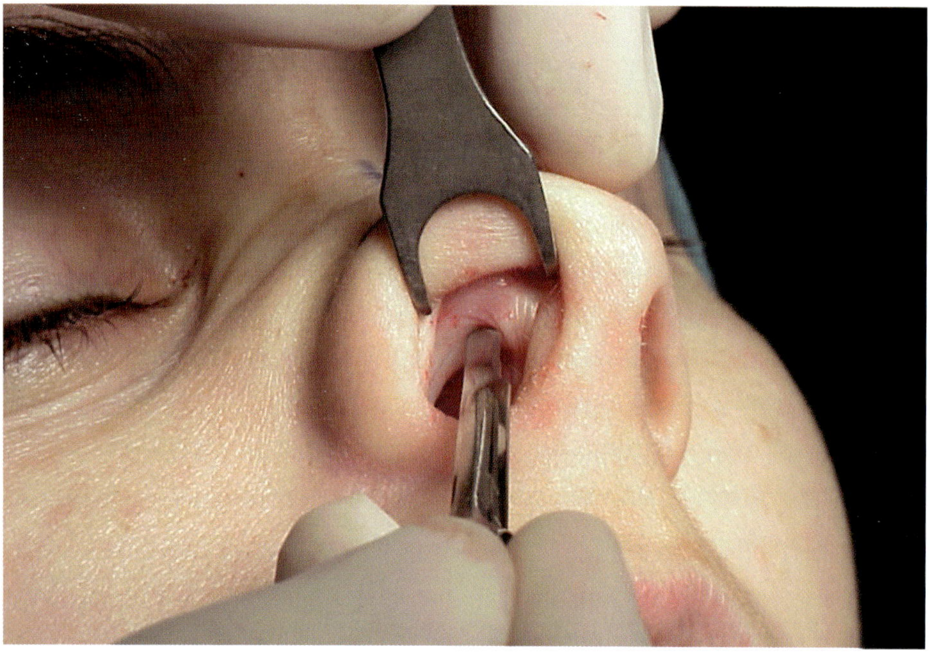

Figure 9: intercartilaginous incision made starting laterally just above the lower margin of the triangular cartilage

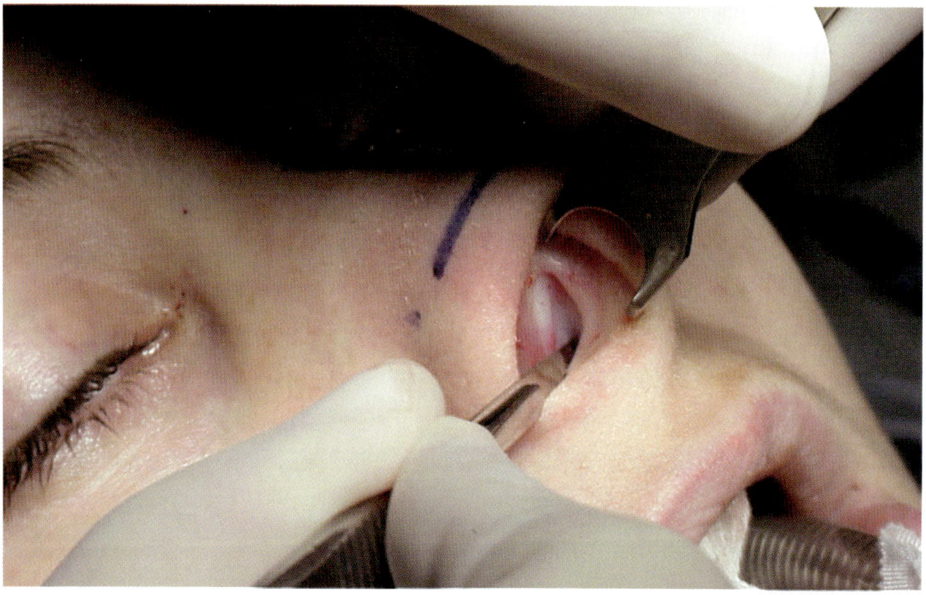

Figure 10: extension of the intercartilaginous incision to the front of the quadrangular septal cartilage

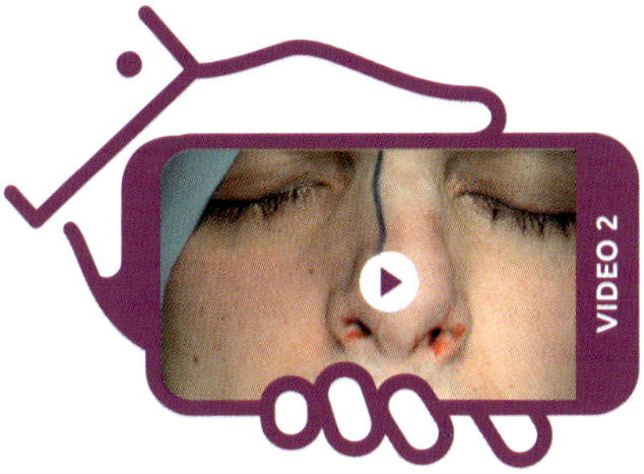

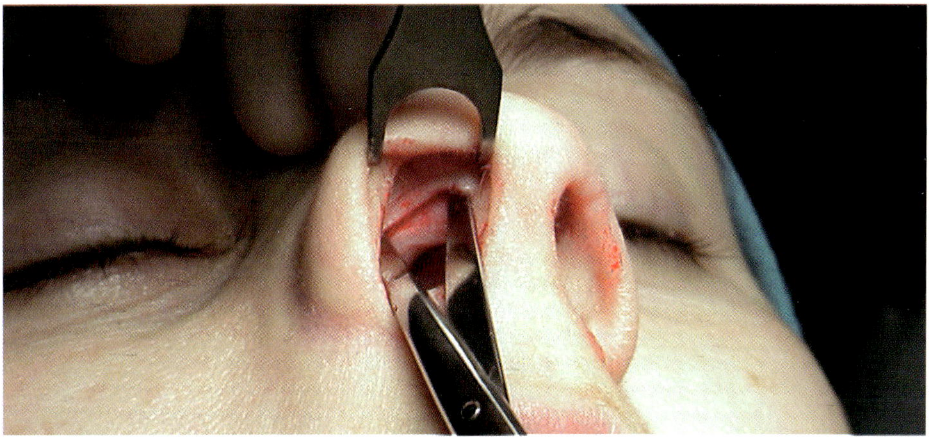

Figure 11: undermining of the nasal dorsum carried out with scissors

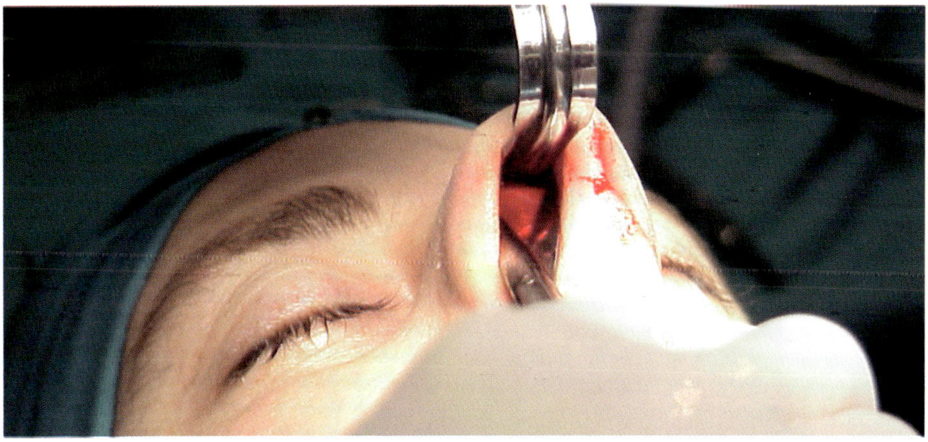

Figure 12: the dissection is wide to allow the introduction of the instruments and the adaptation of the skin to the new shape of the nose

· Hump reduction

The hump is then rasped with Fomon rasps made of widia (video 3) (figs. 13a, b) and with Gasperoni rasps (video 4) (fig. 14) and Rubin rasps (video 5) (fig. 15). The irregularities of the rasped dorsum can be best detected passing the glabella rasp, that can be used both for this reason and to deepen the root of the nose (video 6). The cartilage is precisely cut with direct vision with a Pellegrini scissor (video 7) (figs. 16a, b) and a blade 11 scalpel (video 8) (fig. 17).

Pellegrini nasal dorsal scissors are powerful because they have short branches, have knurling in their surface that make them suitable to cut the cartilage, and have also an optimal angle to permit a direct vision to the septum.

As an alternative to the use of rasp and scissors, a notch can be made at the height of the new profile at the septum - triangular cartilage complex with Mc Indoe scissors (figs. 18a, b), and then an osteotome (1) can be introduced to remove the bony hump. However, this method is less precise because if you make a mistake assessing where to make the notch, or even the inclination of the osteotome, you risk making a big error in setting the new profile. The use of rasps is therefore more precise because it is progressive and it is therefore much more preferred to osteotomy with the chisel.

· Shortening and tilting of the septum

The amount of nose shortening can be easily assessed once the hump has been reduced, and is accomplished removing the caudal part of the septum. To assess how much to shorten and how much to tilt the septum to open the nasolabial angle, the columella is slid to one side of the septum and then is marked out mentally how much to shorten and at what angle. Then with an 11-blade scalpel following the mental mark (video 9), the septum cartilage is shortened along with the chondromucosa of both

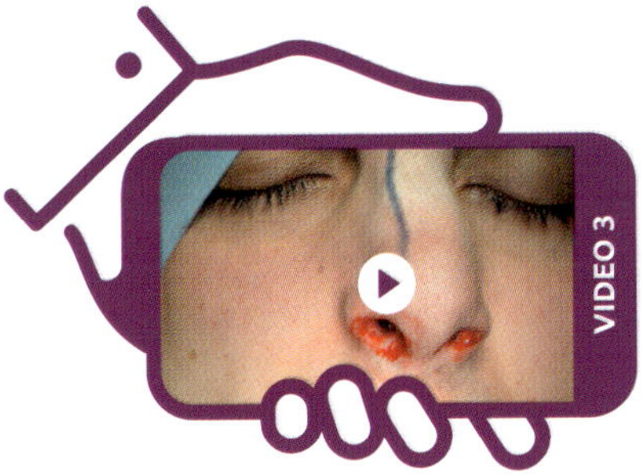

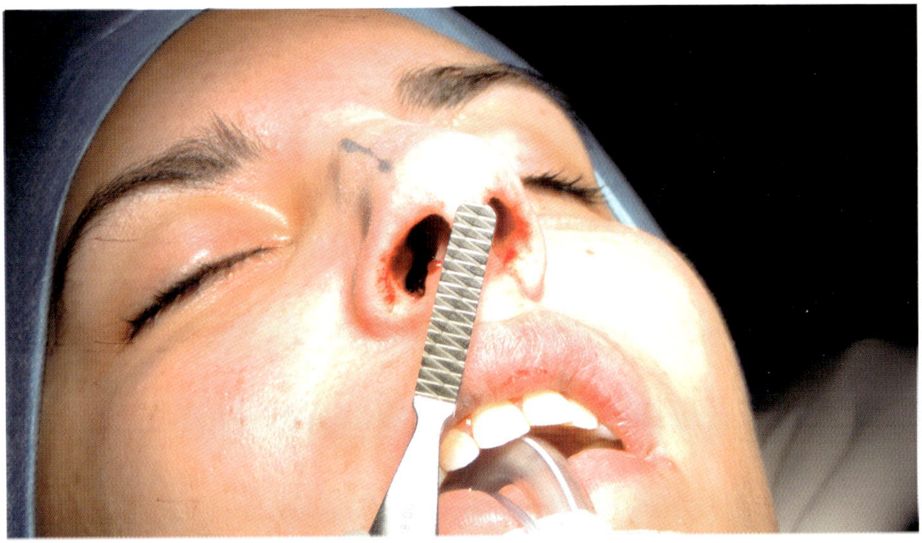

Figure 13a: Fomon rasps made of widia

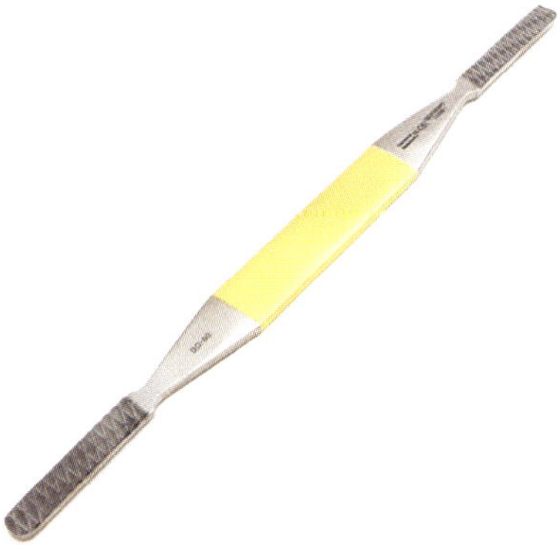

Figure 13b: Fomon rasps made of widia

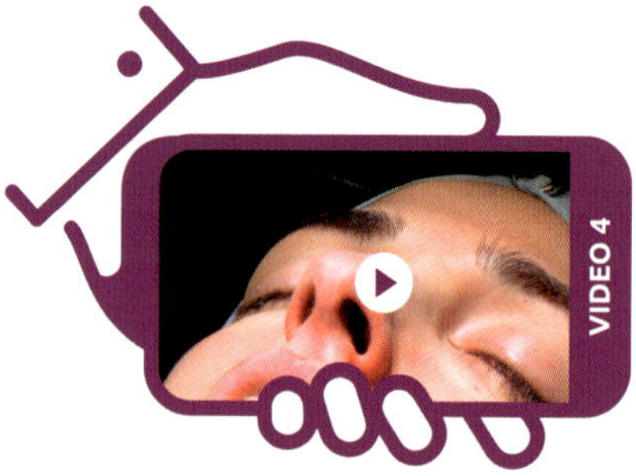

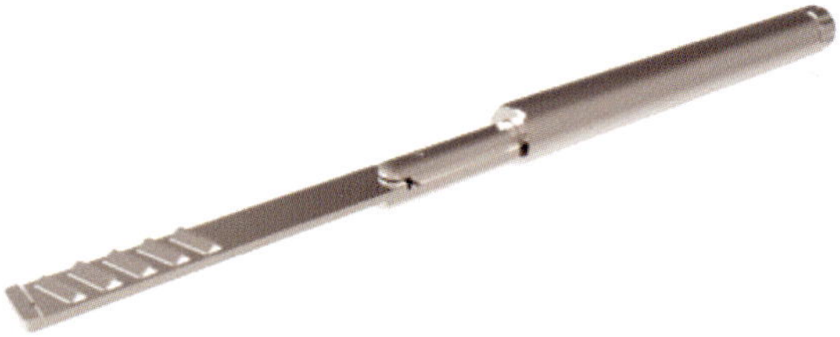

Figure 14: Gasperoni rasp. The cutting edge is suitable for consuming both bone and cartilage and allows a smooth transition between nasal bones and triangular cartilages and septum

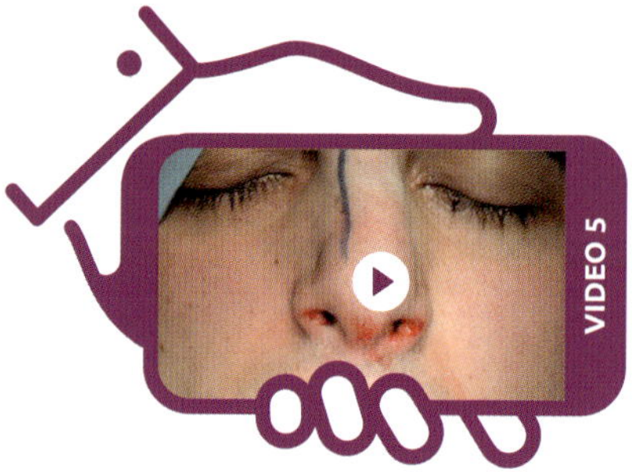

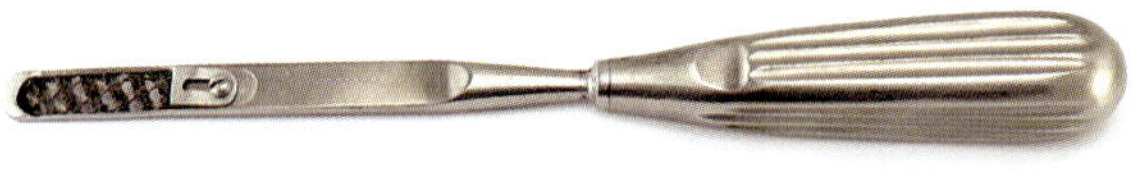

Figure 15: Rubin rasp is also suitable for rasping evenly bone and cartilage

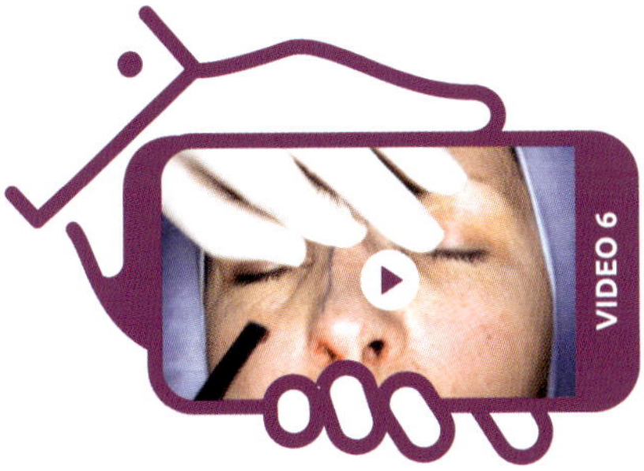

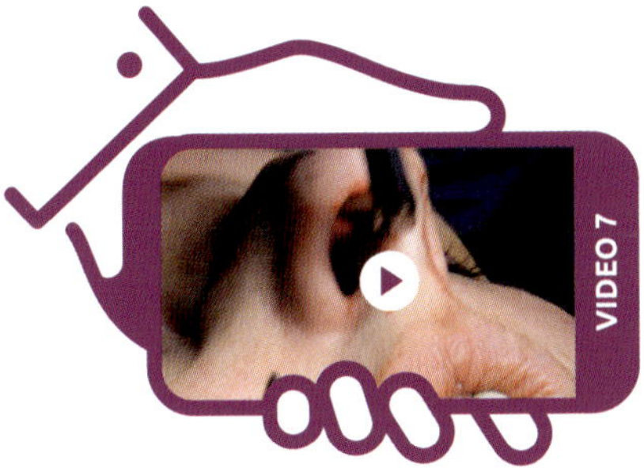

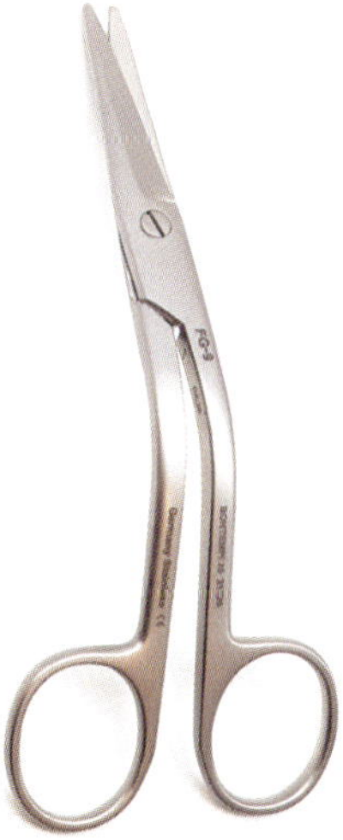

Figure 16a: Pellegrini angled scissors

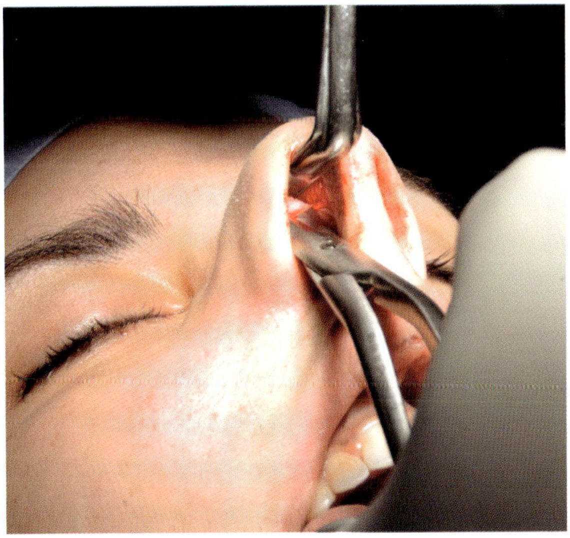

Figure 16b: cartilaginous dorsum reduction with Pellegrini scissors

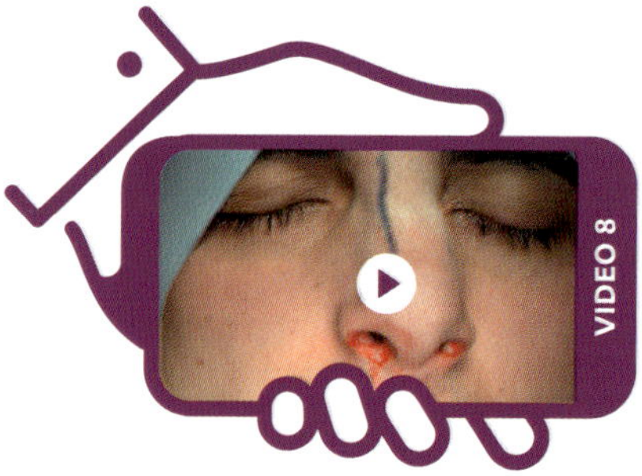

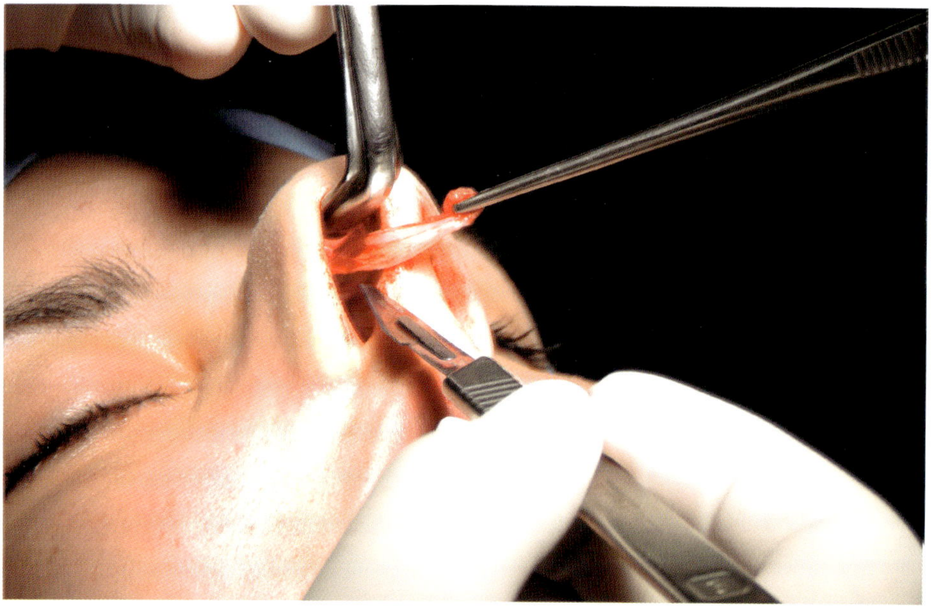

Figure 17: cartilage dorsum reduction using a blade 11-scalpel

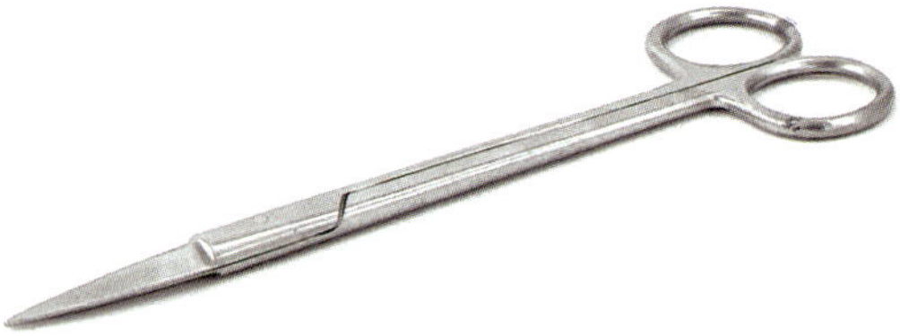

Figure 18a: Mc Indoe scissor

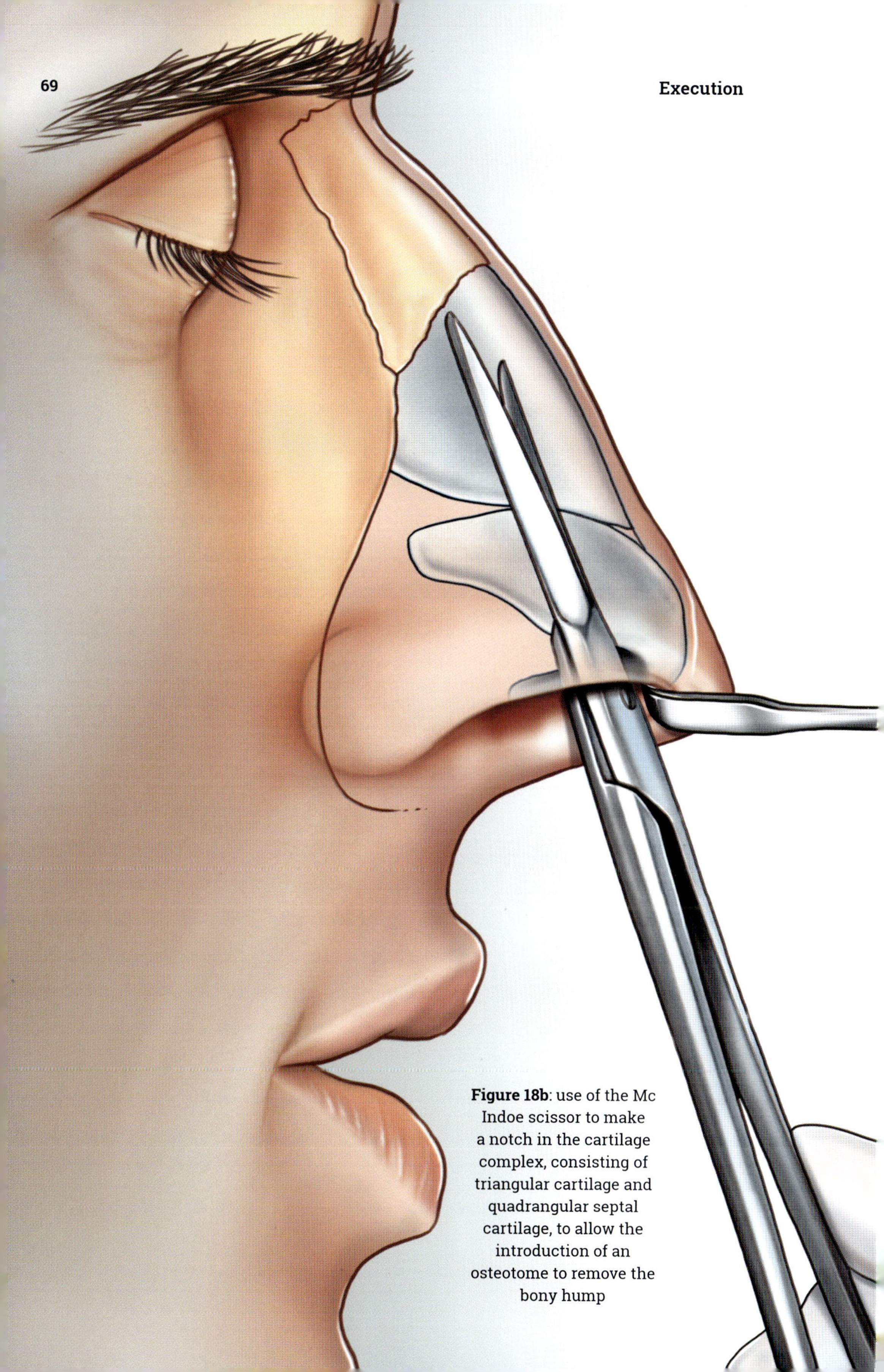

Figure 18b: use of the Mc Indoe scissor to make a notch in the cartilage complex, consisting of triangular cartilage and quadrangular septal cartilage, to allow the introduction of an osteotome to remove the bony hump

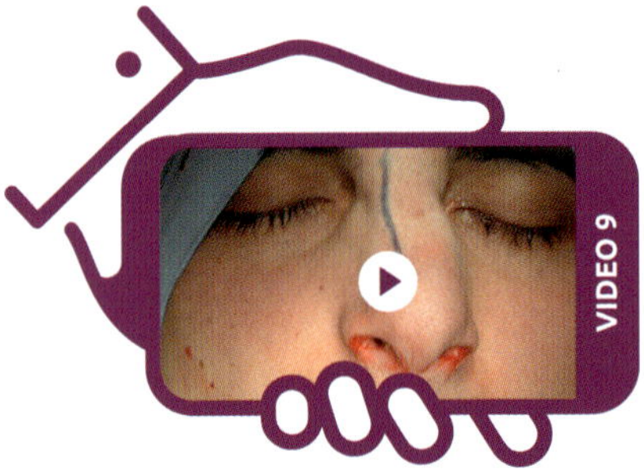

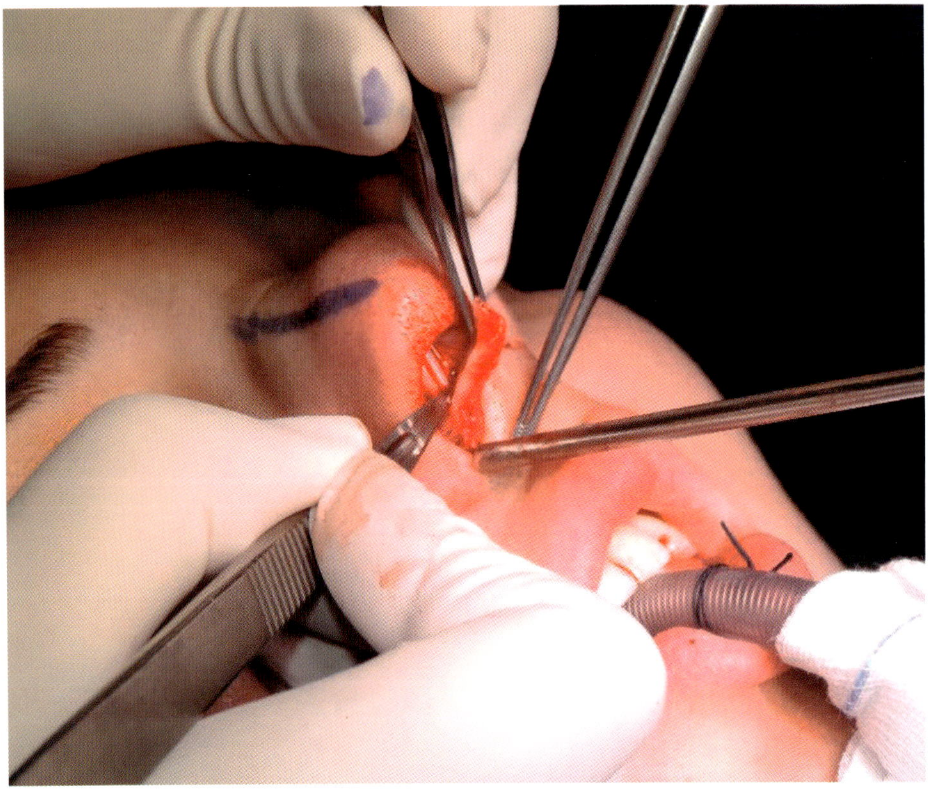

Figure 19: the columella is slid upwards alongside the septum.
Once the desired nasolabial angle and length of the nose are displayed, it is mentally marked how much to shorten the septum and at what angle, and then is possible to proceed shortening the septum with a scalpel

sides (fig. 19). The chondromucosa covering the surface of the cartilaginous septum is sutured to the columella at the end of the operation. If the chondromucosa was left in abundance, the tip would tend to drop postoperatively.

· Tip treatment

The nasal tip is treated with the aim of making it more graceful and in harmony with the nasal dorsum: it should stand out a little on the profile, to give a feeling of the "end of the nose". In reality the tip of the nose is made up of two points that correspond to the domus of the alar cartilages of both sides (fig. 20). The three-quarter line joining the eyebrow to the nasal dorsum should be smooth and end at the domus on the same side (fig. 21) (2).

When observing the tip, it must be determined whether its projection is correct in relation to the dorsum. Therefore, the tip should normally be

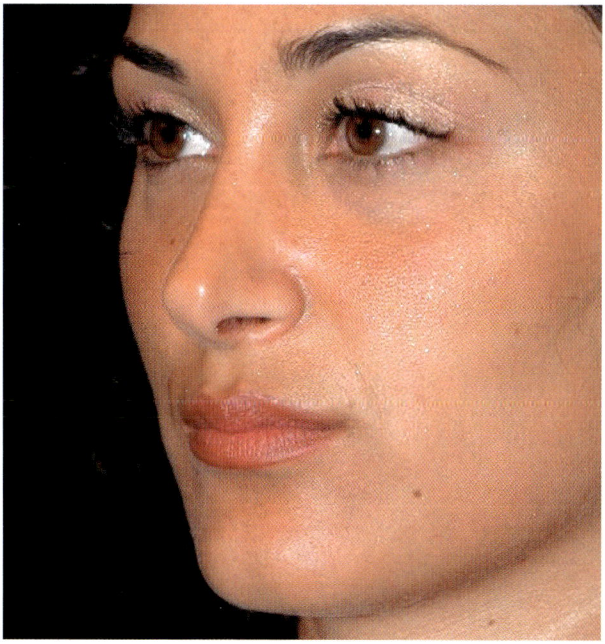

Figure 20: the tip of the Nose is composed of two tips that correspond to the domus of both sides

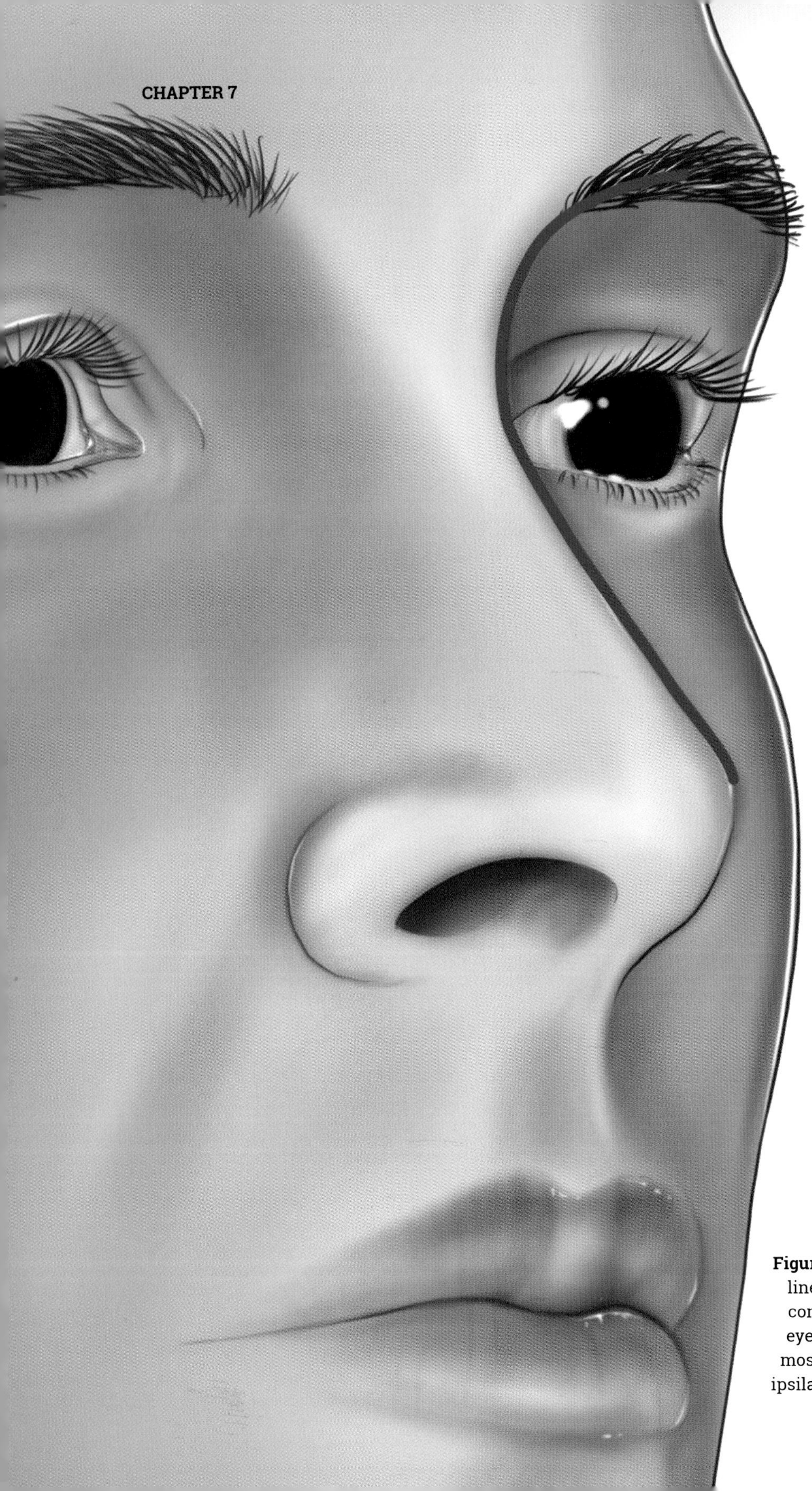

Figure 21: a single line joins with continuity the eyebrow to the most prominent ipsilateral point of the tip

operated after defining the new dorsum or making continuous adjustments to balance the dorsum/tip ratio.

The tip may be normally projected, over-projected or under-projected. The conformation of the alar cartilages can be normal or globular (boxy tip) or even too slim.

To correct an alar cartilage that has a good shape but is only a little bulky in relation to the new nasal pyramid, it is sufficient to trim the cephalic margin of the lateral crus of the alar cartilage to obtain a good result. In this case the Diamond technique (see below) is suitable. If the tip is squared and therefore needs to be narrowed, the Hockey Stick technique is used. If the tip is too projected, a portion of cartilage at the junction of the medial and lateral crus should be resected. If the tip is very globular it may be necessary to expose it through a rim incision, i.e. a marginal incision immediately caudal to the lower margin of the lateral crus and along the anterior margin of the medial crus to expose the cartilage and visually assess what to do.

In the vast majority of cases the technique of choice for tip correction is the hockey stick technique. (3) (figs. 22a, b, c, d). With this technique we obtain a reduction of the cephalic portion of the Alar cartilage, narrowing of the tip and the simultaneous reduction of the angle that the lateral crus forms with the medial crus. If, on the other hand, it is desired to keep this angle almost unchanged or to vary it slightly and it is not necessary to narrow the tip, the Diamond technique (4) is applied (fig. 23). In both cases the amount of cephalic margin of the alar cartilage to be removed is marked from the outside on the skin surface of the nostrils, bearing in mind that a strip of cartilage of at least two millimeters must always be left at the lower margin of the alar cartilage in order to preserve the support function provided by the lateral crus.

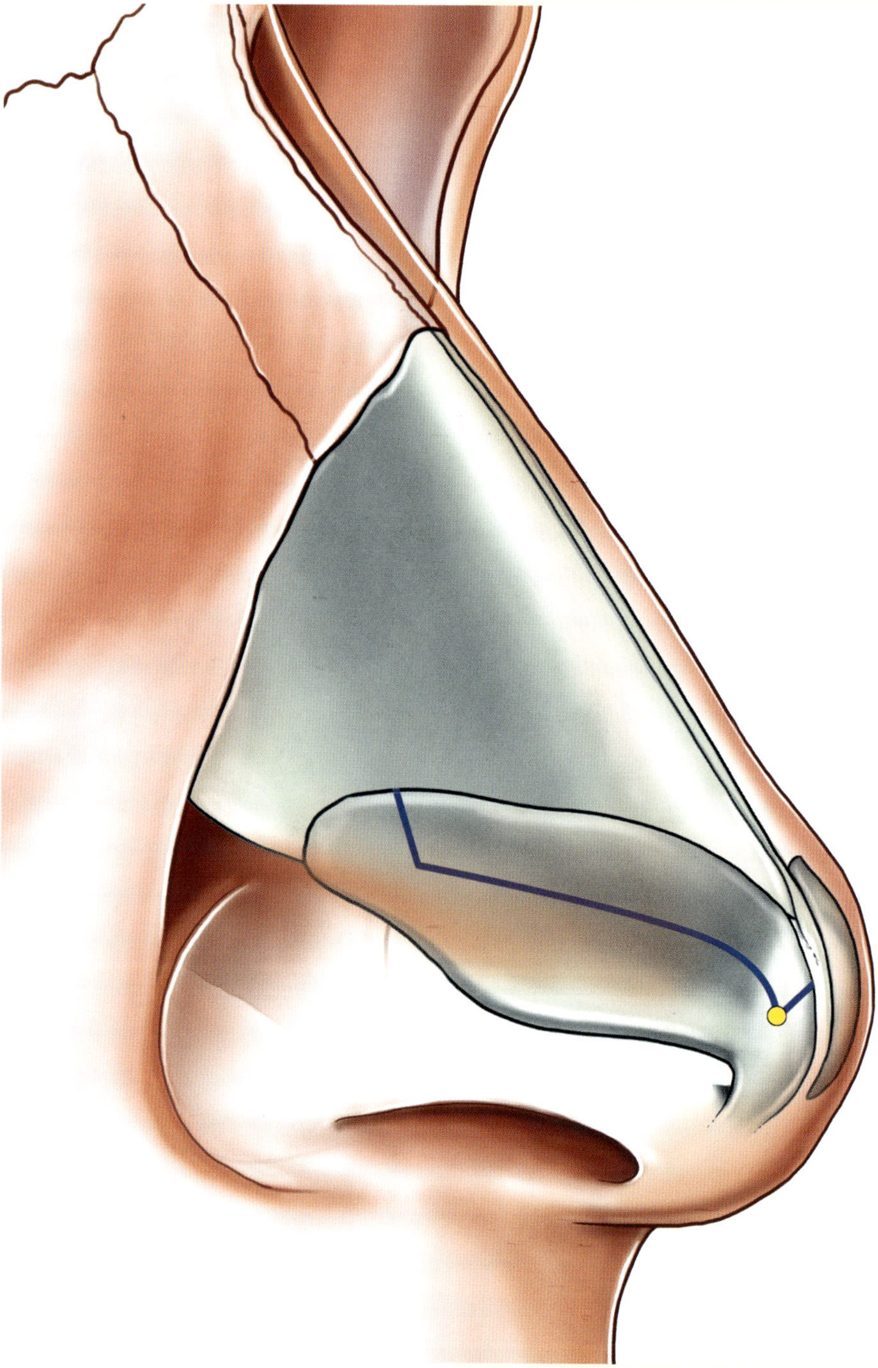

Figure 22a: drawing of the removal of the cephalic margin of the lateral crus of the alar cartilage

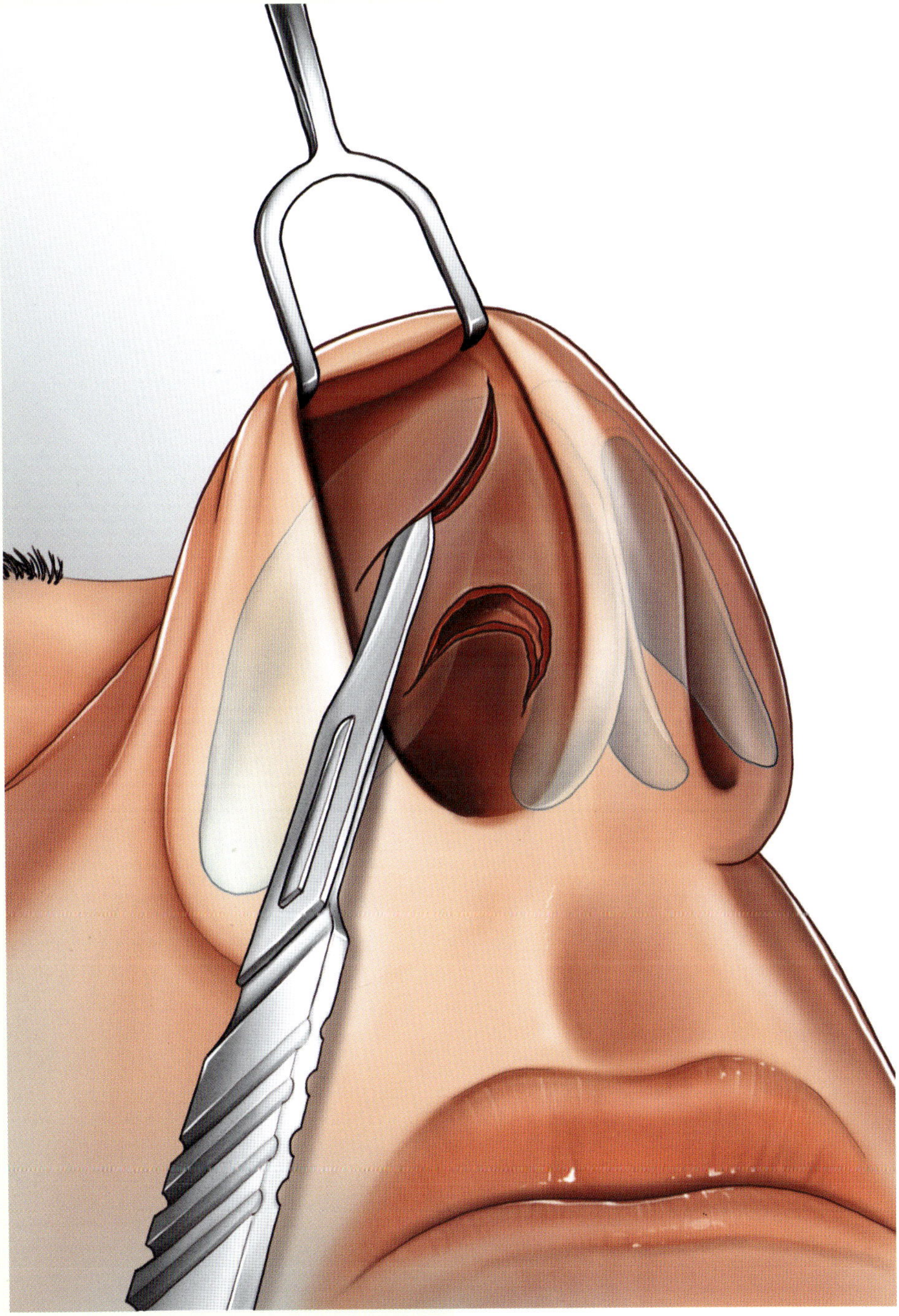

Figure 22b: the hockey stick technique is used to shape the tip removing the cephalic margin of the clare cartilage and at the same time tightening the tip

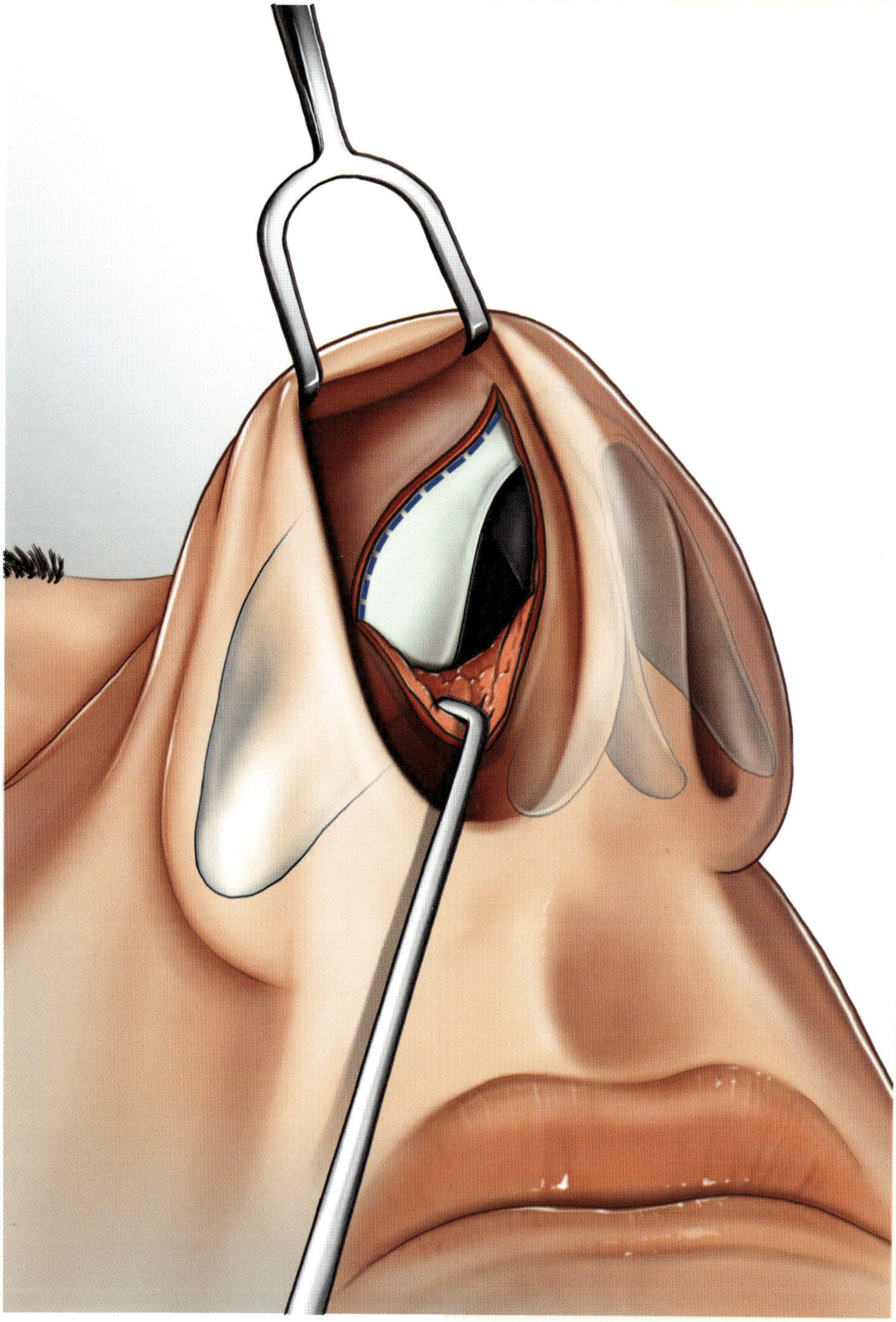

Figure 22c: the portion of exposed cartilage that needs to be removed

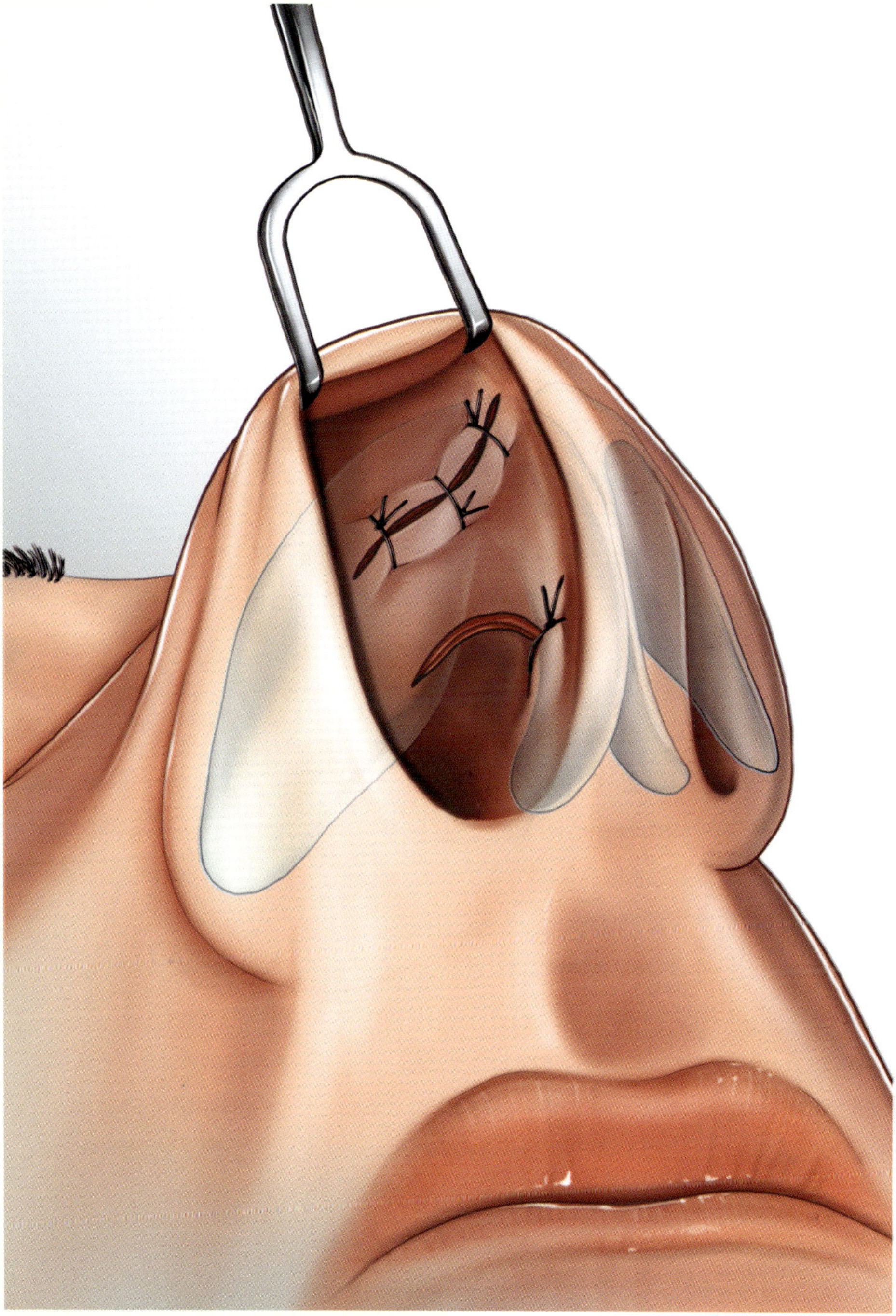

Figure 22d: the carefully sutured incision needed to keep the vestibule's coating intact

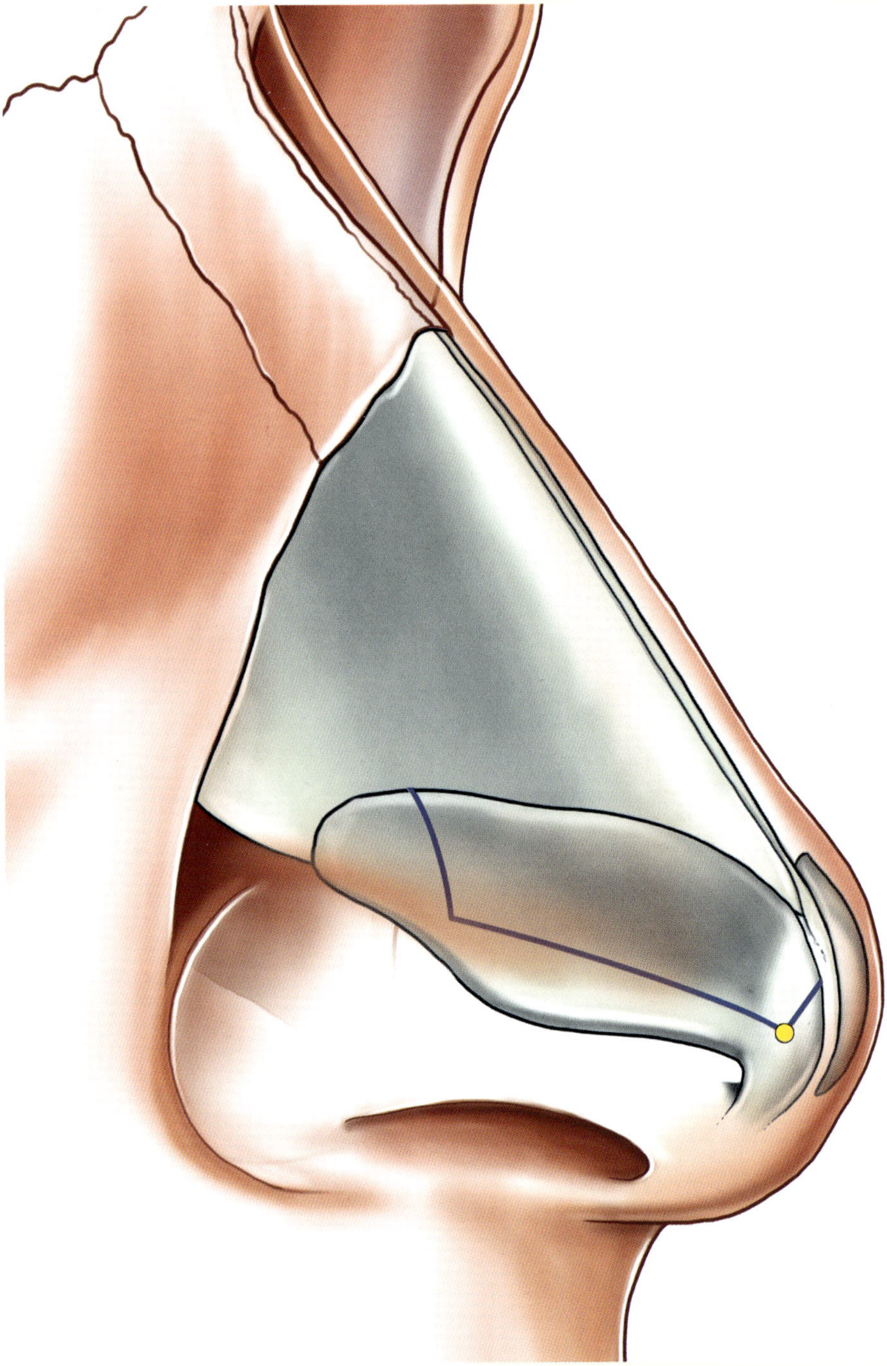

Figure 23: Diamond's technique for reducing the cephalic margin of the lateral crus

How the marking is carried out

First mark the point where the alar cartilage causes a depression on the skin surface of the nostril(video 10). This point constitutes a landmark (fig. 24). I have called this point point D (depression-dimple) and has been the object of many communications at numerous congresses since 1990.

The first times you do your drawing it is convenient to mark the lower margin of the lateral crus of the alar cartilage with the Gasperoni alar

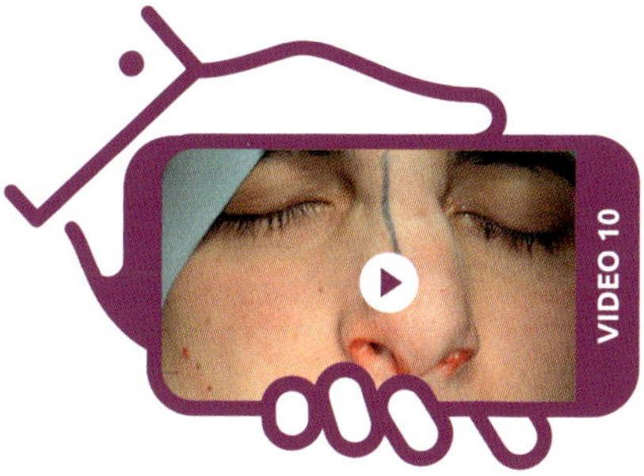

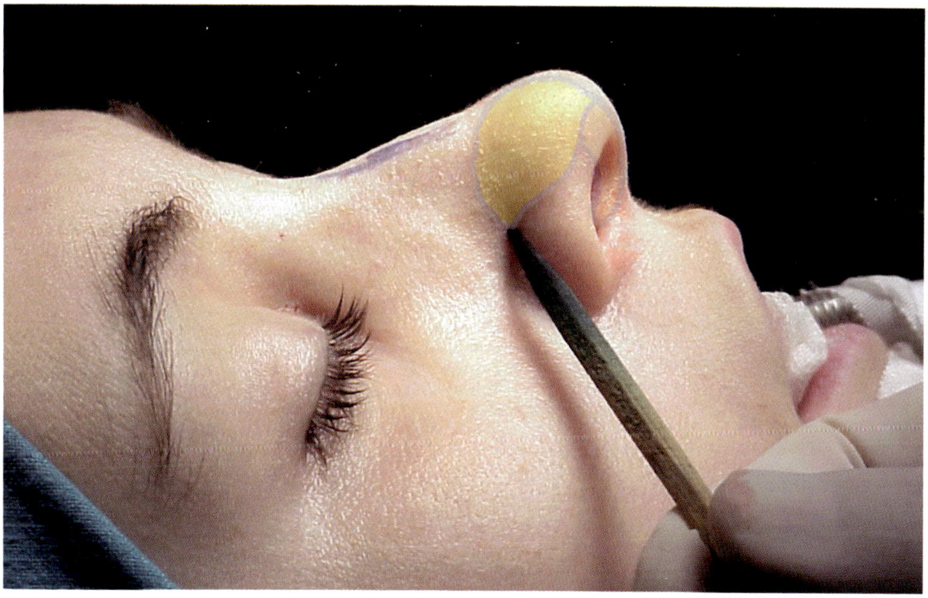

Figure 24: a point is marked where the alar cartilage creates a depression between the ala and the nasal pyramid. This point is a landmark that helps to quantify the portion of Alar cartilage to be removed

demarcator (5). This is done by placing the flat branch of the Gasperoni alar demarcator (fig. 25) inside the nasal vestibule juxtaposing it to the lower margin of the lateral crus of the alar cartilage and then transferring its position on the skin's surface where it is drawn with methylene blue (figg. 26a, b). Once familiar with the technique, this step can be skipped because with experience it becomes intuitive to identify this margin. This maneuver serves to be certain that the planning of the resection of the cephalic margin of the crus lateral of the alar cartilage will be done leaving a lower strip of cartilage of at least 2 millimeters, so that nostril will not collapse.

With the thumb of the left hand (for the right-handed), the normally redundant cephalic part of the nasal tip is hidden and a line is drawn along the thumb starting at about point D and running towards the nasal tip (figs. 27a, b).

Gasperoni alar demarcator is used by placing the flat branch on the marking and squeezing. Start at the lateral portion of the marking going towards the tip (figs. 27c, d, e). The notched branch will mark a line on the inner side of the cartilage. A 15 blade will be used to make a full-thickness incision of the lining of the vestibule and cartilage along this line, taking care not to go deep into the skin.

The medial apex of the drawing can end in a straight line (Diamond technique) (7.4) (fig. 23) or curving towards the domus (hockey stick technique) (7.3) (figs. 22a, b, c). The latter is applied when you want to narrow the tip, and also involves a certain degree of closure of the dihedral angle that the Ala makes with the nasal axis: basically, you narrow the tip and the Ala rotates slightly upwards.

The domus is the most projected point located on the inner side of the nostril, and is marked with the tip of a scissor (fig. 28).

The incision, with a 15-blade scalpel, along the pattern transferred from outside to inside the nostril with Gasperoni forceps, begins near the domus

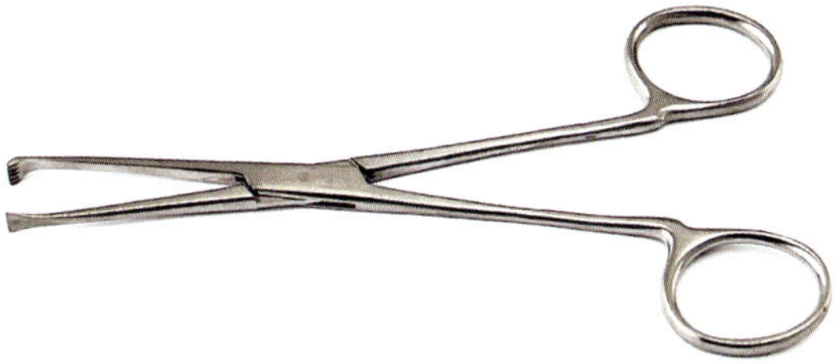

Figure 25: Gasperoni forceps

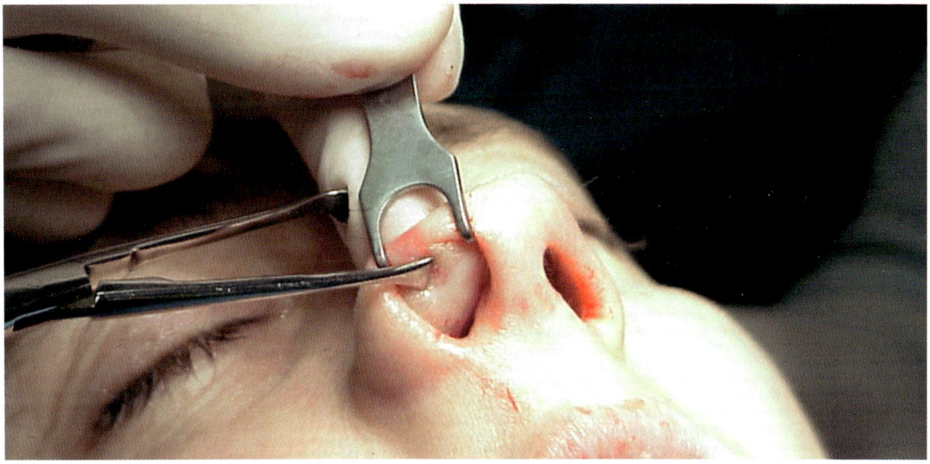

Figure 26a: the flat branch of the Gasperoni forceps fig. 7.25 a is placed on the lower margin of the lateral crus of the alar cartilage. It is used to transfer its position on the outer surface of the nostril

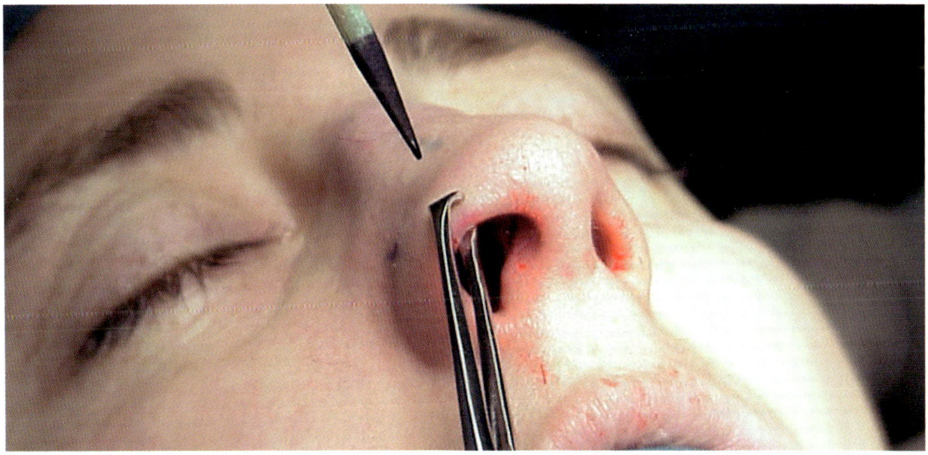

Figure 26b: the lower margin of the lateral crus cartilage is marked on the skin surface using methylene blue

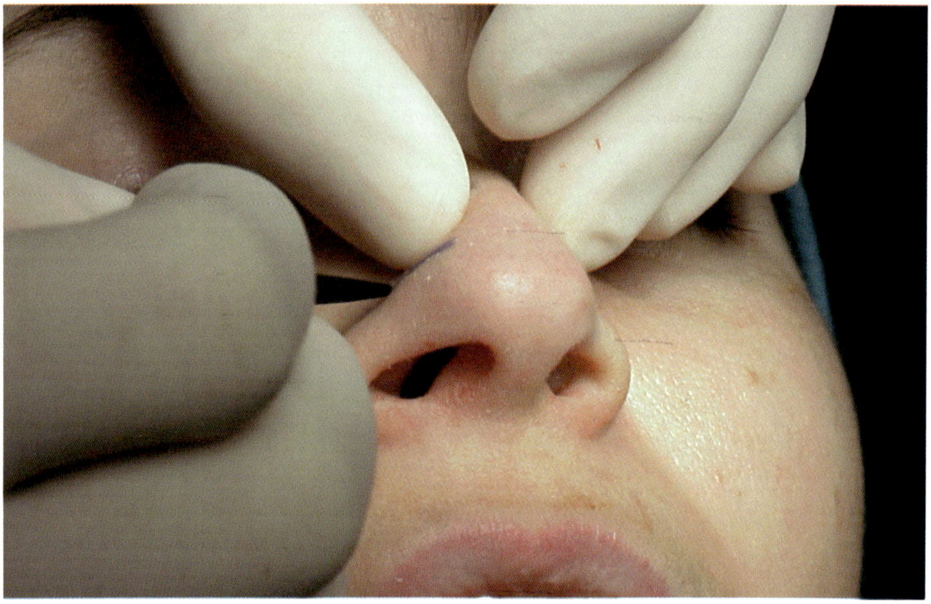

Figure 27a: covering with the thumb the redundancy of the alar cartilage that makes the tip too full, a line is marked going towards the most projected part of the tip that will be coincident with the domus

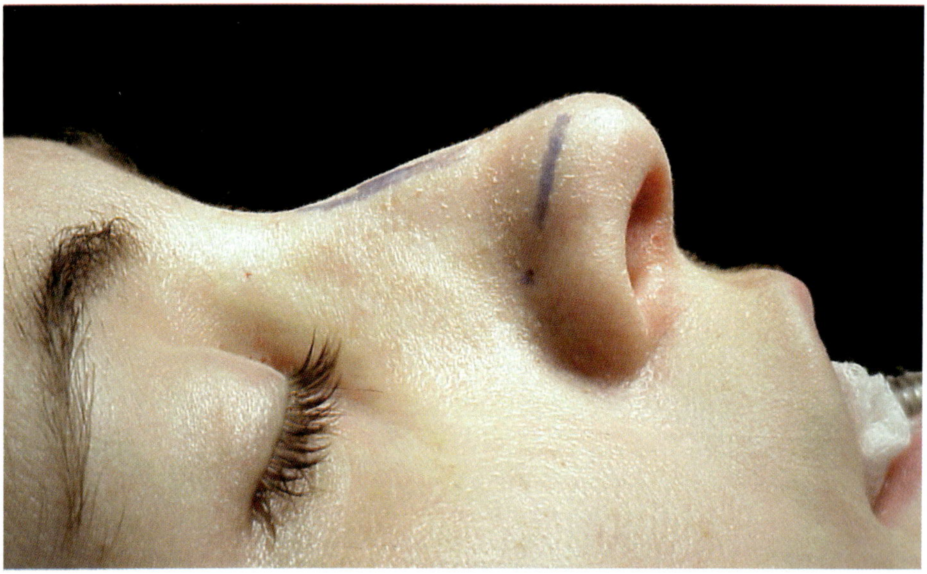

Figure 27b: completed drawing of the lower limit of the excision of the cephalic margin of the lateral crus of the alar cartilage

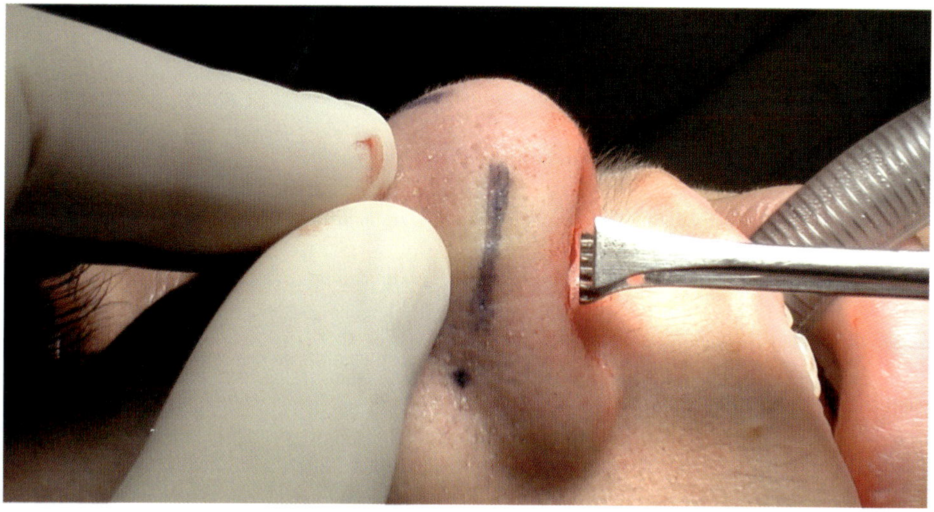

Figure 27c: Gasperoni forceps that has a flat branch and an indented branch. It is used to transfer the drawings made on the skin of the nostril to its inner side

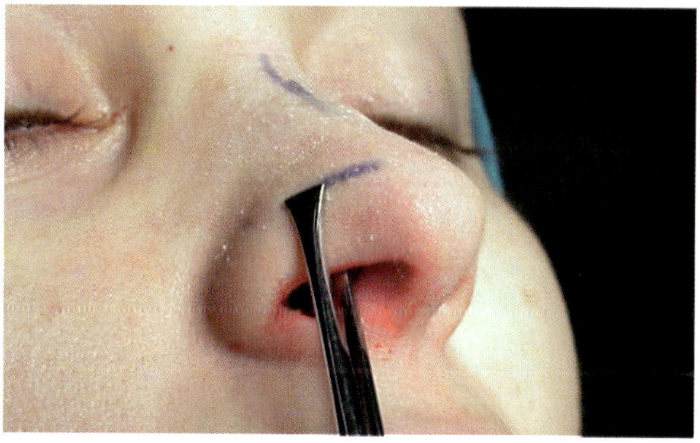

Figure 27d: the drawing is transferred to the internal side with the Gasperoni forceps starting laterally

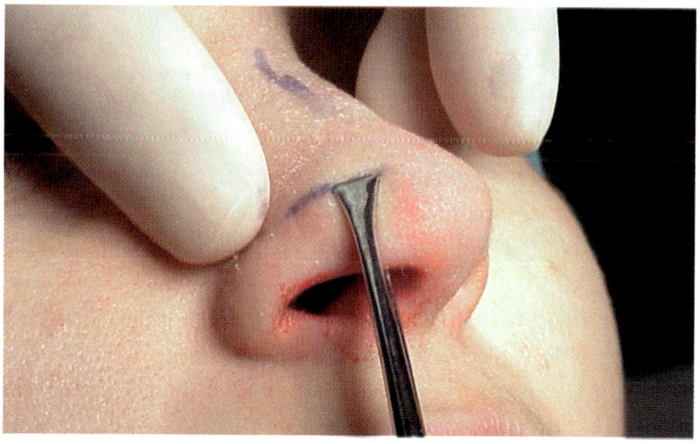

Figure 27e: the transfer to the inner side is completed by proceeding towards the domus

and continues laterally along the line that has been chosen. With the scalpel the vestibular skin and cartilage are incised (fig. 29). The vestibular skin is hooked (fig. 30) and is undermined in a cephalic direction from the lateral crus with pointed scissors (fig. 31a). The cephalic strip of cartilage that is going to be removed is then undermined from the overlying skin and then removed with the scissors and, when approaching the domus, where more precision is needed, an 11-blade scalpel is used (fig. 32) (video 11).

In the majority of cases, the dorsum is reduced and thus the profile is lowered. This leads to a loss of projection of the tip because the support of the septum is lost, so its shape changes from a isosceles triangle to an almost equilateral triangle. This change must be observed and, if the base of the nostrils becomes too wide it must be narrowed. To some extent retraction of the nostrils always occurs. This retraction may be sufficient to make the shape of the triangle of the nasal tip in harmony with the new nose, so a reduction of the nostrils is often not advisable, even if it seems necessary. The reason for the gull-wing opening of the nostrils is the difficulty to adapt to the new shape due to the connections between the lateral crura and the skin that impede their sliding so the shape is some what maintained (fig. 33). To a lesser extent, the connections with the vestibular skin also prevent the lateral crus cartilage from sliding laterally, hindering the desired change in shape of the tip. If further adjustments are not required, it is possible to go on with the trans-cartilaginous sutures made to reduce the cephalic part of the lateral crus of the alar cartilages (video 12).

If the nostrils have opened too wide, the dihedral angle between the lateral and medial crus becomes too wide. To reduce it, the caudal strip of the lateral crus of the alar cartilage is undermined from the skin to allow it to slide laterally. With this maneuver the ala can collapse slightly closing the angle (figs. 34a, b). If the closure is not sufficient, a small amount of the lateral apex of the lateral crus is removed so that it may slide laterally

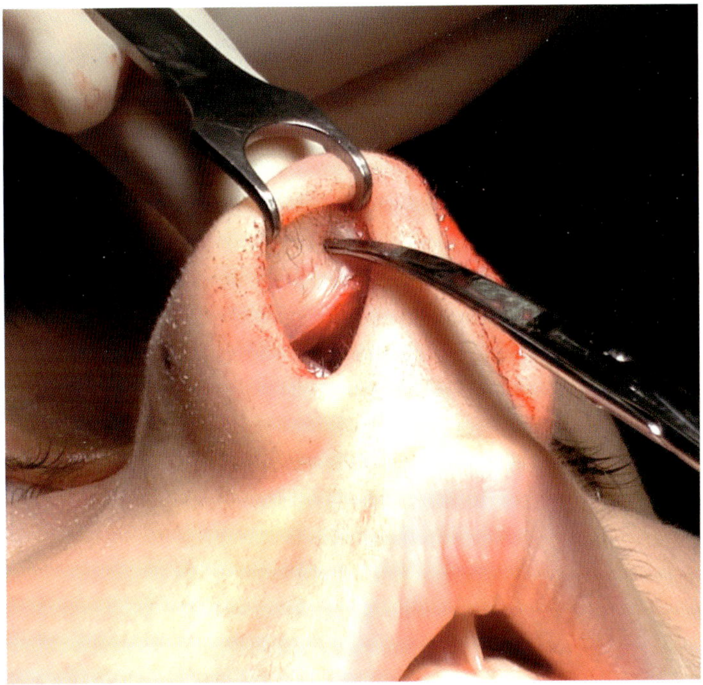

Figure 28: the tip of the scissors is slid upwards ending in the recess that corresponds to the domus

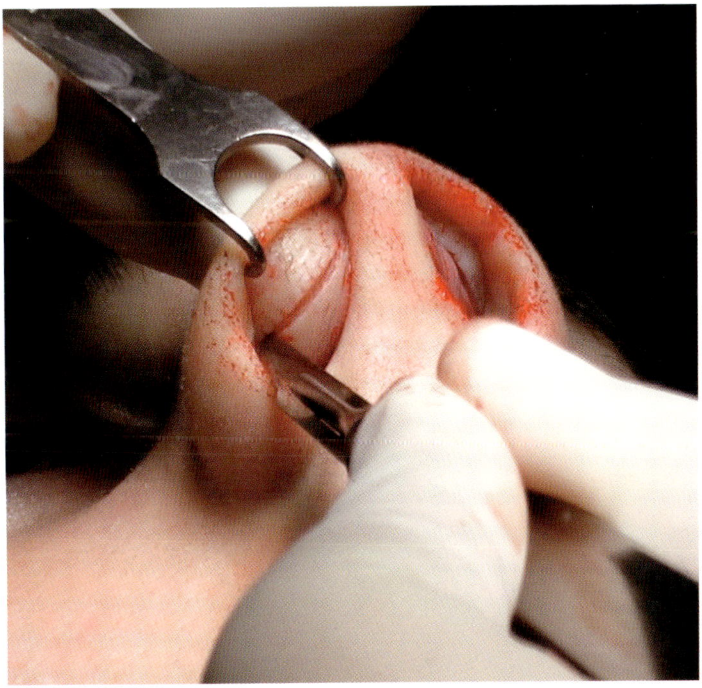

Figure 29: Incision of the skin and cartilage

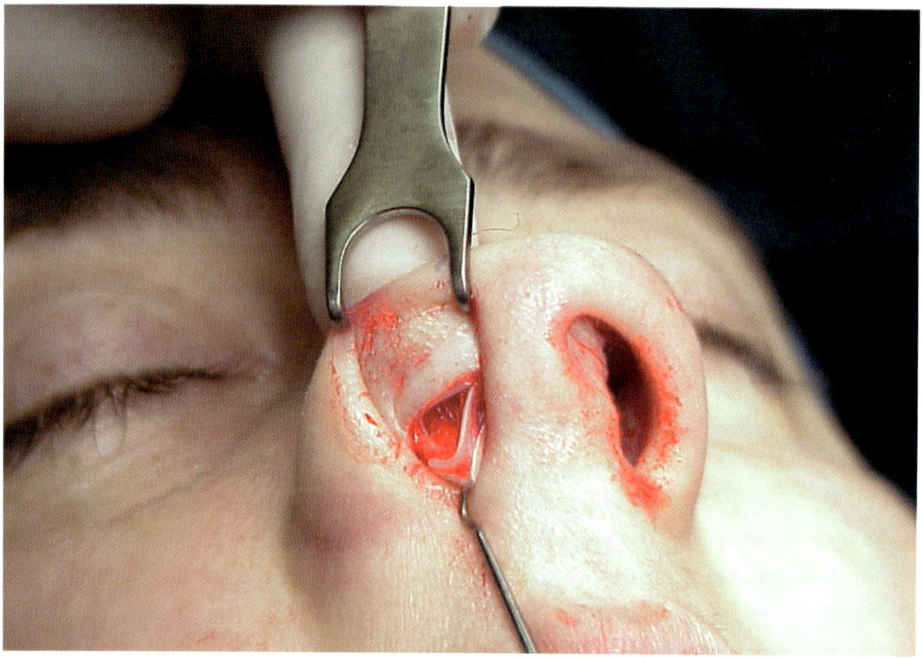

Figure 30: the vestibular skin cephalic at incision clasped with a hook

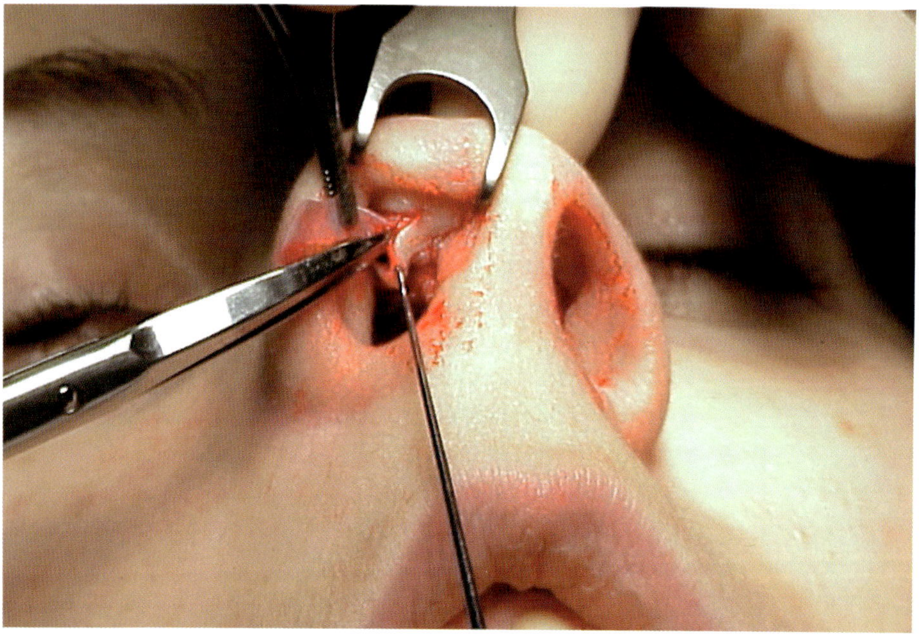

Figure 31: the cartilage is undermined with pointed scissors

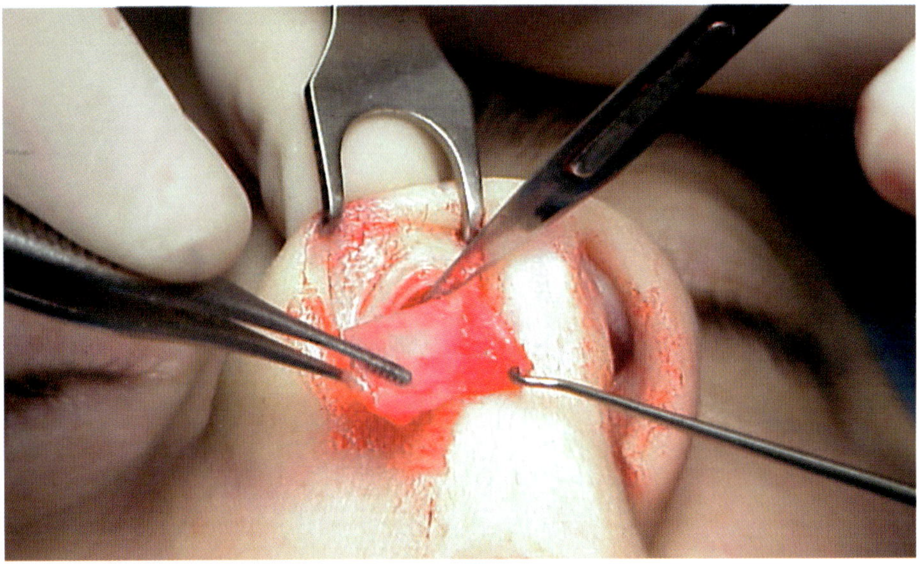

Figure 32: near the domus, a blade-11 scalpel allows precise cartilage removal

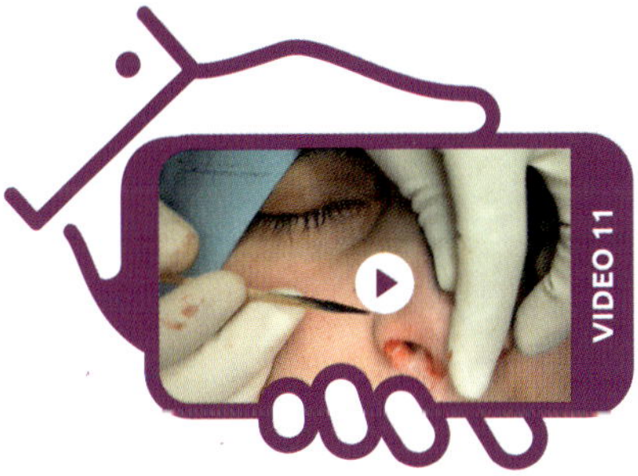

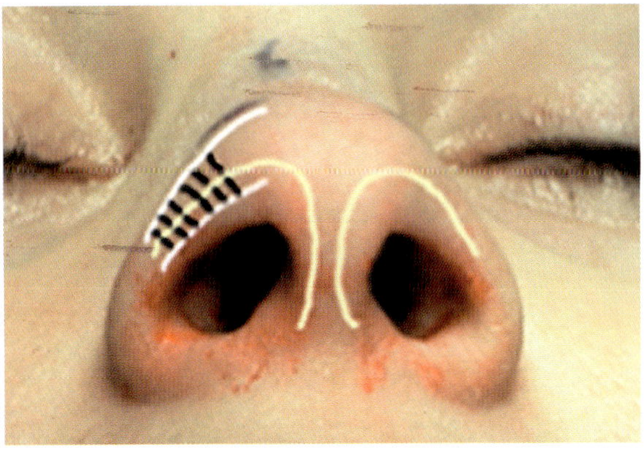

Figure 33: the connections between the lateral crus and the skin prevent the cartilage from sliding in relation to the skin. As the tip is less projected, the nostrils widen like gull wings

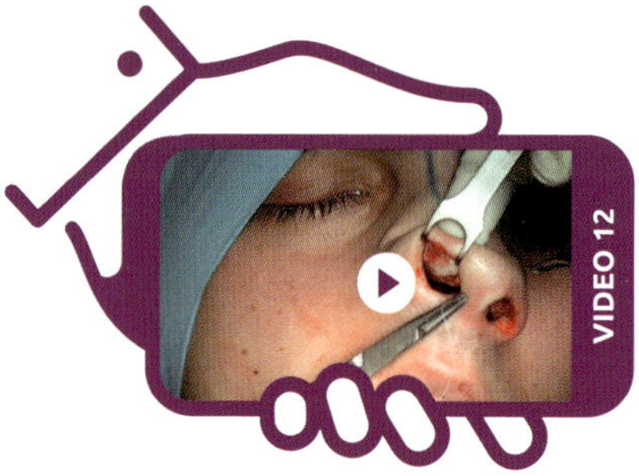

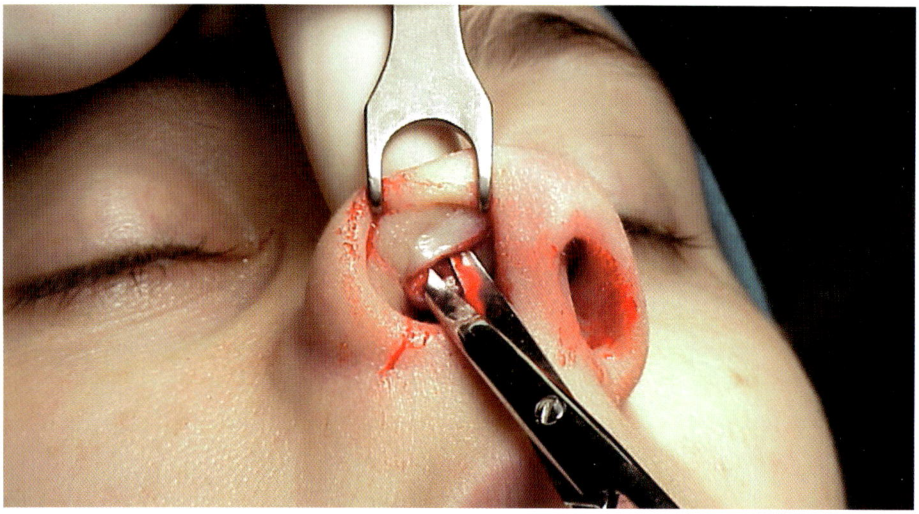

Figure 34a: undermining the caudal stripe of the lateral crus in order to allow its lateral shift

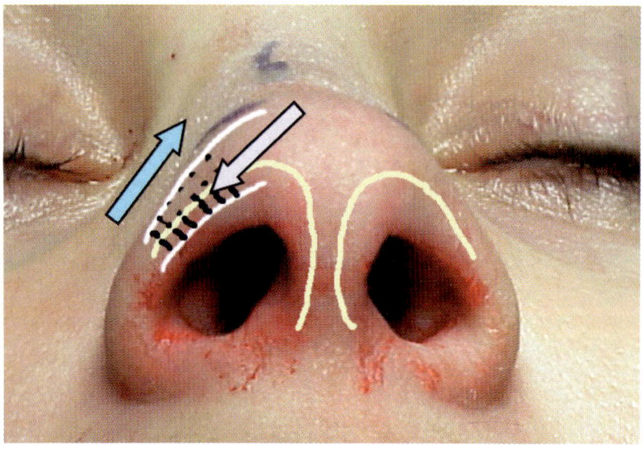

Figure 34b: diagram of the cartilage sliding in relation to the skin

closing the dihedral angle formed by the medial and lateral crus (6) (figs. 35a, b, c) (video 13). Only in rare cases the continuity of the vestibular skin at the inferior margin of the lateral crus of the alar cartilage still constitutes an obstacle to this movement, and so it must be incised to allow a freer movement of the lateral crus (fig. 35d).

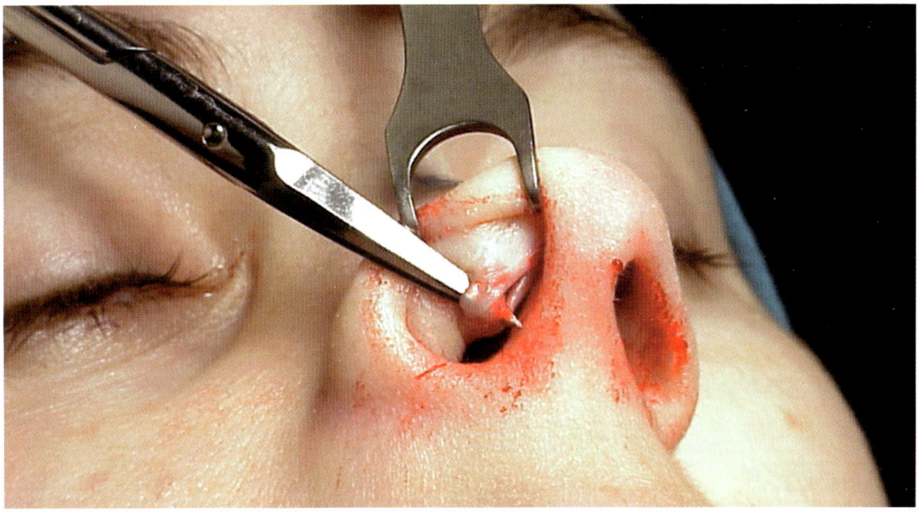

Figure 35a: exposure of the tail of the lateral crus of the alar cartilage

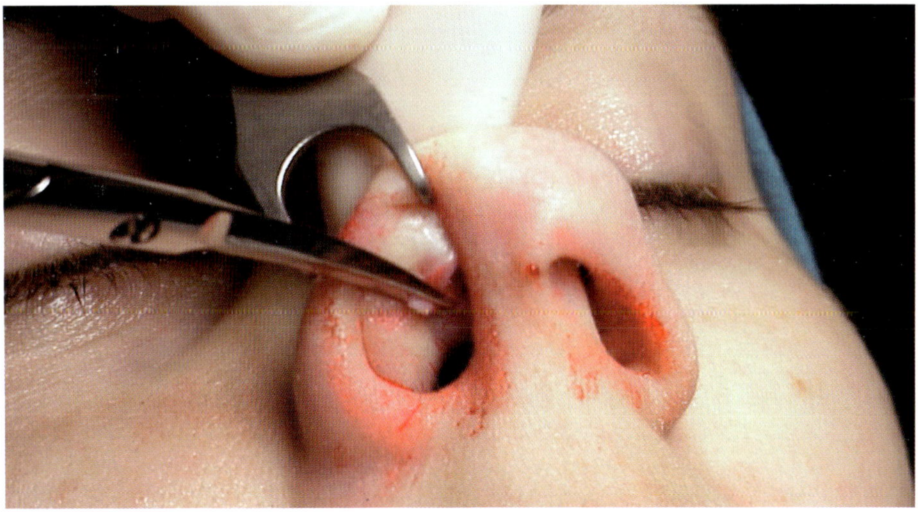

Figure 35b: removal of a small amount of cartilage from the tail of the alar cartilage

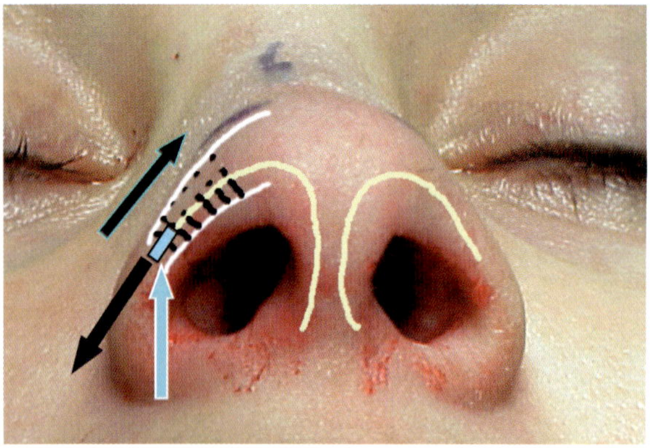

Figure 35c: very effective change in the position of the lateral crus in relation to the skin. The cartilage slides in a lateral direction

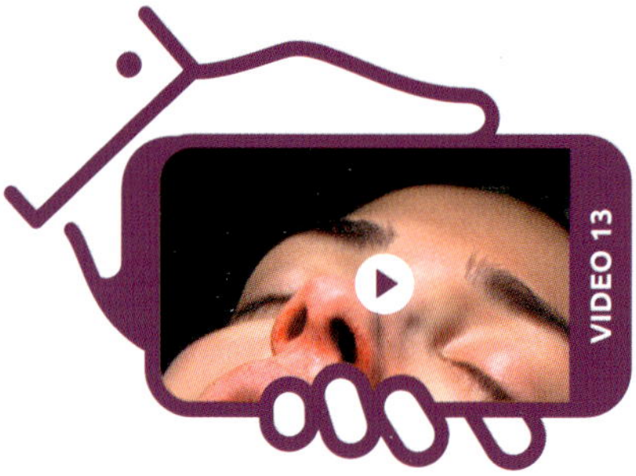

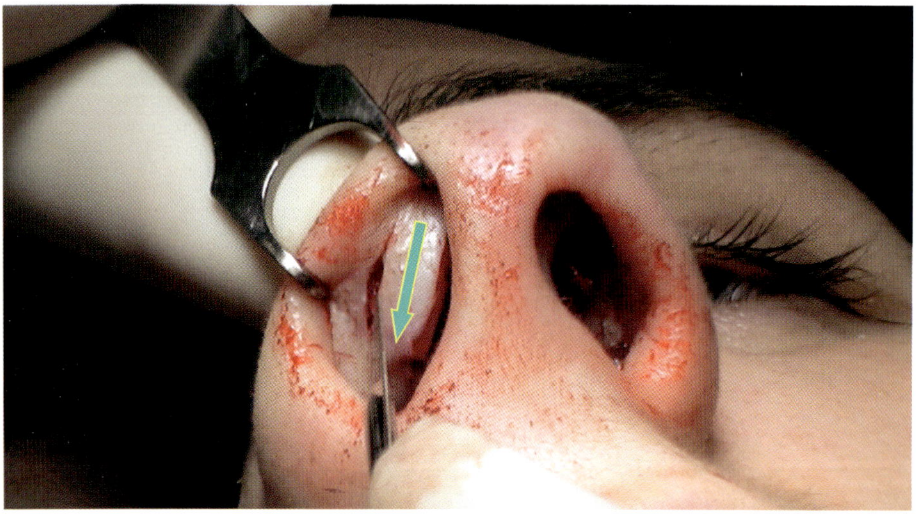

Figure 35d: if the lateral the lateral crus sliding is restrained by its connection with the skin of the vestibule, an incision can be made along the lower edge of the cartilage to render the lateral crus more mobile

The foot of the nostril should now be observed, and if it widens and rounds off too much resulting in a negroid nostril, its shaping (fig. 36a) is done at the end of the surgery, with the dressing already on, before applying the plaster of fracture restraint. (see also chapter 11 “Shaping the base of the nostrils”) (figs. 36b, c, d).
The choice of modelling the base of the nostrils as the last surgical step, is dictated by the need to assess its appropriateness, and the width of the vestibular skin wedge to be removed, only after all other components of the nose have changed definitively.

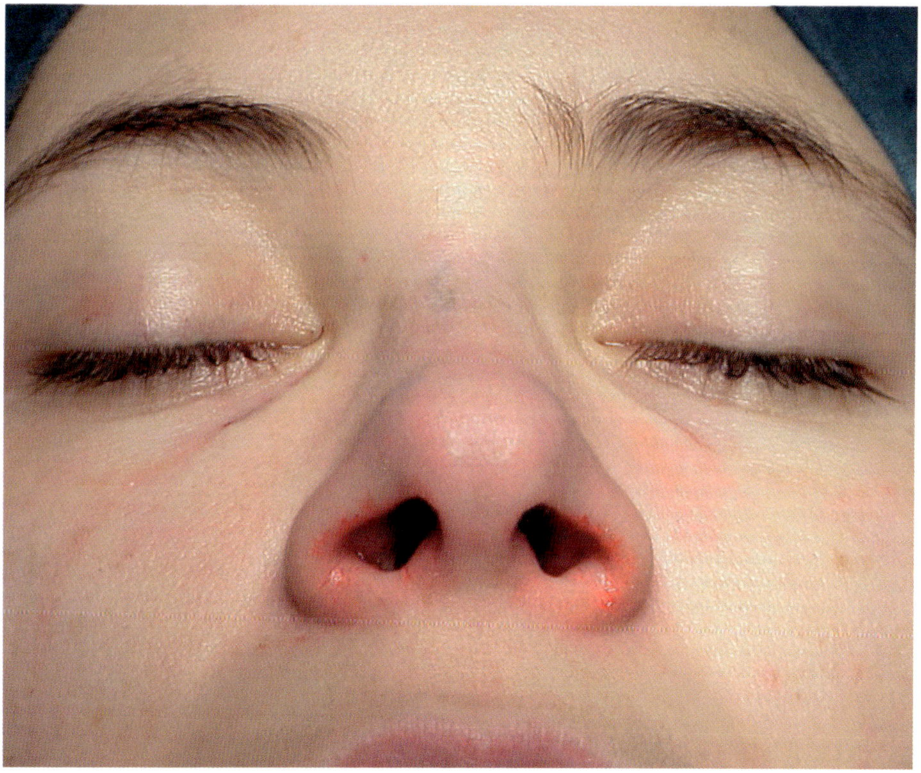

Figure 36a: enlargement of the nostrils due to decreased projection of the tip

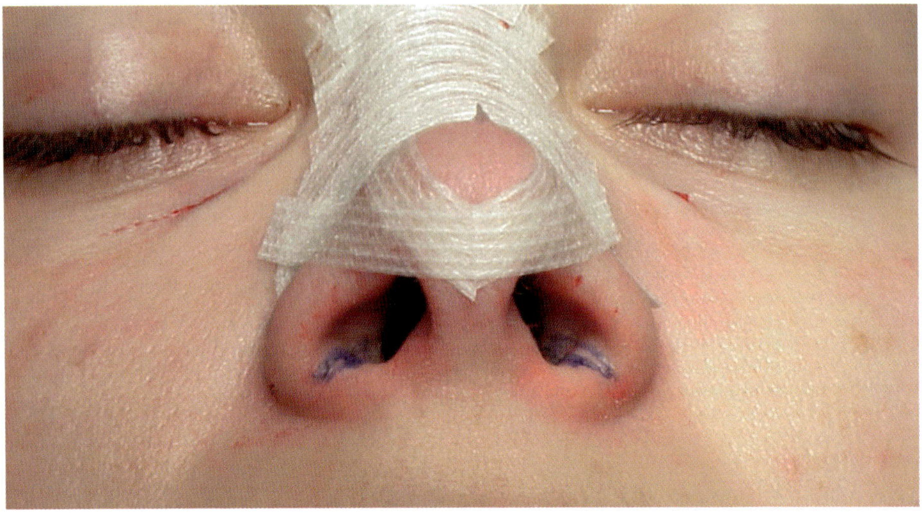

Figure 36b: drawing of the wedge-shaped excision involving the vestibule and part of the foot of the nostril. (Sheehan's technique) This drawing should be done slightly below the point where the internal curvature begins in order to preserve the roundness of the nostril. If it would be done exactly where the curvature begins, an angle would form and therefore the outline of the nostril would no longer be rounded

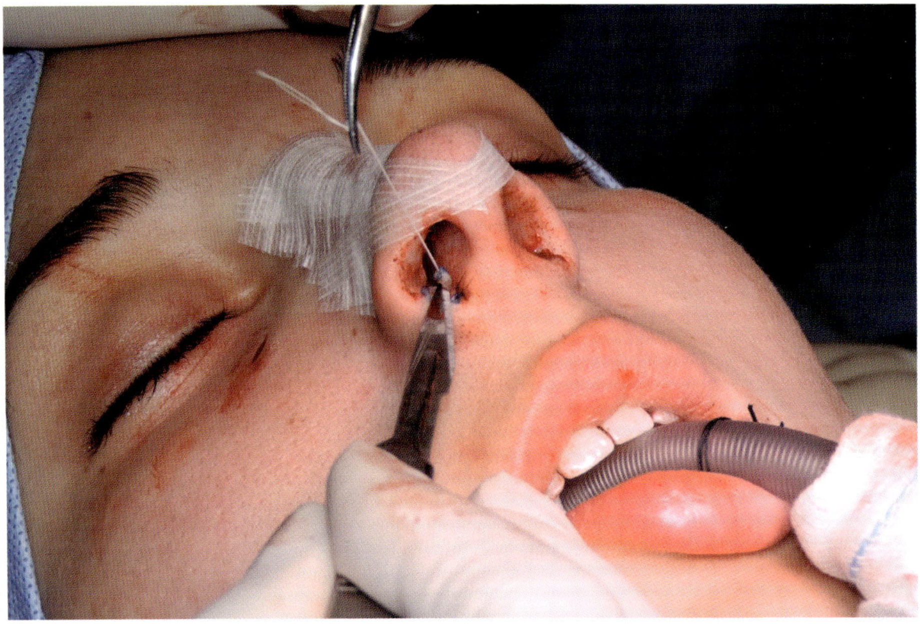

Figure 36c: to facilitate the removal, a stitch is placed in the center of the wedge of skin to be incised with a blade-11 scalpel and then removed

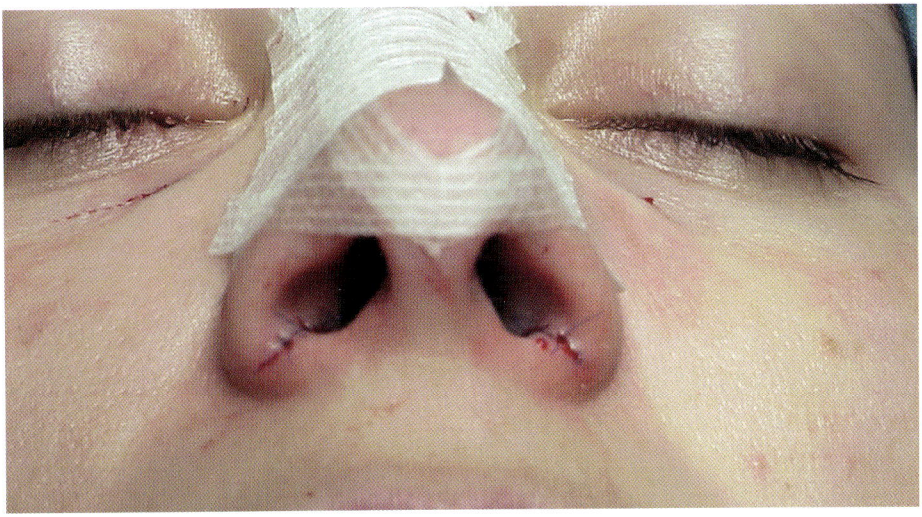

Figure 36d: reduction of the foot of the nostril achieved preserving the roundness of the nostril

The poorly projected tip

Diamond and hockey stick techniques are applicable in most cases. They are both slightly reductive or do not significantly change the projection. However, it can happen that the tip needs more projection instead.

When an increase in projection is required, an exposure of the alar cartilage through a marginal incision may be the first choice. The vestibular skin is incised caudally to the inferior margin of the alar cartilage. Laterally this incision follows the inferior margin of the lateral crus and medially follows the anterior margin of the medial crus along the columella. (figs. 37a, b).

A small point is located on the anterior margin of the alar cartilage, inferiorly to the junction between the lateral and medial crus, that I have called Deneb (see chapter 6) (fig. 38). This pin-point is a landmark which allows to operate exposing the cartilages of the tip from a single nostril without fear of not mastering asymmetries. In fact, joining the point (that

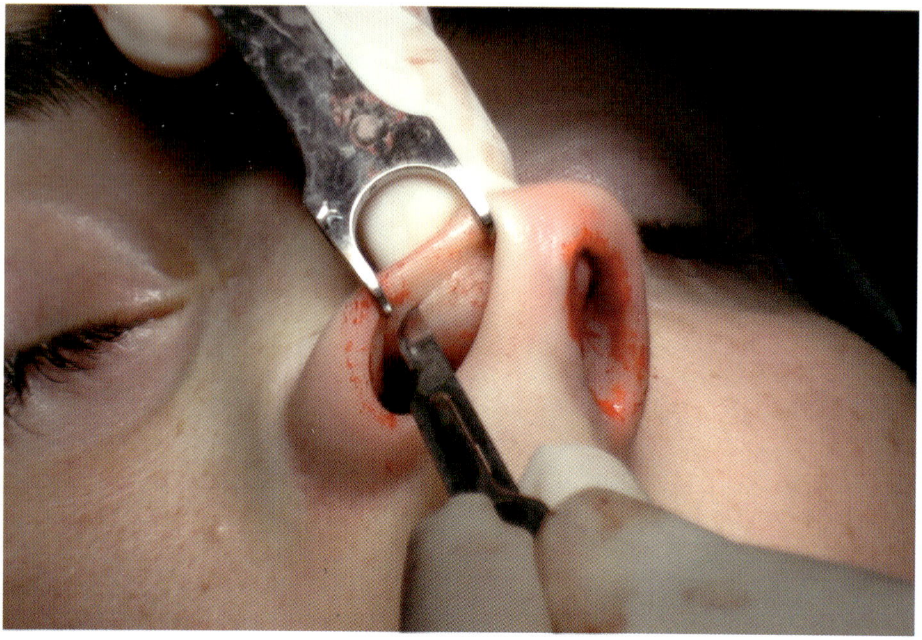

Figure 37a: marginal incision caudal to the lateral crus

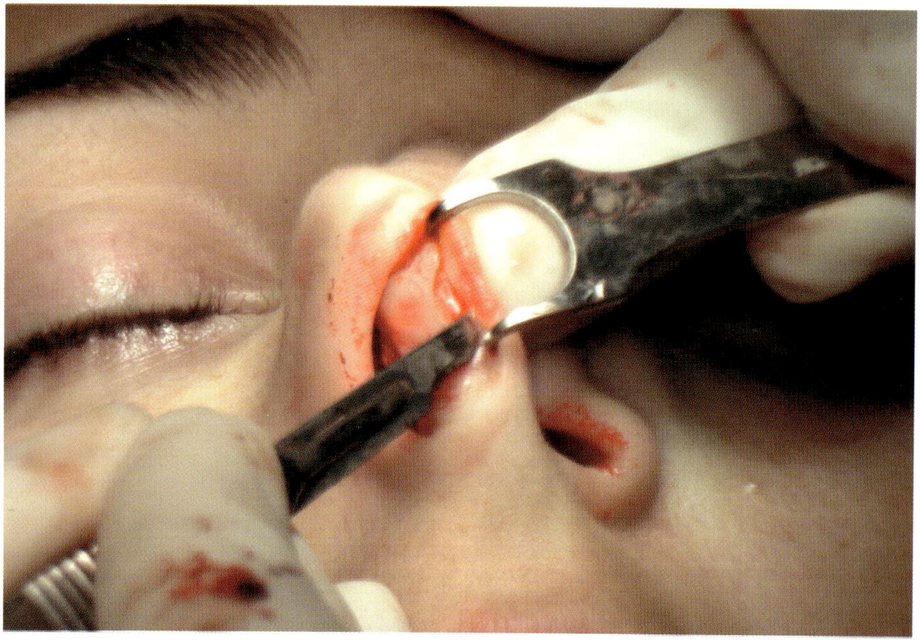

Figure 37b: marginal incision along the columella

I named Deneb) of one side with that of the other side permits to be sure that no asymmetry is being created. This stitch enable the sculpture of the tip or the placement of grafts being sure of maintaining or creating a symmetry of the tip (fig. 39). The identification of the Deneb point makes the open technique almost always superfluous. The open technique was first proposed by Rethi in 1929 (7) (fig. 40) and then modified by Goodman (8) with a broken incision at the columella, and is now back in vogue and simply called "open".
Stabilization of the Deneb point with a stitch (I use vicryl rapid 5-0), allows to approximate to the desired extent both lateral crura of the alar cartilages (fig. 41). The more the two lateral crura of the alar cartilages are approximated the more the tip becomes projected and slimmer. Once the Deneb point has been stabilized and a more projected tip obtained, the desired portion of the cephalic margin of the lateral crus can be removed to reduce the redundancy of the nostril (fig. 41b). Increased projection of the tip by bringing the medial crus together was proposed by Berson in 1948 (9) (figs. 42a, b, c, d).

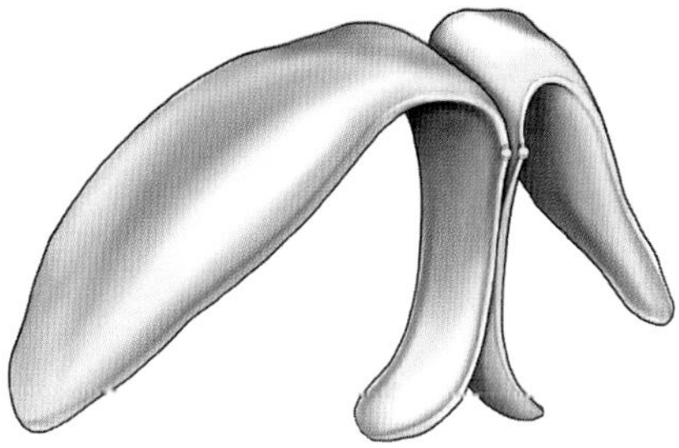

Figure 38: on the anterior margin of the crus medialis, just below the domus there is a very small dot that I have named Deneb, after the brightest star in the swan constellation

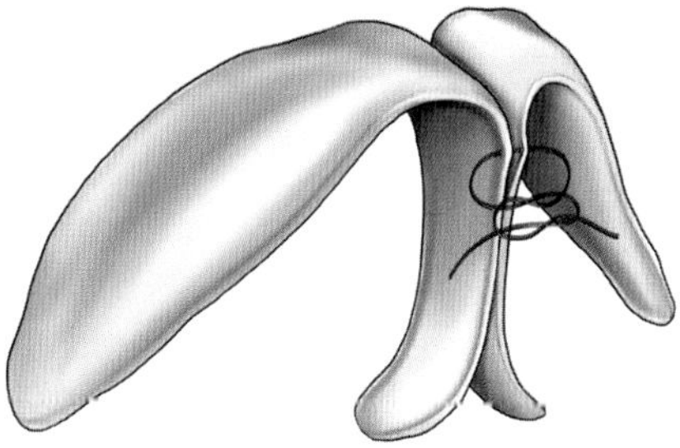

Figure 39: stabilizing Deneb with a stitch allows to expose the alar cartilages from one nostril only. Then it is possible to proceed with the chosen technique, be it the Ponti technique or grafting or another one, with no fear of producing asymmetry

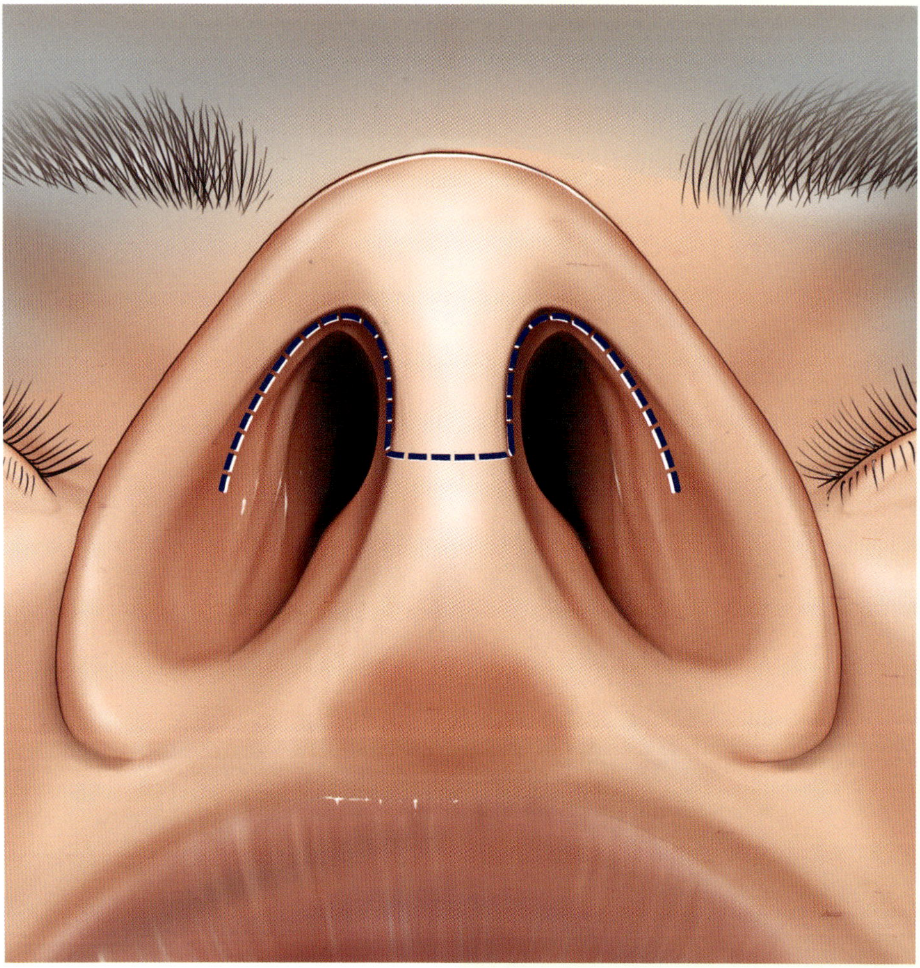

Figure 40: Rethi's incision in 1931 modified by Goodman in 1961, now back in fashion under the generic name of open technique

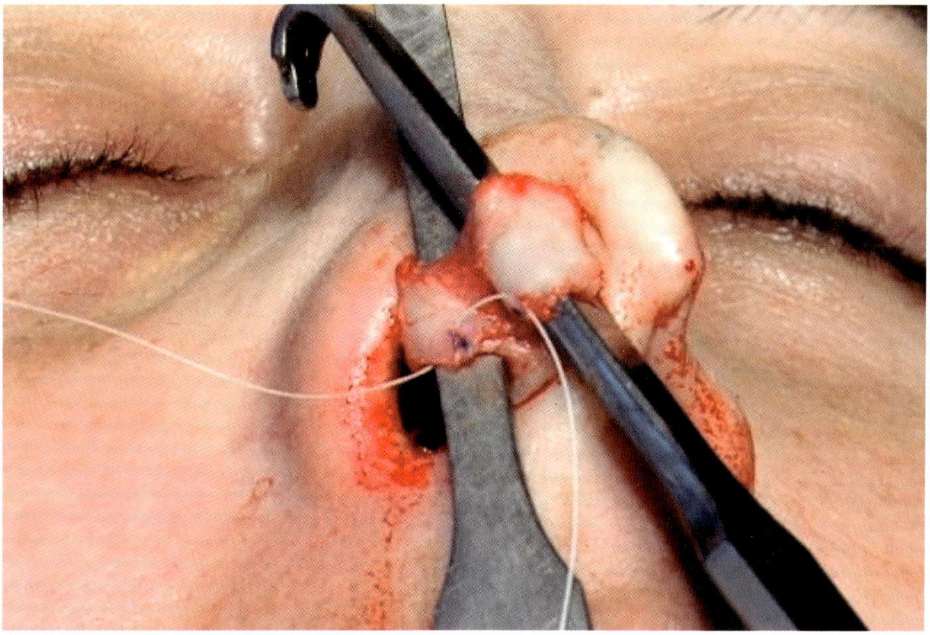

Figure 41a: approximation of the Deneb points of the alar cartilages

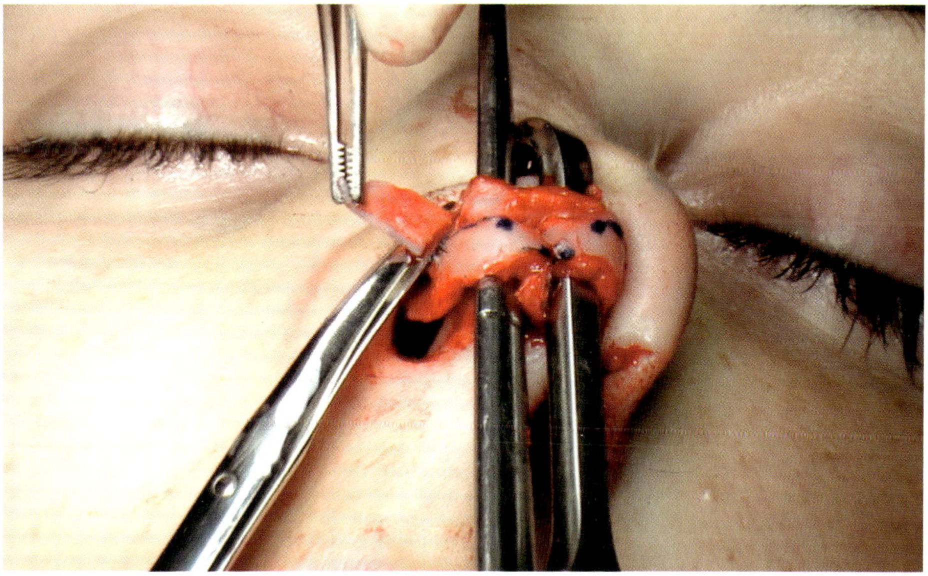

Figure 41b: excision of the cephalic margin of the lateral crus to make the lateral crus smaller in its cephalic portion. The two domus and the points called Deneb are marked with methylene blue.

Ponti's Butterfly Technique (10) is also suitable to obtain greater tip projection. With the Ponti Technique the alar cartilages are interrupted lateral to the domus and the medial stumps are brought together centrally to form a butterfly-wing cartilaginous tip. From this characteristic the Ponti technique takes the name of butterfly technique (figs. 43a, b, c, d, e, f, g, h, i). The increase in tip projection obtained with the Ponti technique depends on the amount of cartilage belonging to the lateral crus that, once sutured to the contralateral one, will become an extension of the medial crus.

As an alternative to the Ponti technique, a graft can be taken from the septum, opened into a Y shape so that the two oblique branches of the Y reproduce the shape of the tip as in the Ponti butterfly technique. The vertical branch of the Y is inserted between the medial crura. The depth of insertion of the vertical branch of the Y between the medial crura determines the greater or lesser projection of the tip (fig. 44a) This is the "fleur de lys" technique of Tessier (11) which may be applied in rhinoplasties with a negroid tip, in which the alar cartilages normally have little consistency and therefore changing their shape does not lead to appreciable tip modification. In these cases, however, the cartilage of the septum is rather thick and lends itself to be sculpted into a Y and still be strong enough to support the nasal tip (figs. 44b, c). If necessary a graft can be placed between the branches of the Y to keep them open (fig. 44d).

Other types of grafts may be used to increase the projection of the tip, but with slightly different effects. Onlay grafts and Sheen's shield (12) do not project as the techniques just described, so are used more to change the shape of the tip, making it more defined than to project it more.

Onlay grafts (figs. 45a, b) are grafts that are placed at the tip above the domus to make it more defined. (13) Cartilage taken from the septum can

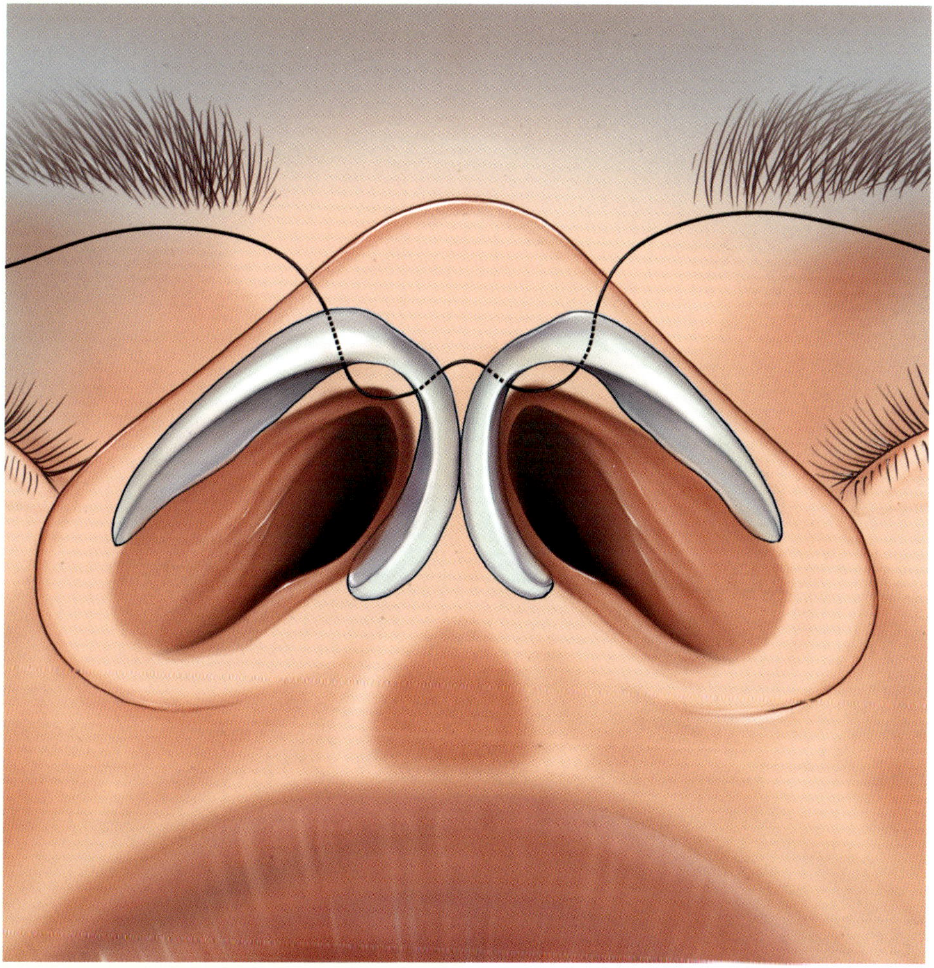

Figure 42a: Berson technique. The cartilage belonging to the lateral crus is picked up on the median line, resulting in prolongation of the medial crus that enhances the tip projection

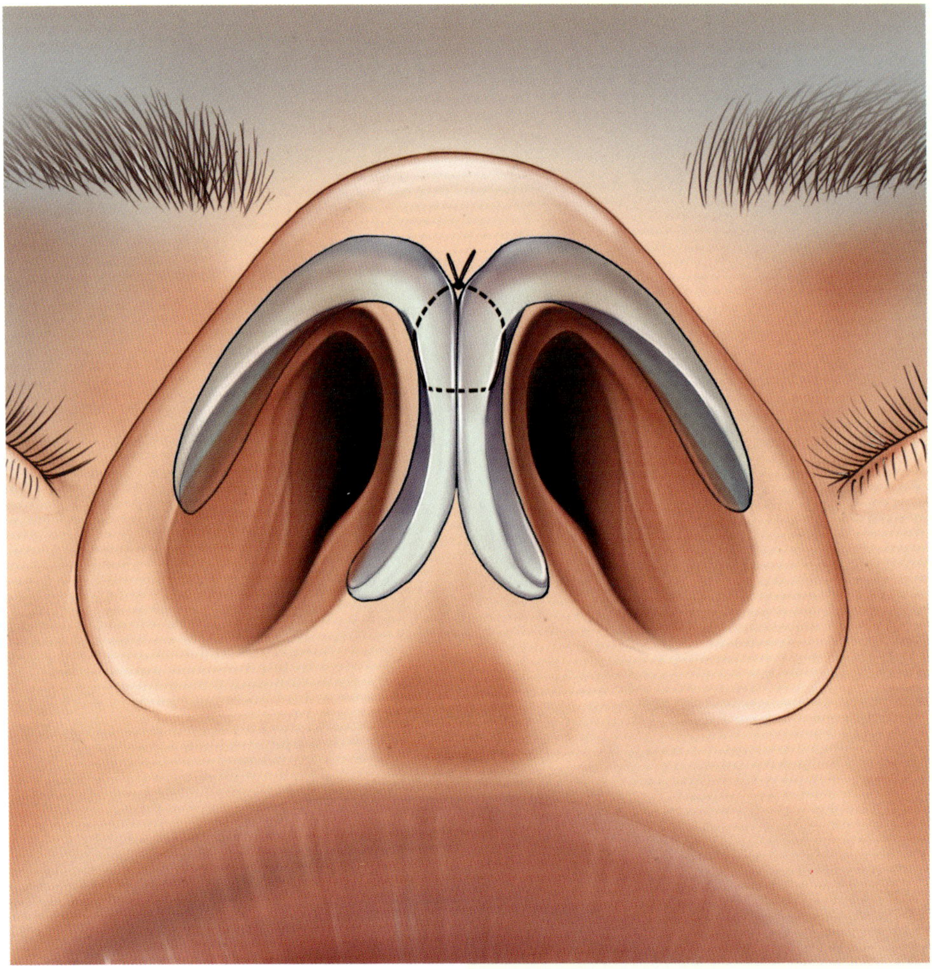

Figure 42b: approximation of the cartilages along the medial line using the Berson technique.

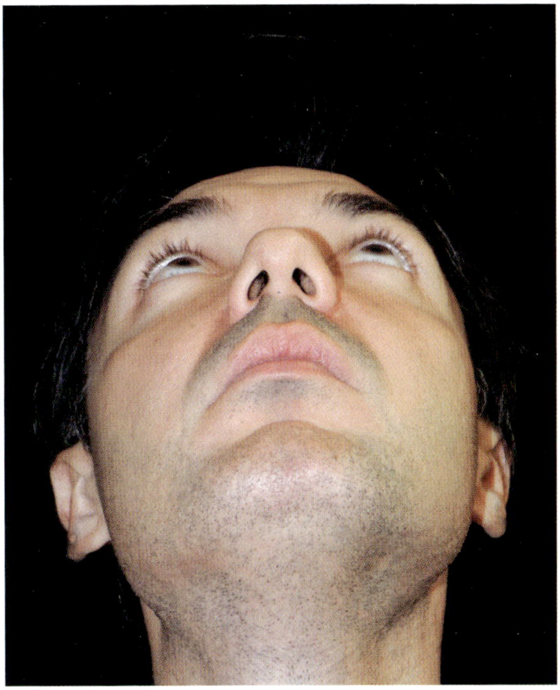

Figure 42c: tip that needs to be treated with the Berson technique in order to increase its projection

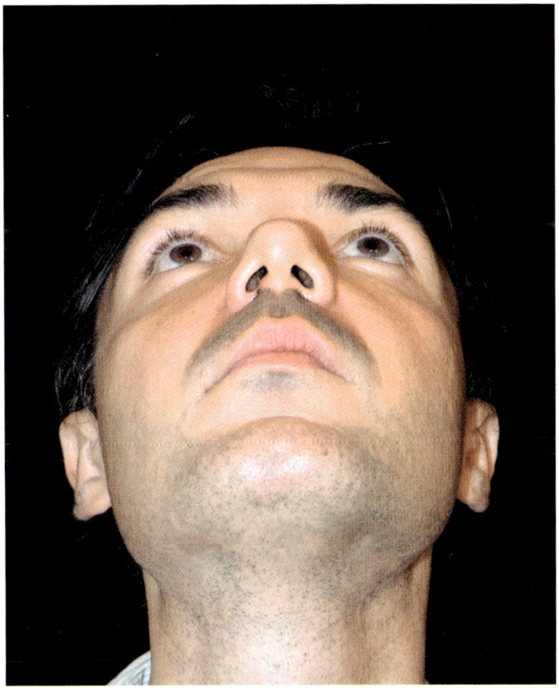

Figure 42d: postoperative look at the tip after the Berson tecnique

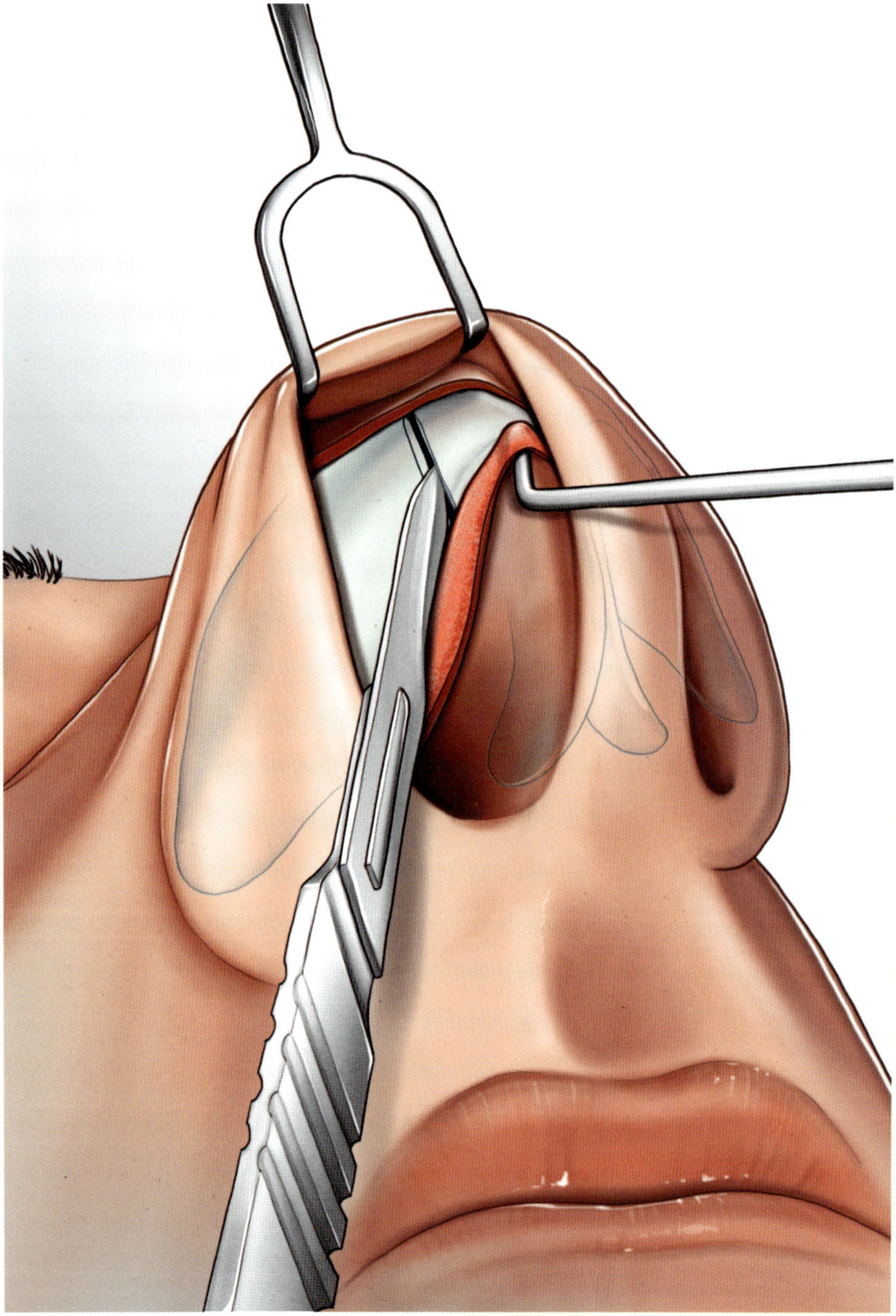

Figure 43a: Ponti technique. With the hook at the domus, the incision is performed laterally

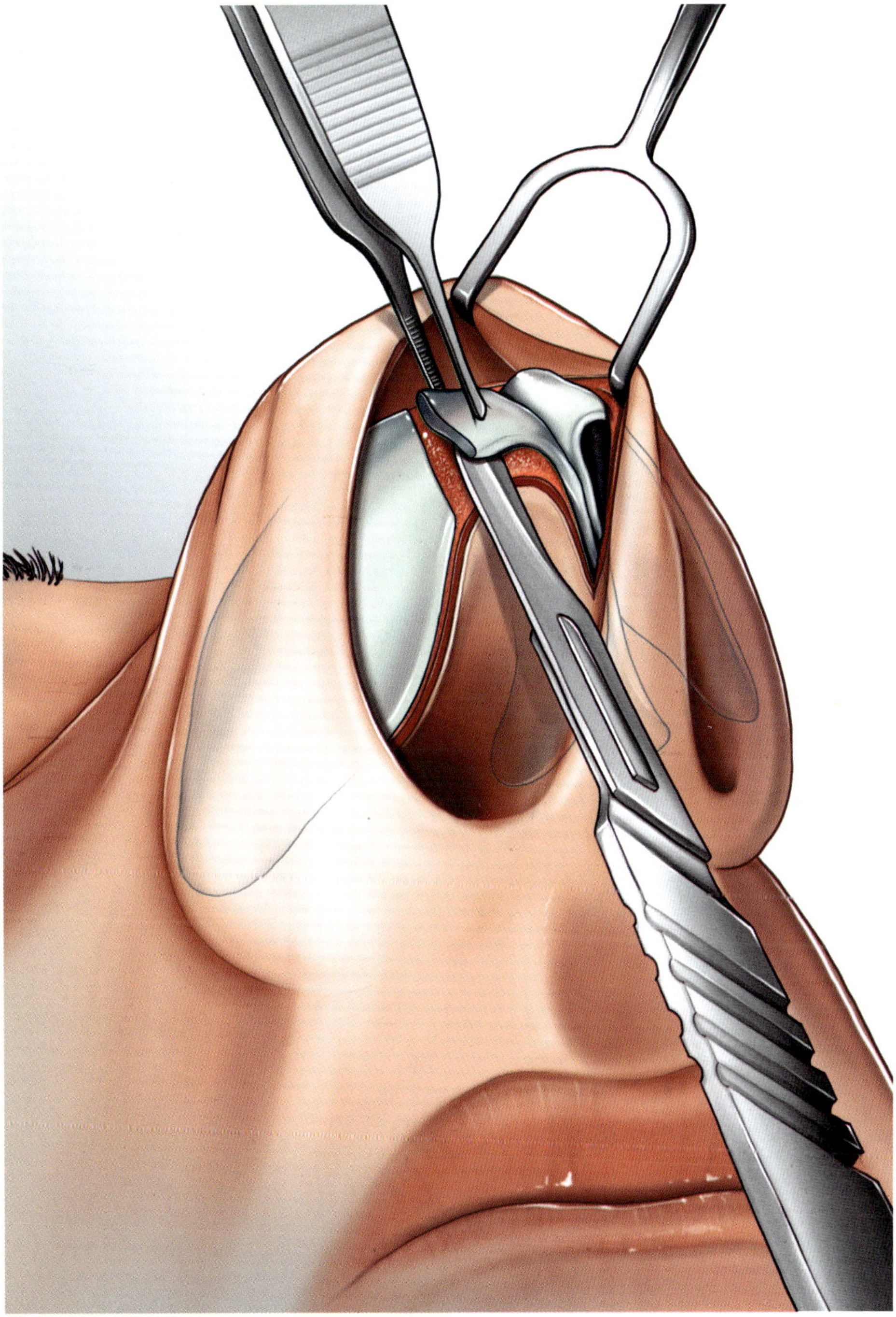

Figure 43b: Ponti technique. Lifting of the medial stumps of the lateral crus

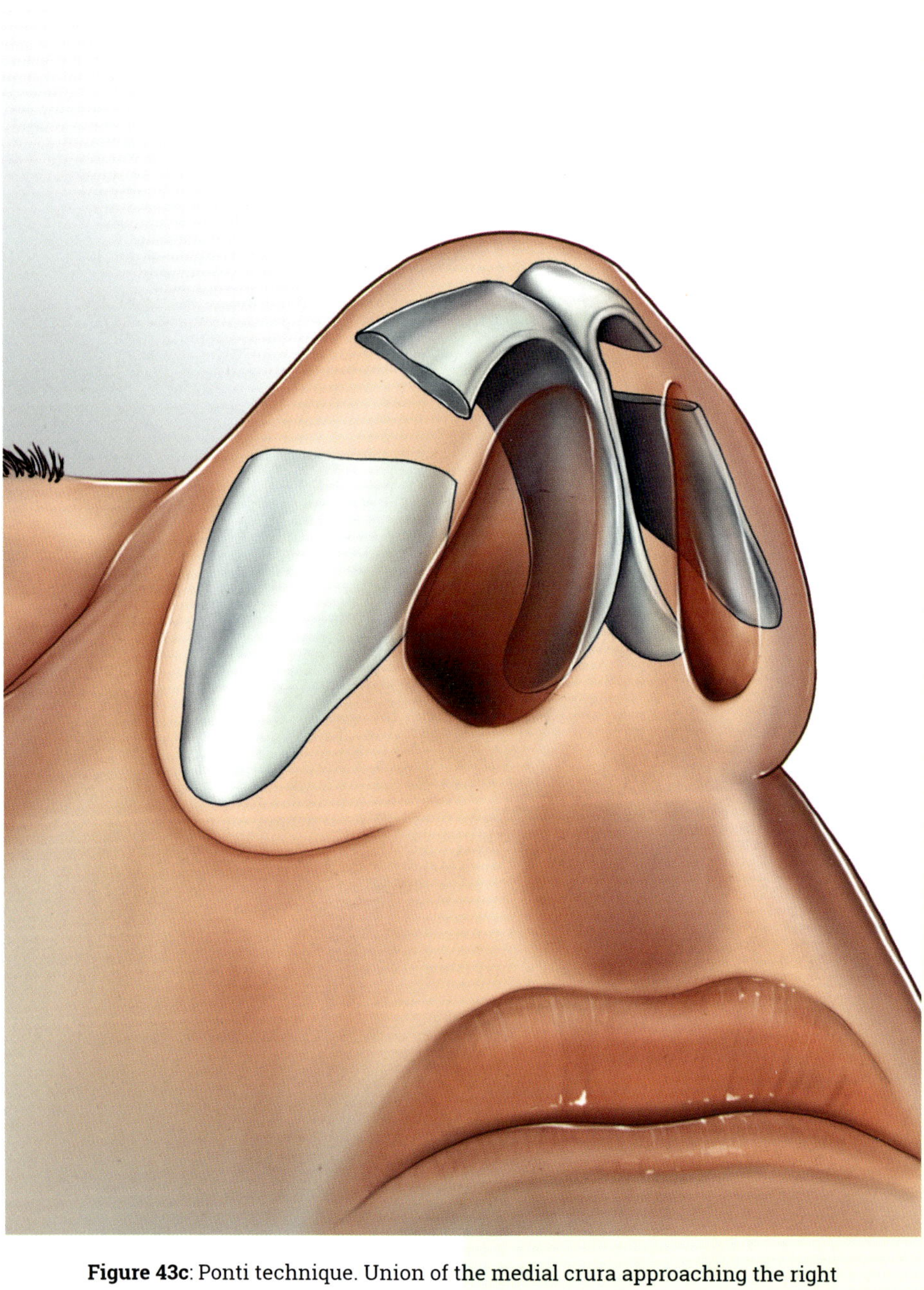

Figure 43c: Ponti technique. Union of the medial crura approaching the right and left domus towards the midline leaving a butterfly-shaped opening of the cartilages, hence the name butterfly technique given to the Ponti tecnique

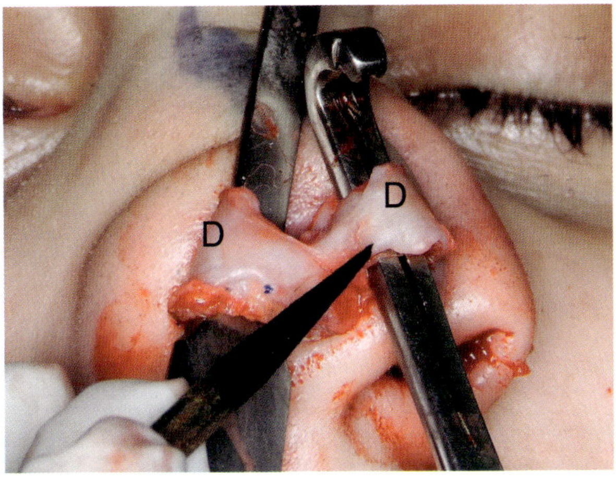

Figure 43d: cartilages exposed at the right of the columella. Both domus are marked with a D. On the right the Deneb point has been marked with methylene blue, on the left is being marked. Just lateral to the left Deneb it is also observable just anterior to the domus a tip of the cartilage

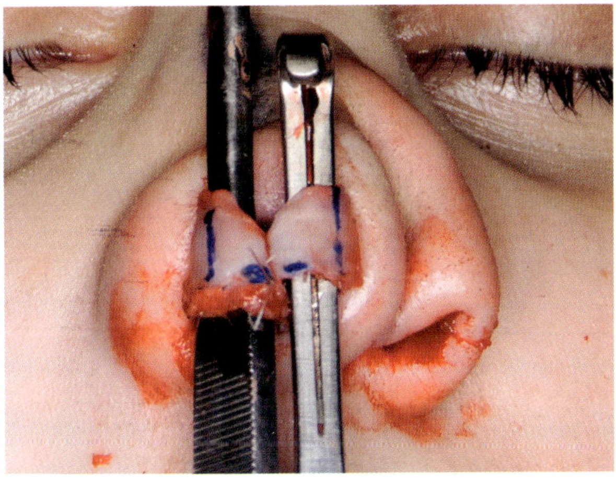

Figure 43e: the two Deneb points are joined to ensure symmetry, even without an open exposure. The butterfly is outlined with methylene blue

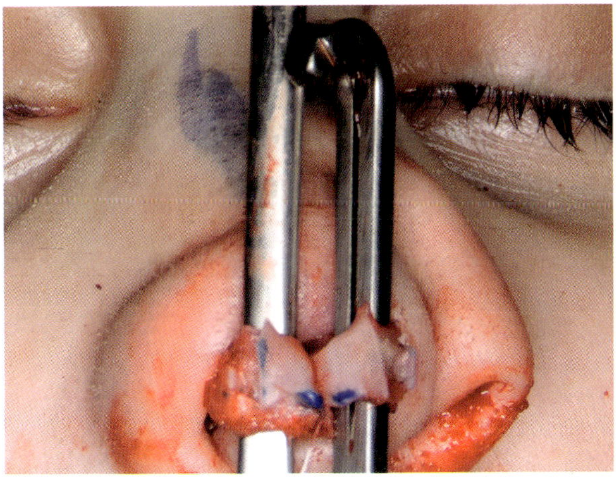

Figure 43f: the wings of the Butterfly are undermined from the vestibular skin

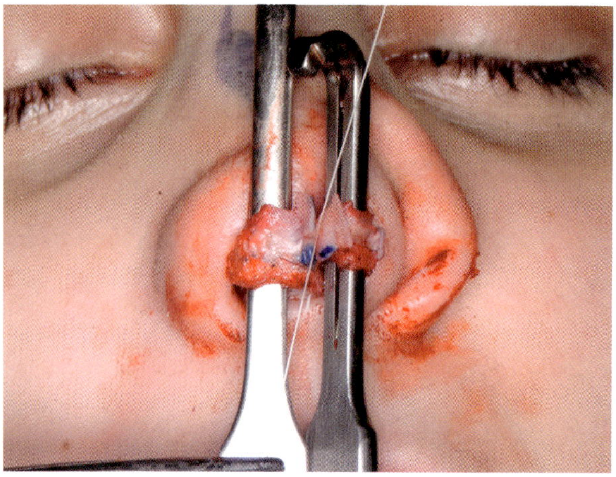

Figure 43g: a stitch whose ends are in the middle of the alae is passed

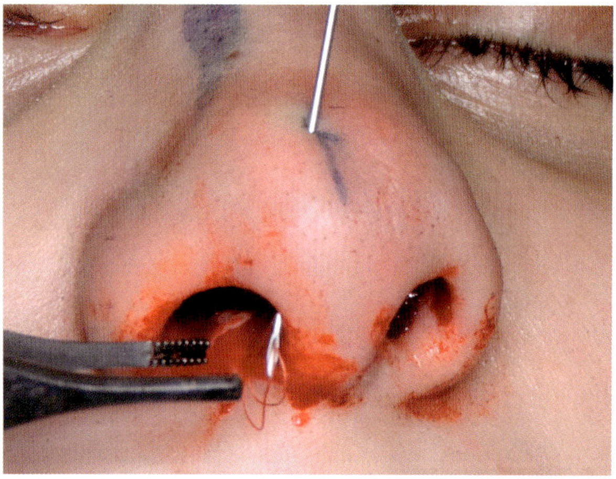

Figure 43h: the stitch is passed into a syringe needle so that it exits exactly in the center of the nasal lobule

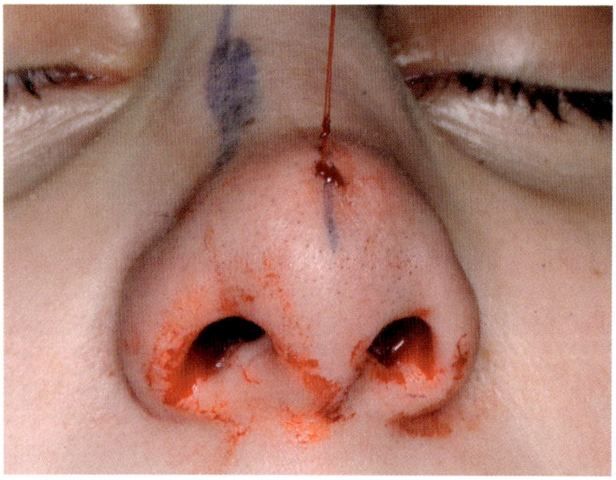

Figure 43i: the stitch is pulled to keep the cartilages in the center and to facilitate the suturing of the incisions inside the vestibule

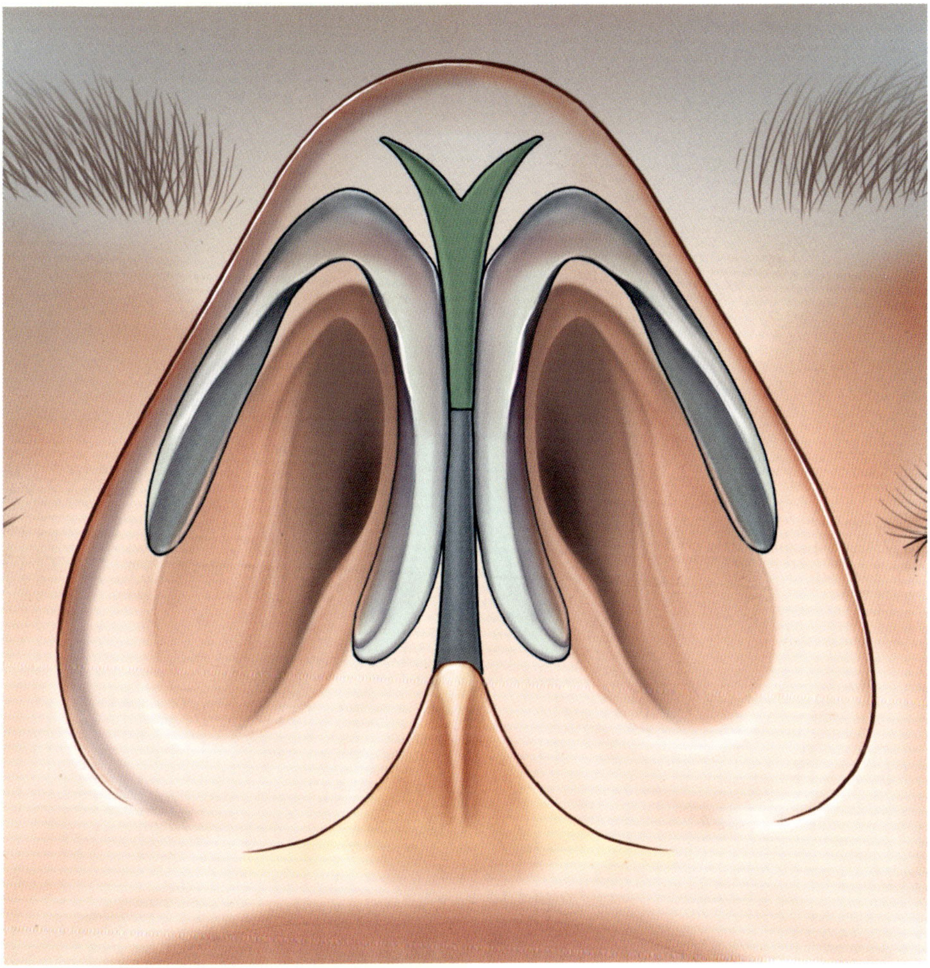

Figure 44a: Y-technique. Increase of the projection by inserting a graft taken from the septum between the medial crura and opened in a Y shape to reproduce Ponti's butterfly. This is feasible in negroid noses in which the septal cartilage is generally thick and therefore it can be opened to form a Y. In these noses, in fact, the alar cartilages have little consistency and their modelling is not very effective in changing the shape of the tip

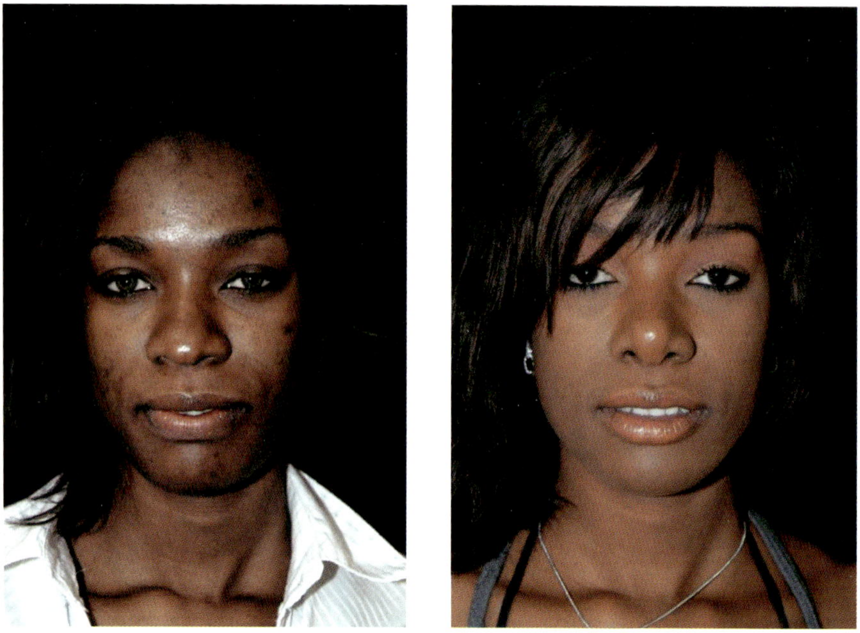

Figure 44b: a patient in which a Y graft was used to reproduce the butterfly of Ponti

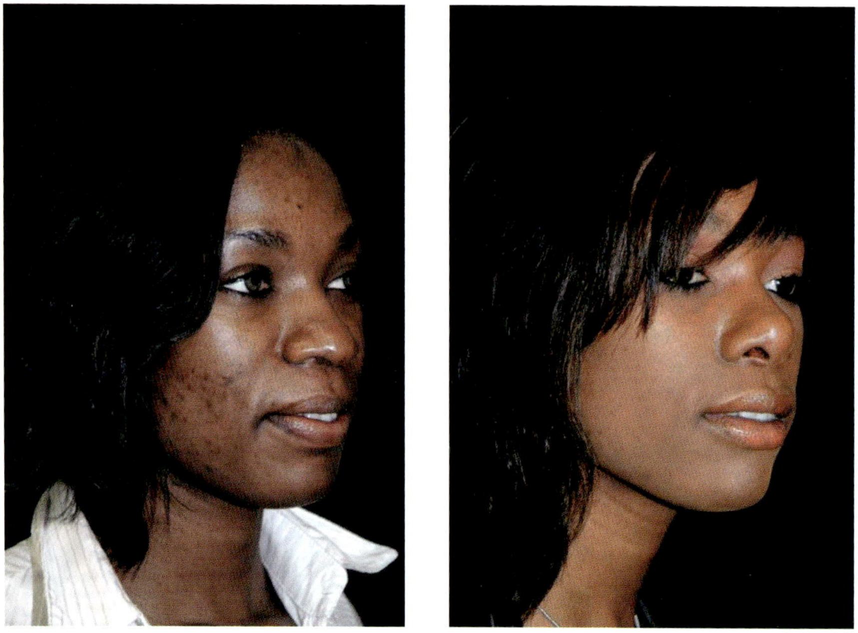

Figure 44c: three-quarter view of the tip correction using the "fleur de lys" technique by Tessier

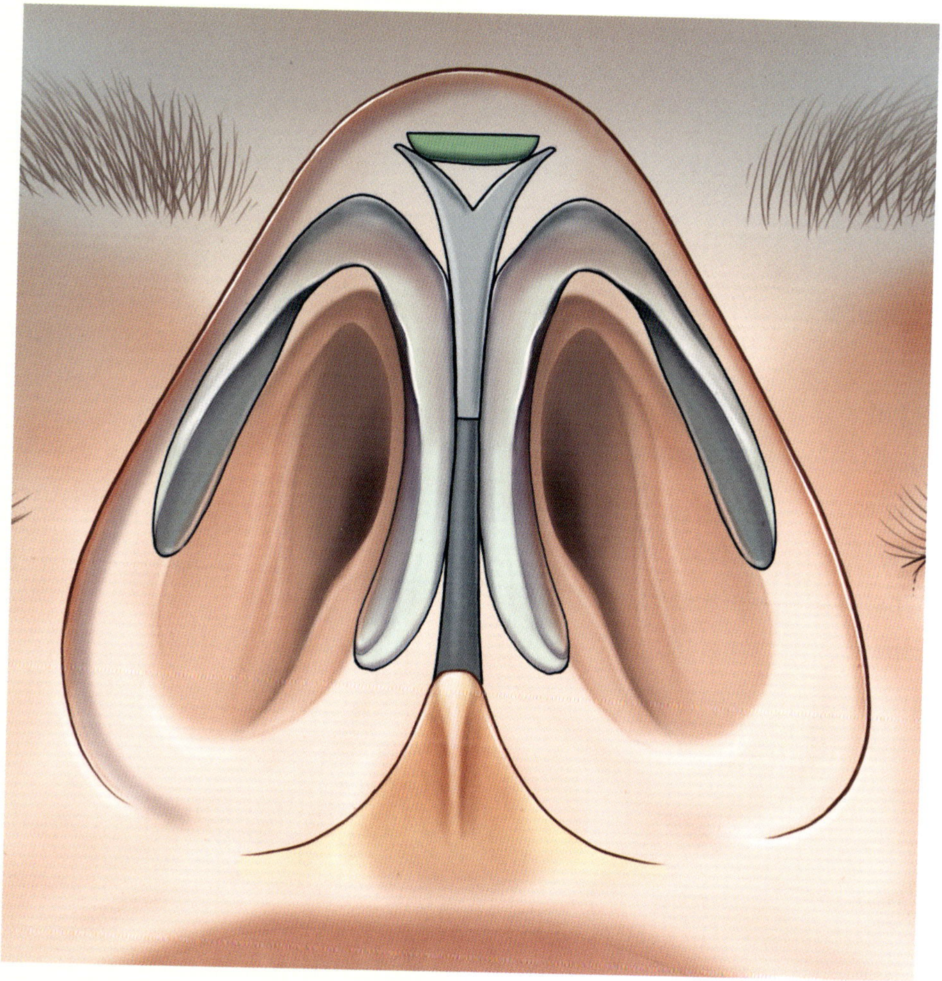

Figure 44d: a cartilage graft can help to keep the Y open

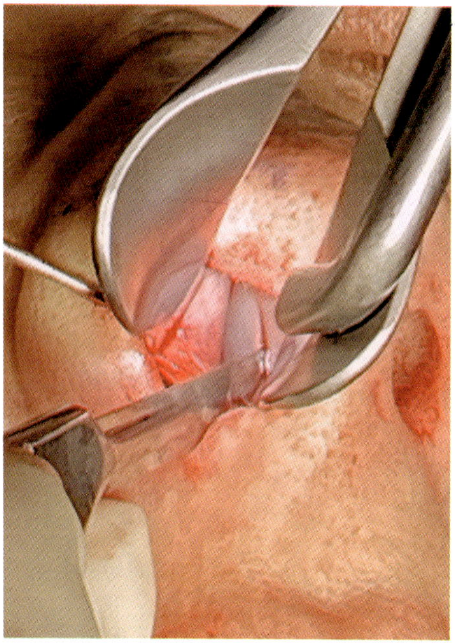

Figure 46b: septum undermining
on the right side and incision with number
15 scalpel blade

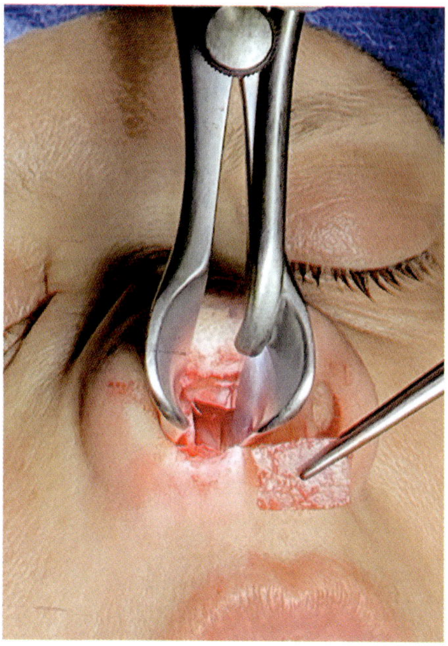

Figure 46c: cartilage graft to be
to be sculpted according to Sheen
in a shield shape

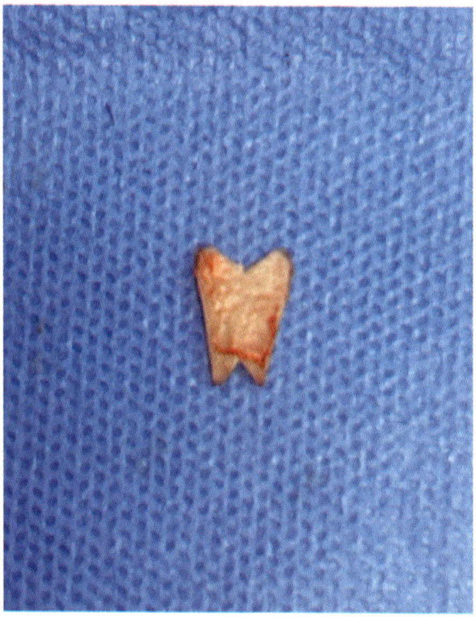

Figure 46d: septal cartilage shield shaped
according to Sheen

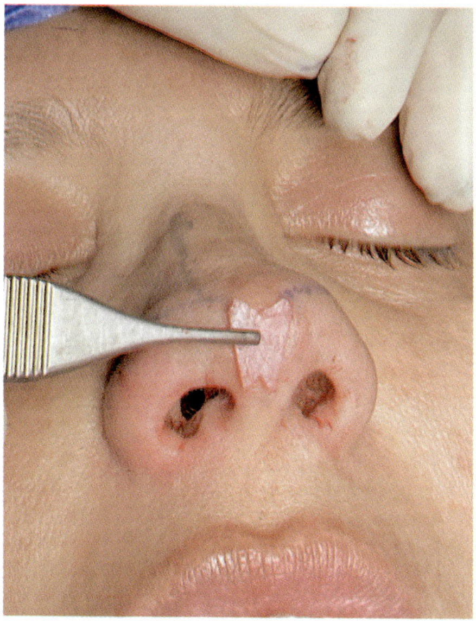

Figure 46e: predicted position for the tip
graft according to Sheen

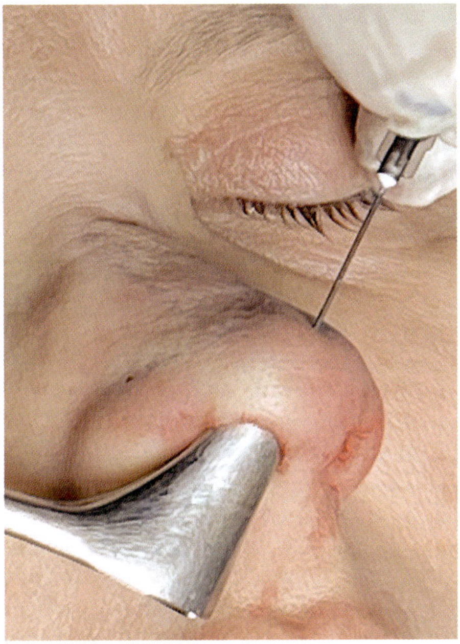

Figure 46f: after creating a pocket for the graft a suture thread is passed with the aid of a syringe needle

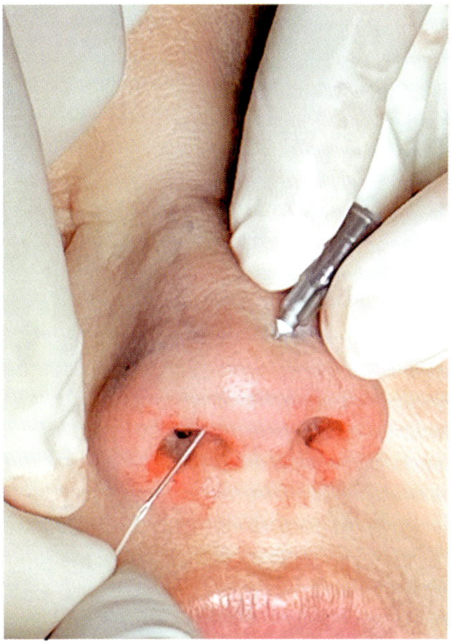

Figure 46g: the two ends of the stitch are passed through the needle so that the graft may be positioned with the correct orientation

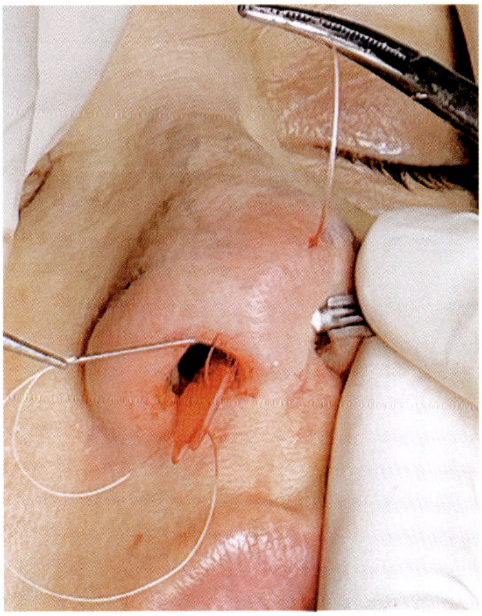

Figure 46h: after a first stitch, a second one is passed to facilitate a more precise positioning

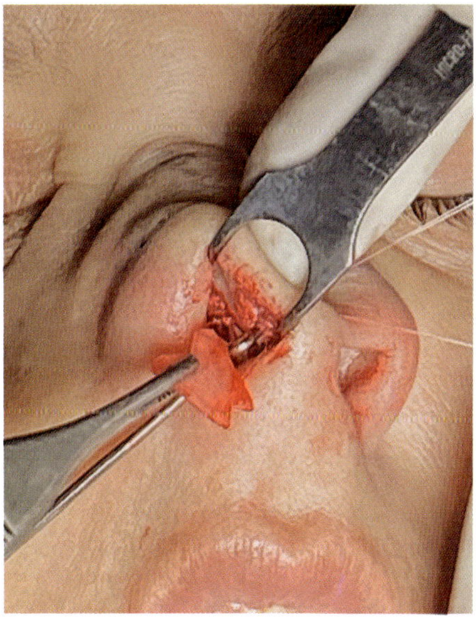

Figure 46i: the graft is inserted in the desired position pulling the stitches

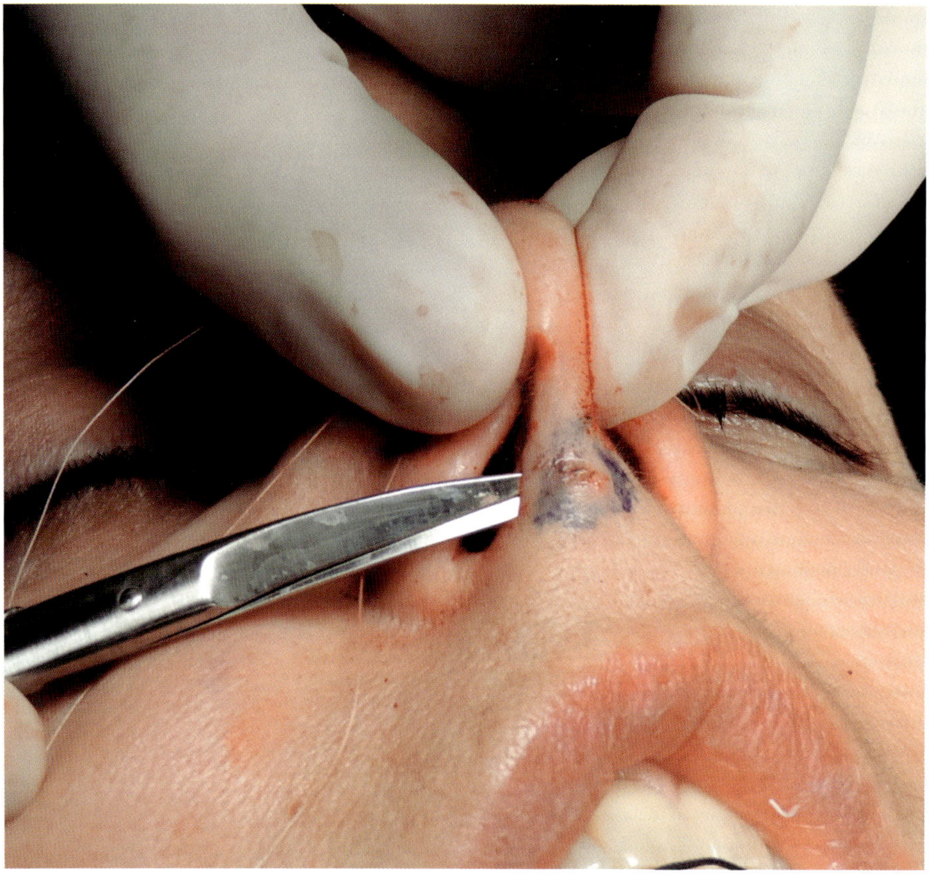

Figure 47a: the creation of a subcutaneous pocket for the cartilage graft

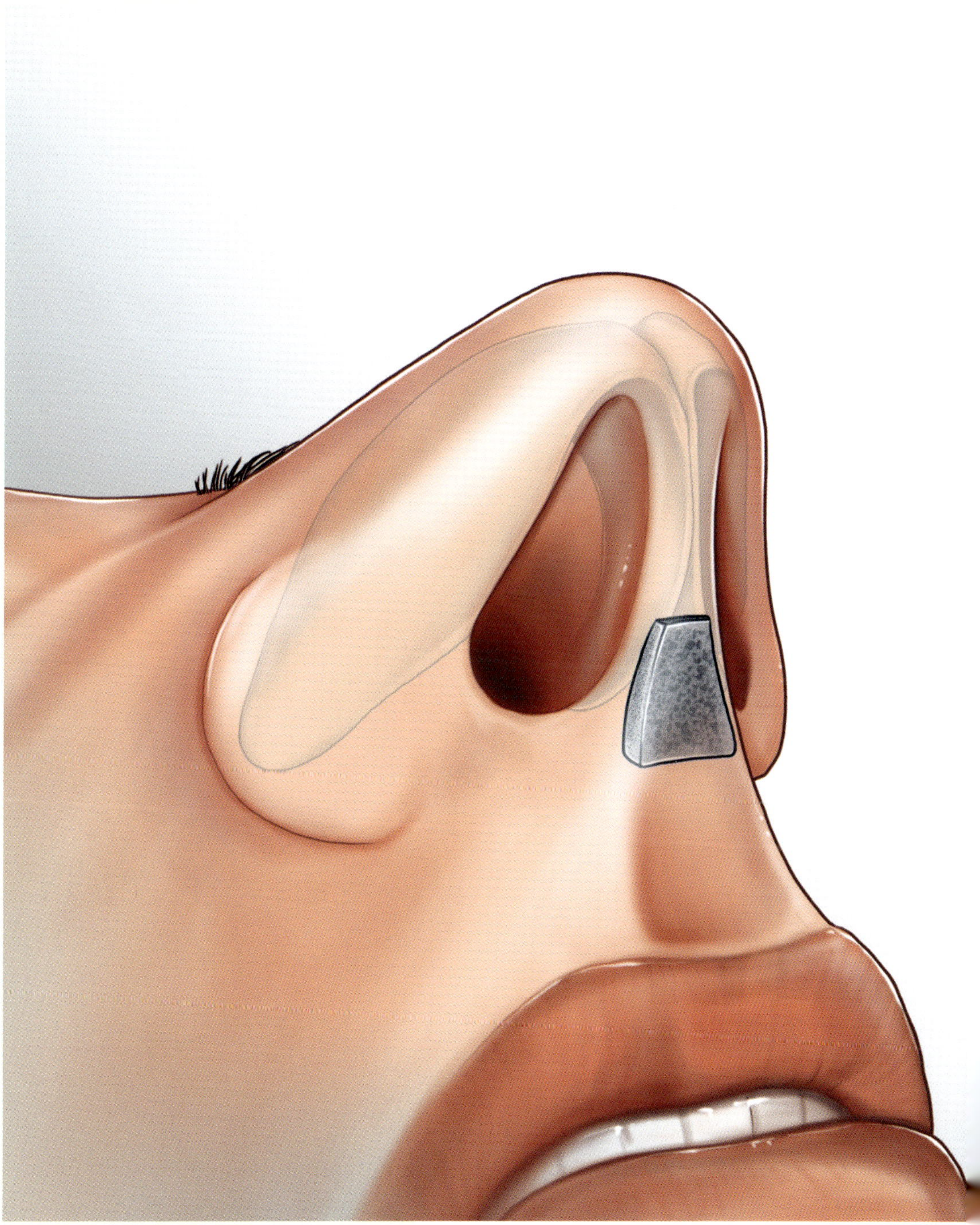

Figure 47b: the placement of grafts at the base of the medial crus increases a little bit the projection of the tip

Over-projected tip

In cases where the tip is too projected, a marginal Incision is made (figs. 37a, b), the cartilages are exposed from one nostril; the Deneb point is identified and the medial crus are stabilized with a stitch (fig. 41a). Once the medial crus have been stabilized it is possible to decide how much of the domus, lateral crus and medial crus to remove. One stitch can be placed lower to Deneb to maintain symmetry, even if it should also be removed to reduce the tip. Removing this portion of cartilage decreases the projection. (fig. 48a). The medial crura are then opened at the level of the tip to give a butterfly-wing shape similar to that of Ponti's technique (figs. 48b; 49a, b, c; 50a, b; 51). If it is not possible to keep the medial crura open, a cartilage graft can be placed between them to stabilize the butterfly shape of the tip (fig. 51).

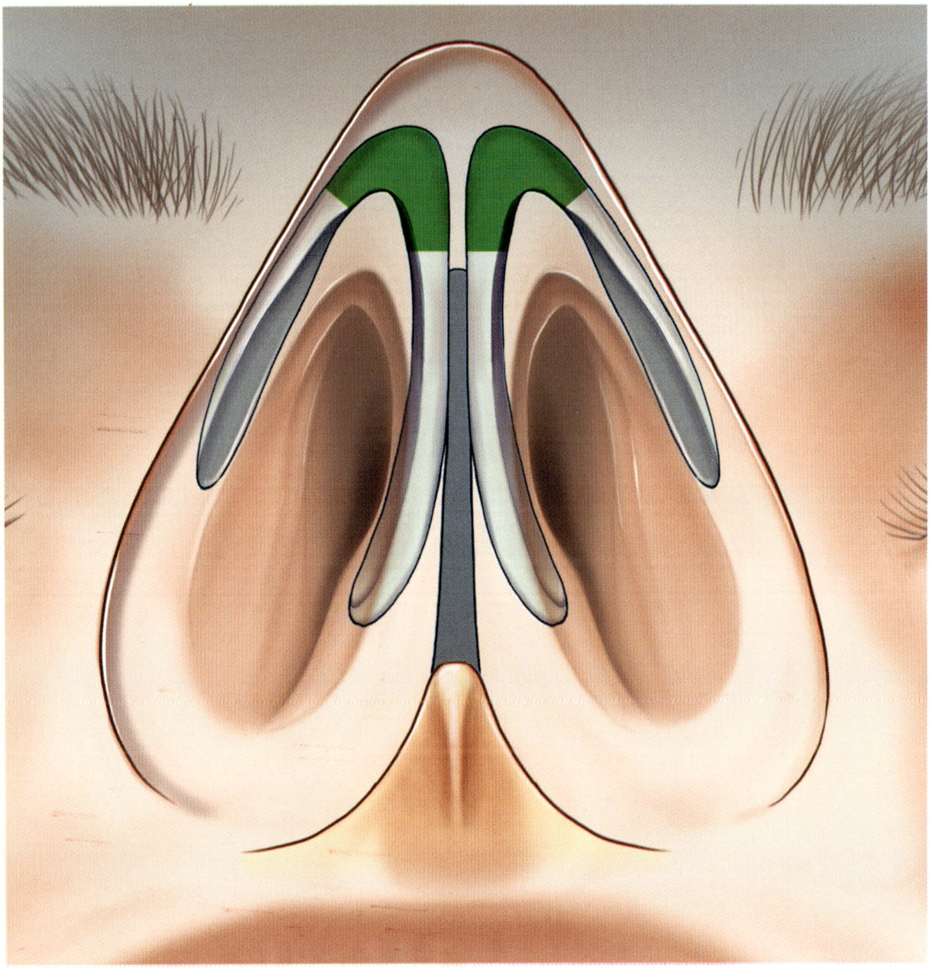

Figure 48a: resection of the domus, part of the lateral and medial crus

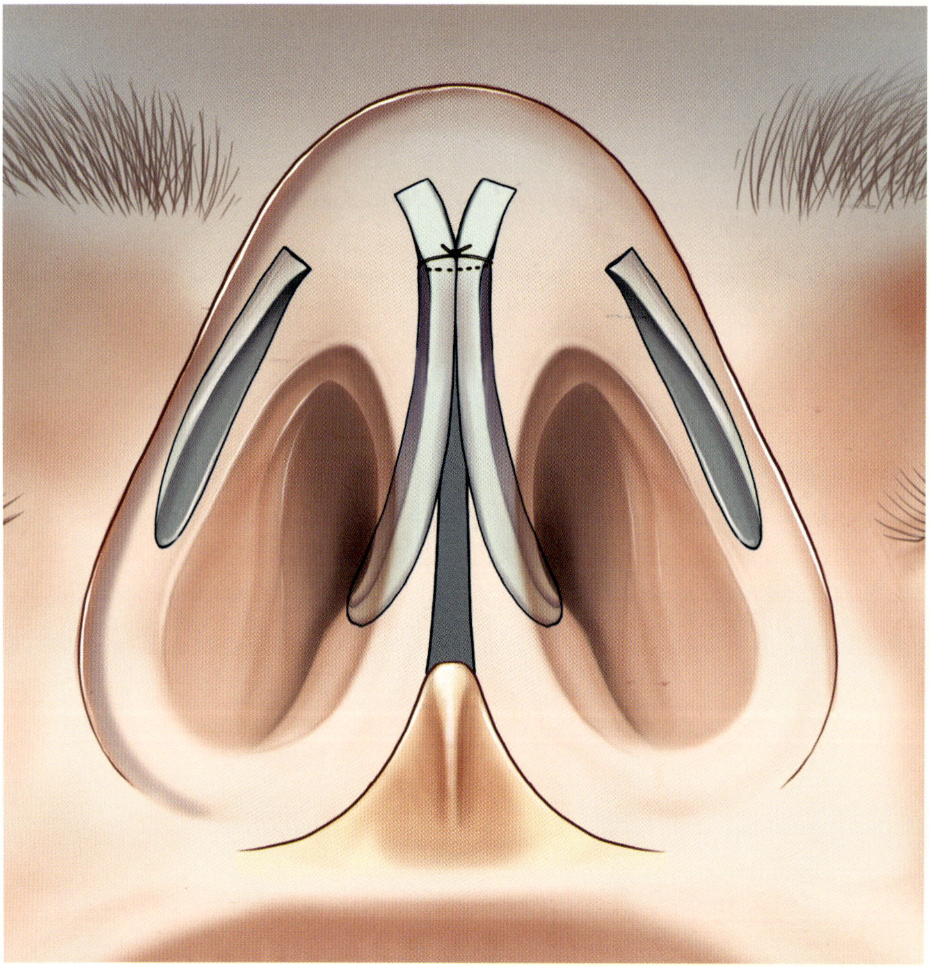

Figure 48b: opening of the medial crura to simulate Ponti's butterfly

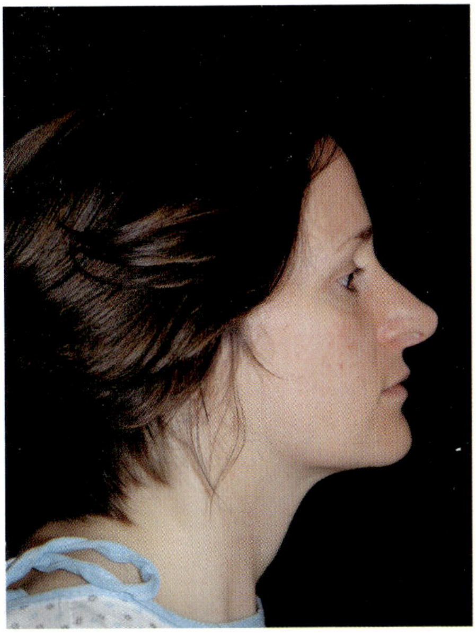

Figure 49 a: preop of a secondary case in which the Domus was amputated and a Ponti Butterfly simulated.
See case 6, chapter 21

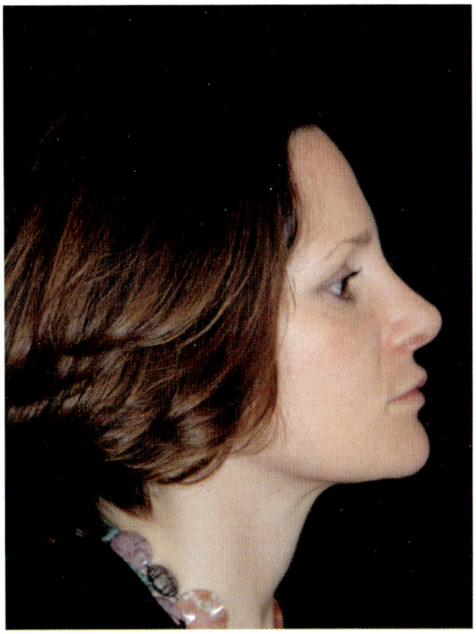

Figure 49b: postoperative

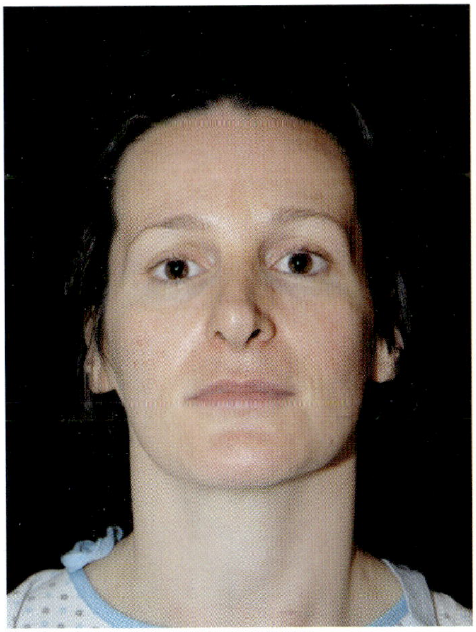

Figure 49c: front preoperative

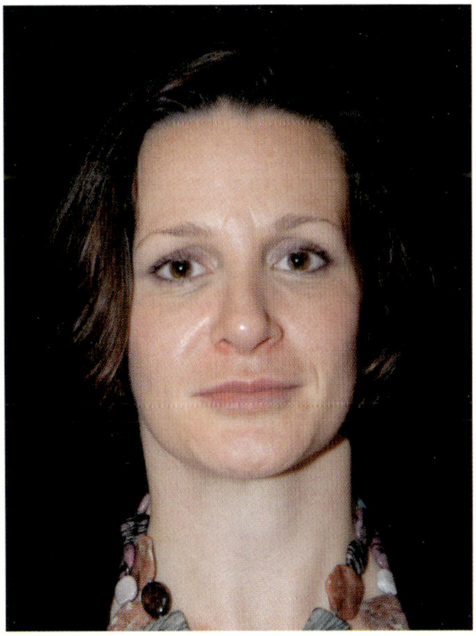

Figura 49d: postoperative

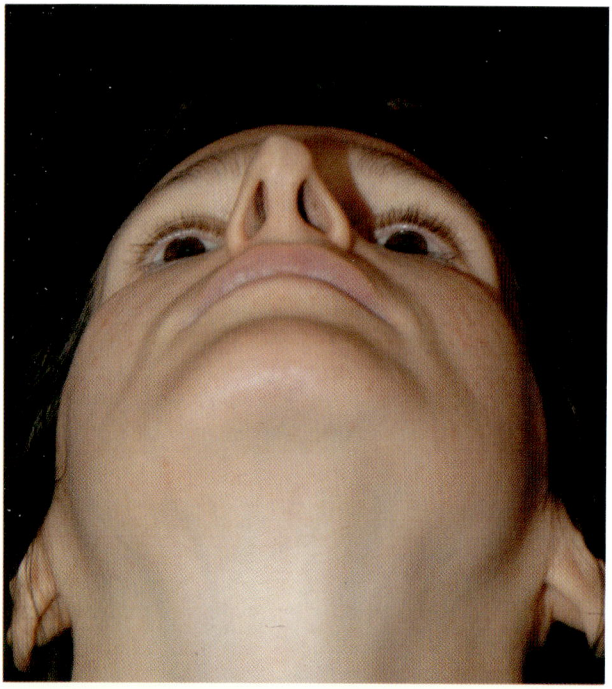

Figure 50a: preoperative, view from below

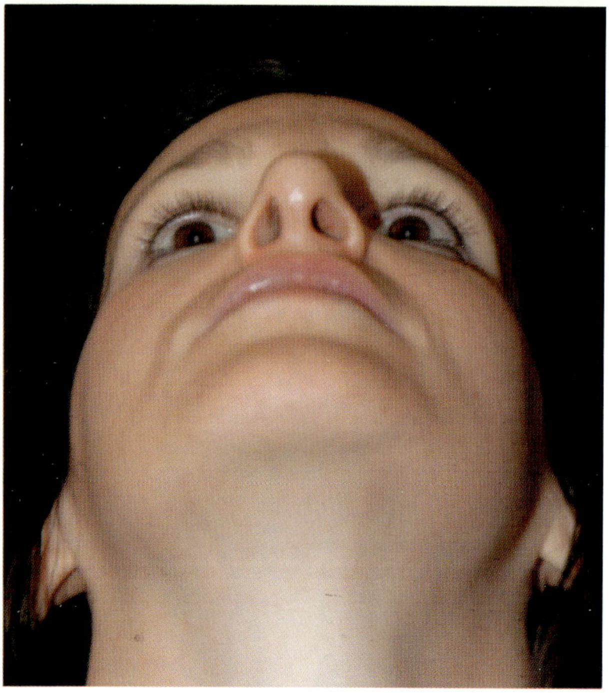

Figure 50b: postoperatively, view from below

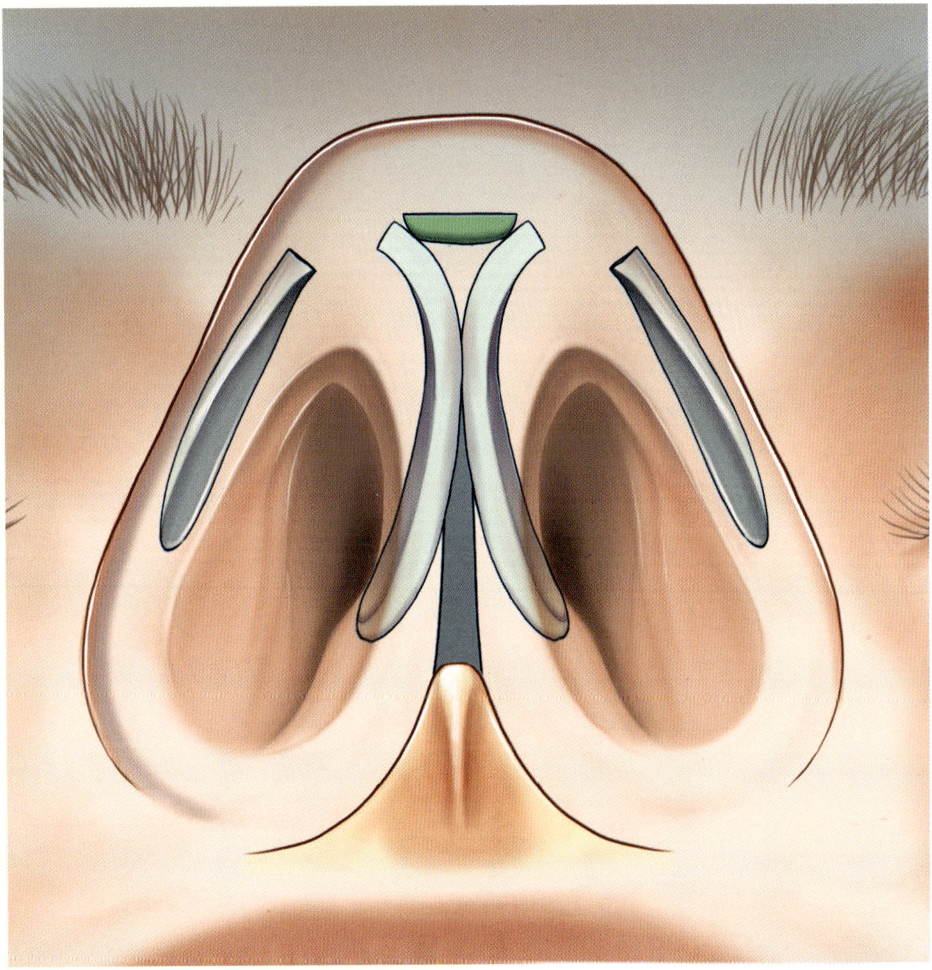

Figure 51: insertion of a cartilage graft between the open medial crura so as to simulate a butterfly wing as in the technique conceived by Ponti

References

1. Pitanguy I. Aesthetic Plastic Surgery of head and body. Berlin Springer Verlag, 1981; p. 263.

2. Sheen Jack H, Aethetic Rhinoplasty. The C.V. Mosby Cpmpany , St Louis 1978; p. 57.

3. Rees, T D Aesthetic Plastic Surgery Vol 1. W.B. Saunders Company 1980; p.187.

4. Diamond, H. :Rhynoplasty techniques. Surg. Clin. North Am, 1971. 51:317.

5. Gasperoni et al, A new alar demarcator to facilitate the intercartilagineous approach to tip plasty, Annals of the International Symposium Recent Advances in Plastic Surgery (Raps 90), 1990; p. 609-613.

6. Jost G : Boxy tip and Bulky tip. Rhinoplasty Problems and Controversies, a discussion with the experts. The C. V. Mosby Company St. Louis- Washington DC – Toronto 1988.

7. Rethi, A : Plastische Neobildung der Nase. Chirurg 1929; 1:165.

8. Goodman JB: Arch Otolaringol 1961; 74:636.

9. Berson MI: Atlas of Plastic Surgery. London William Heinemann, 1948.

10. Ponti L. : Surgery of the Nasal Tip. A modification of the Goldman Technique. Excerpta Medica International Congress Series No.216, 1969.

11. Tessier P La rhinoplastie esthetique G.M. de France, 1968; 75.28.

12. Sheen JH, Sheen AP. Aesthetic Rhinoplasty, 2nd edn. St.Louis Quality Medical Publishing.

13. Peck GC Techniques in Aesthetic Rhinoplasty , Gower Medical Publishing, New York NY.

CHAPTER 8

Septoplasty

When a deviation of the nasal septum is present, it has to be corrected for two reasons: firstly, to solve or avoid functional problems in the future, and secondly for aesthetic reasons. It would not be possible to build a straight nose on a crooked septum. Often the septum that has grown crooked has guided the growth of the nose by pushing it to one side leading not only to a deviation of the septum but also of the whole pyramid (figs. 1a, b).

Deviations of the nasal septum can be divided into posterior to the complete growth of the nose and prior to it.

Cases of malformation are beyond the scope of this book.

Deviations posterior to the complete growth of the nose are of traumatic

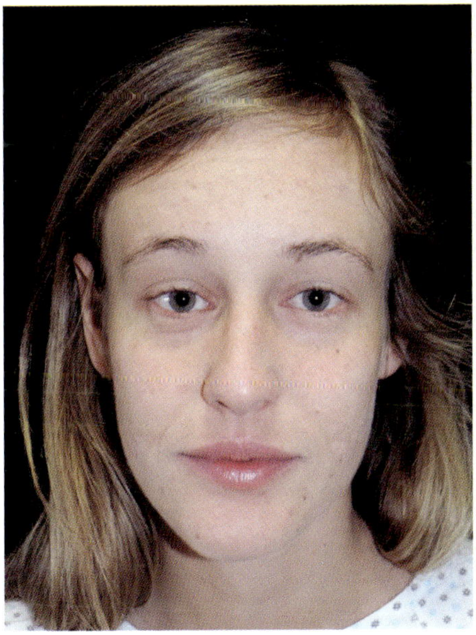

Figure 1a: right pyramidal displacement

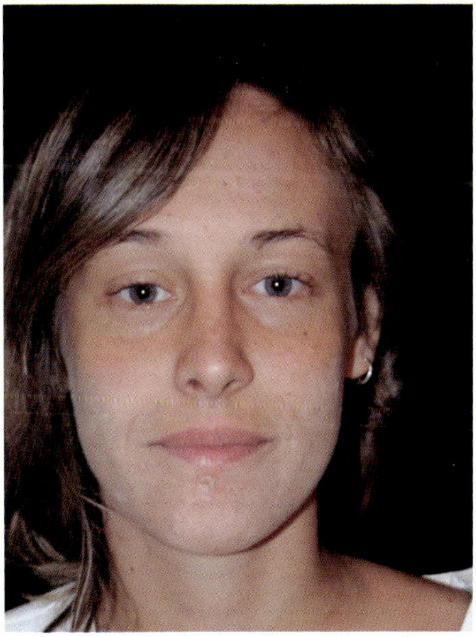

Figure 1b: pyramidal displacement corrected with rhinoseptoplasty

origin. In these cases we deal with structures that have grown normally, and therefore rather symmetric and fairly well aligned, and that have undergone a deviation only after the end of their growth. Basically, the various components are normal but out of place, so it is sufficient to put them back in their normal position with a corrective surgery.

Deviations that have taken place prior to the complete growth of the nose are more complex because the structures have grown with different thrusts, due to the displacement of the growth plates, and therefore the bone and cartilage components of the nose have acquired abnormal and asymmetrical shapes and curvatures.

In most cases the deviation is to the left, i.e. the base of the septum occupies the left nasal fossa, while the upper part of the septum goes to the opposite side and therefore from the outside a deviation to the right is observable. Therefore it is more correct and more descriptive to say left-convex deviation. The reason why the deviation of the septum in most cases is left-convex is that with childbirth the nose is crushed by the rotational movement that takes place in the birth canal; the quadrangular cartilage is dislocated as a consequence of this movement and also the growth plates of septal bones are dislocated, leading to an offset future growth of its both cartilaginous and bony part.

Septoplasty often has to be performed to ensure that the nose is functionally efficient and aesthetically straight. The septum is examined and the part that needs to be corrected is identified. The deviation can be anterior, posterior or both, affecting multiple Cottle areas (see chapter 4), so it can be more or less complex.

Standard access

From the intercartilaginous access that extends to the caudal margin of the septum, as in the rhinoplasty derived from Joseph taken into consideration in this book, the access to the septum is wide and convenient. To begin the subperichondral undermining an incision of the perichondrium from the concave part of the septum is made, and with an elevator the perichondrium can be undermined over the whole of the deviated portion (fig. 2). The undermining can then extend posteriorly to raise the periosteum of the perpendicular lamina of the ethmoid and vomer (fig. 3). In the anterior portion of the vomer the undermining must be done starting posteriorly in anterior direction. If it is made from the front to

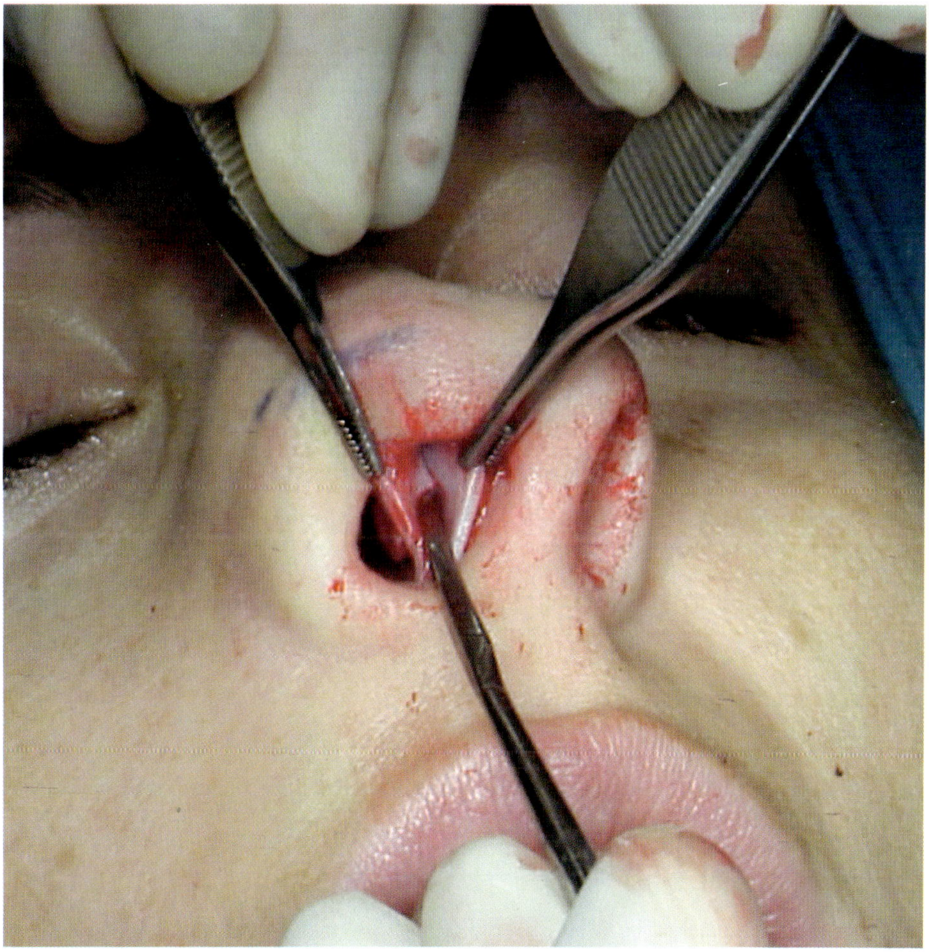

Figure 2: from the incision at the caudal margin of the septum, the mucoperichondrium is elevated on the concave side

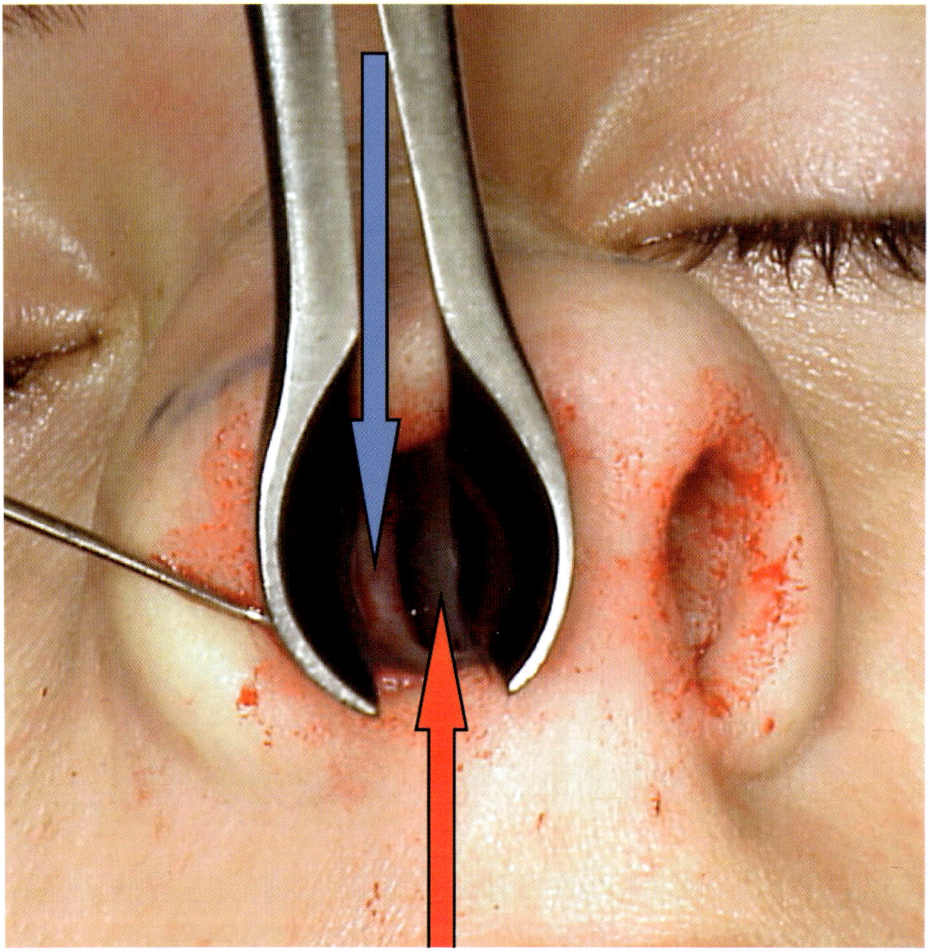

Figure 3: elevated mucoperichondrium (blue arrow) permits the vision of the septum (red arrow) allowing to reach the vomer and the ethmoid's perpendicular lamina

back, the movement of the elevator risks to traumatize the Nasopalatine Nerve which is at the base of the Premaxilla. An injury to this nerve leads to paresthesia or anesthesia of the incisor teeth, which are included in the premaxilla. Once the mucoperichondrium has been elevated from the concave side of the septum, it can be elevated on the convex side. The Killian speculum is then be inserted with its branches under the perichondrium of both sides, making it easy to see the whole septum (fig. 4). When

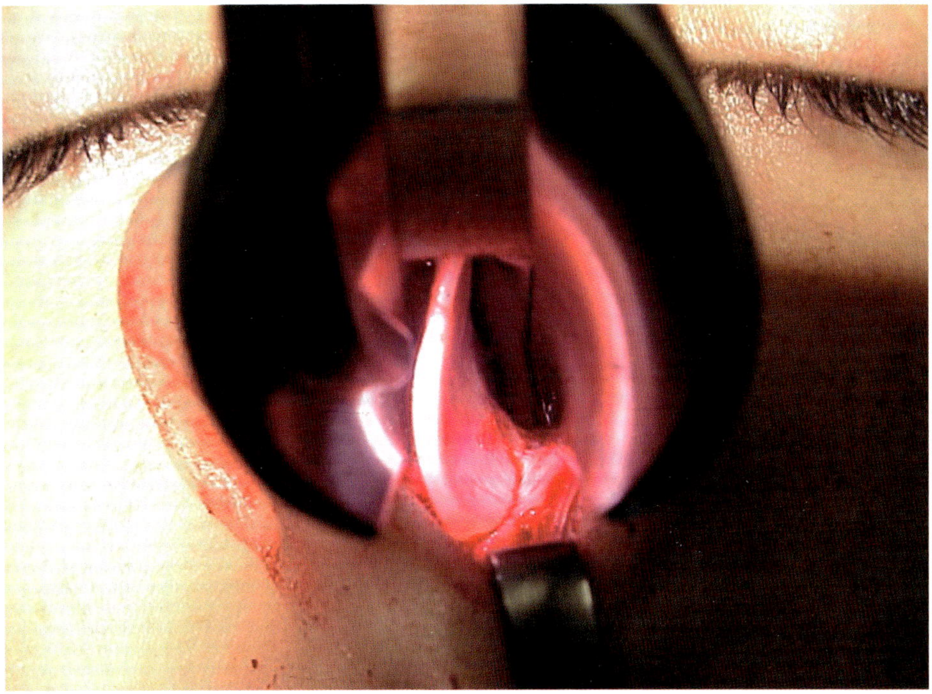

Figure 4: the septum is visualized inserting a Killian speculum under the perichondrium. Obstruction of the left nasal fossa is well appreciated

removing the deviated portions of the septum it is necessary to be as conservative as possible, compatibly with the unblocking of the nasal cavities. It is more convenient to start from the concave side because it is easier to undermine. It is important that the chondromucosa remains intact on at least one side to avoid perforation of the septum. Undermining on the convex side may be difficult at angles and spurs where lesions of the chondromucosa may occur. In order to prevent perforation of the septum it is good practice to leave as much as possible cartilage of the quadrangular lamina and bone, so that re-epithelialization can take place along their surface.

The septum must be rigid to provide a good support for the nasal dorsum and the tip, and to allow the turbinates to correctly perform their funcross branch with two fingers (figs. 7a, b). The posterior portion of the septum, consisting of the perpendicular lamina of the Ethmoid, articulates with the vomer and therefore the chisel used to disengage the vomer from its base can be pushed further back to disengage also the perpendicular lamina of the Ethmoid from its base. The deviated portion of bone is then removed with a Hartmann forceps (fig. 7c). Sometimes, if only the posterior septum (fig. 8) is deviated, a Killian septoplasty can be performed: the septum is undermined on one side only; before the deviation, an incision is made on the cartilaginous septum, a MacKenty elevator is introduced (fig. 9) , and the contralateral chondromucosa and periosteum is

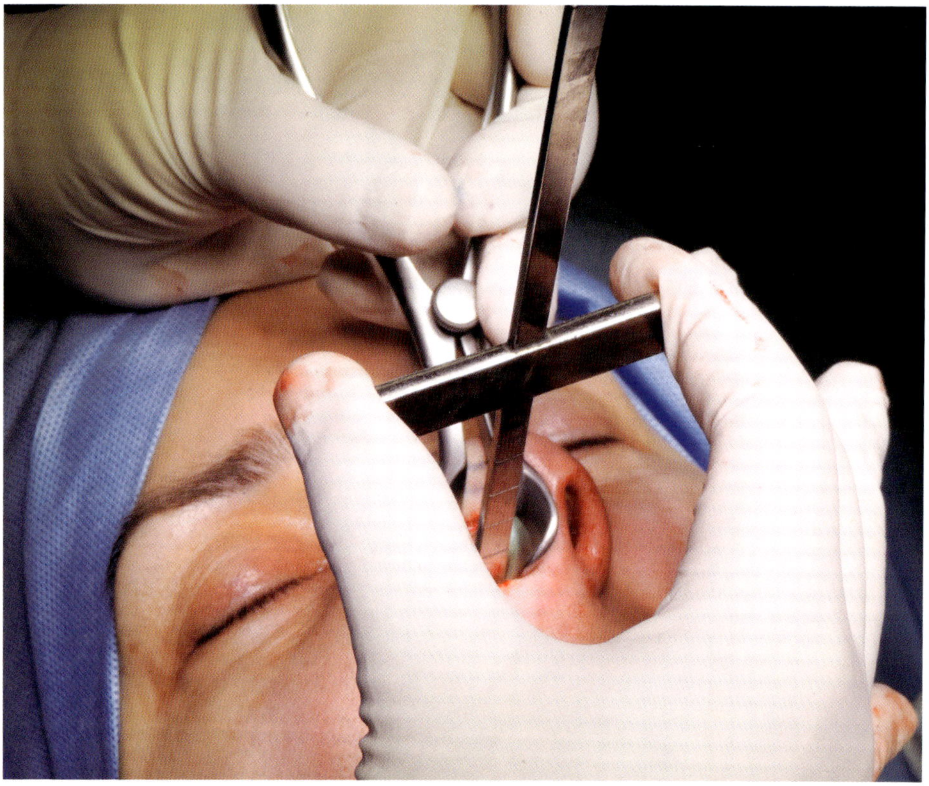

Figure 7a: the deviated bone is first fractured with a Cottle's cross chisel and then removed with a Hartmann forceps

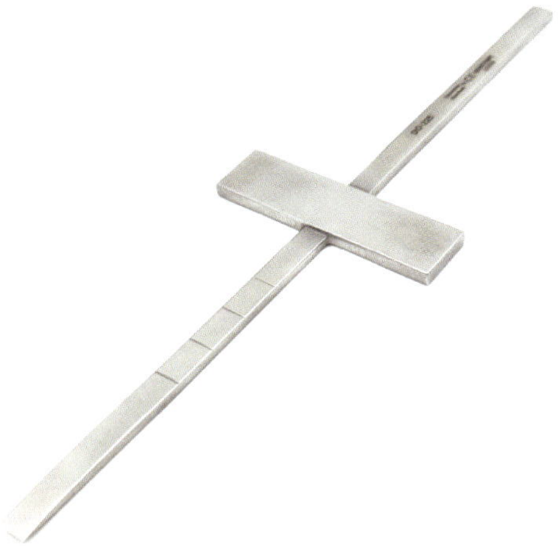

Figure 7b: Cottle cross chisel

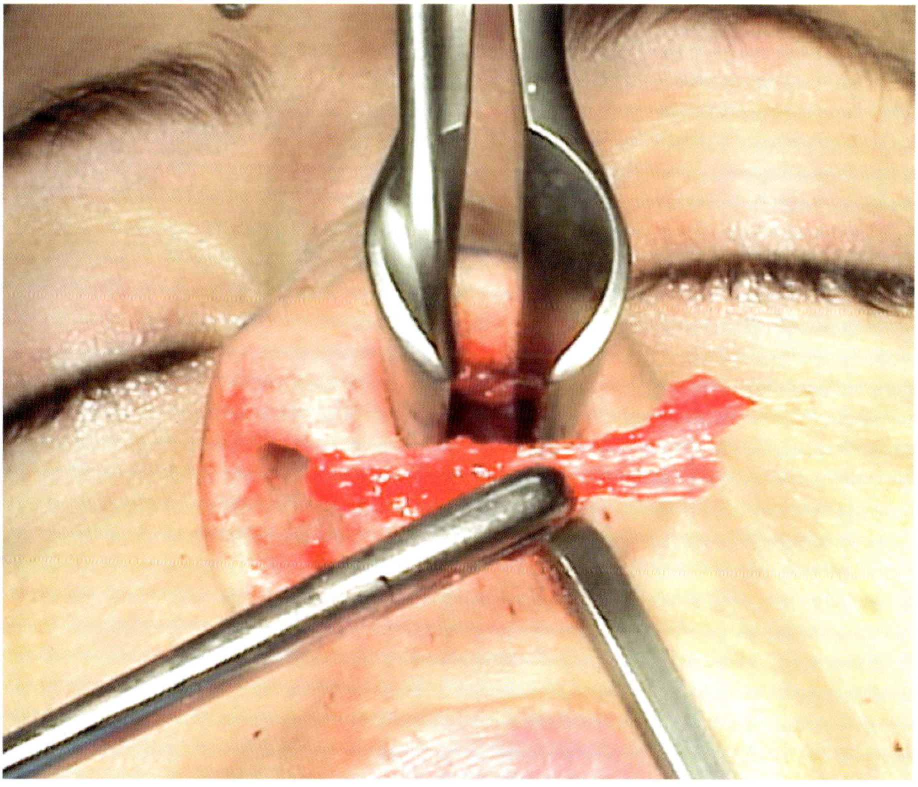

Figure 7c: the lower part of the septum, consisting of the vomer and perpendicular lamina of the ethmoid, is removed with the Hartmann septum forceps

undermined. The deviated bony part is then dislocated and removed with Hartmann's forceps (figs. 10a, b, c).
Anterior cartilaginous deviations are corrected with serial incisions from the concave side (fig. 11), or with the use of Rubin's morselizer forceps (fig. 12a) which has a branch with a squared surface that has the function of weakening the cartilage without completely incising it (fig. 12b).
The concave part, weakened by these methods, can be straightened and locked in place by means of an Ash forceps (fig. 13a) and kept straight with transfixed stitches on the septum (figs. 13b, c). Sometimes, especially when the septum has a clear straight fracture line, the Swinging Door technique can also be used. This technique consists in undermining from one side only, make a full-thickness incision at the level of the cartilage fold, or if needed, even removal of the cartilage responsible for the fold.

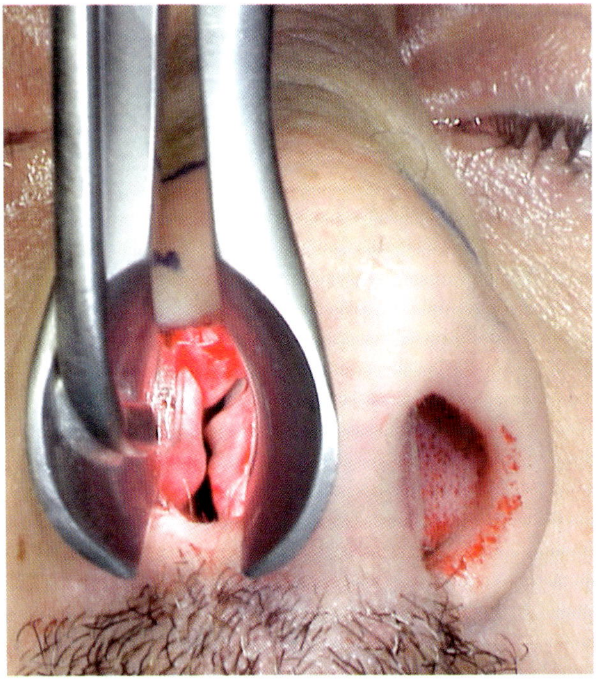

Figure 8: posterior septal spur obstructing the right nasal fossa. The Killian technique can be used in such cases

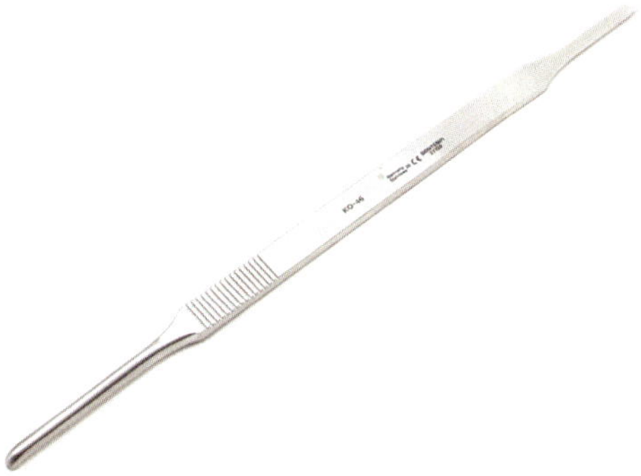

Figure 9: MacKenty's elevator

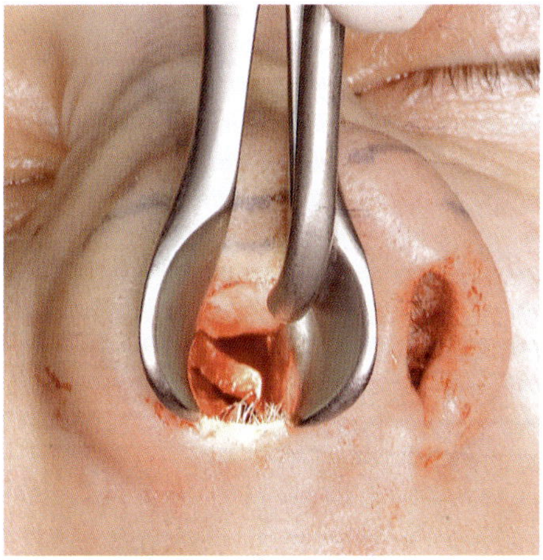

Figure 10a: deviated portion of the perpendicular ethmoid lamina dislocated with the MacKenty elevator

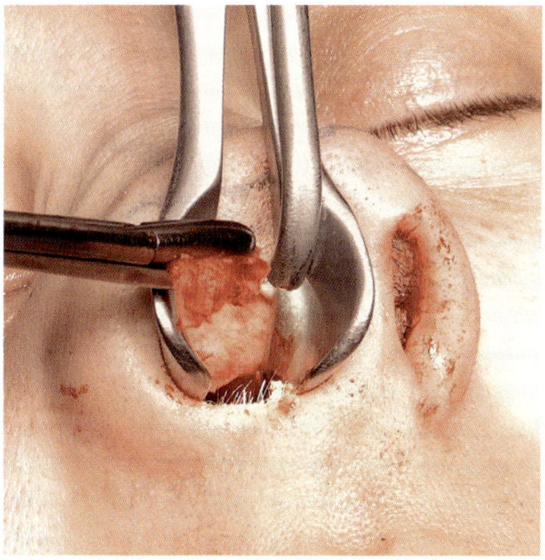

Figure 10b: excision of a fragment of the dislocated ethmoid with Hartmann's forceps

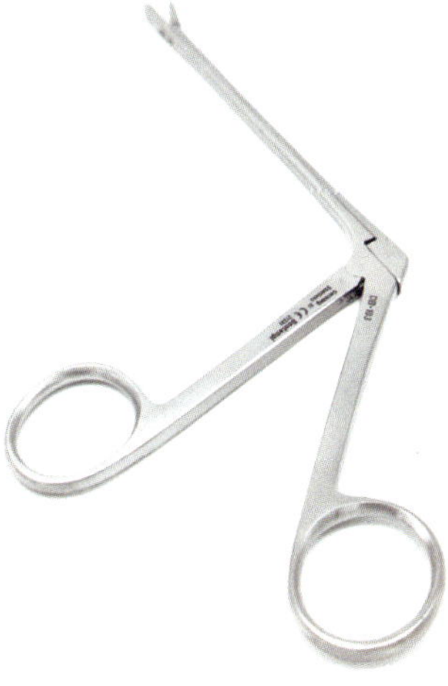

Figure 10c: Hartmann's rongeur forceps

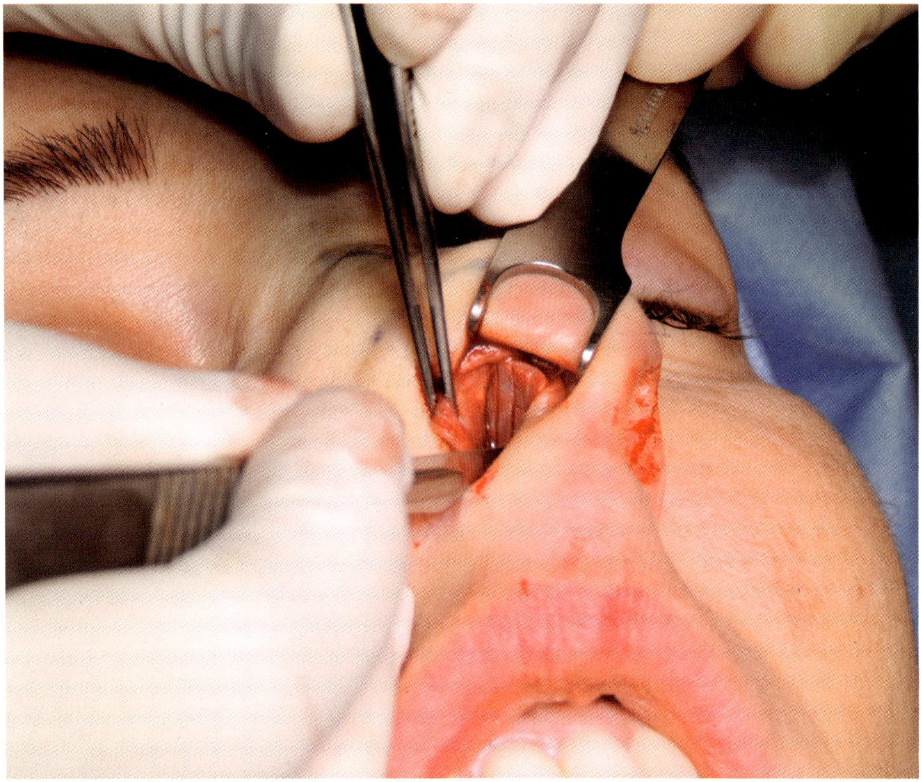

Figure 11: serial incisions from the concave side to straighten the anterior septum

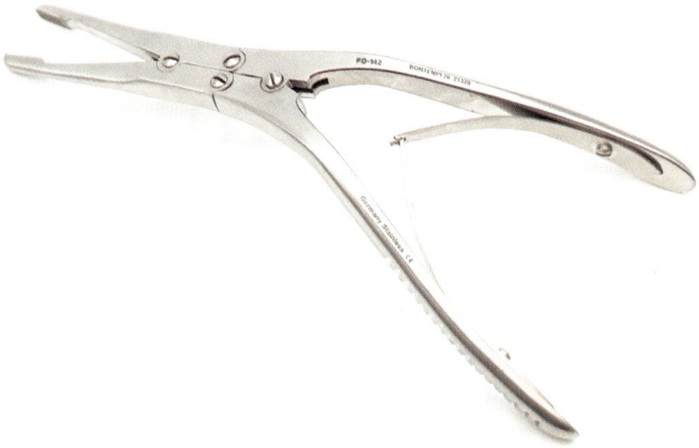

Figure 12a: Rubin's morselizer forceps

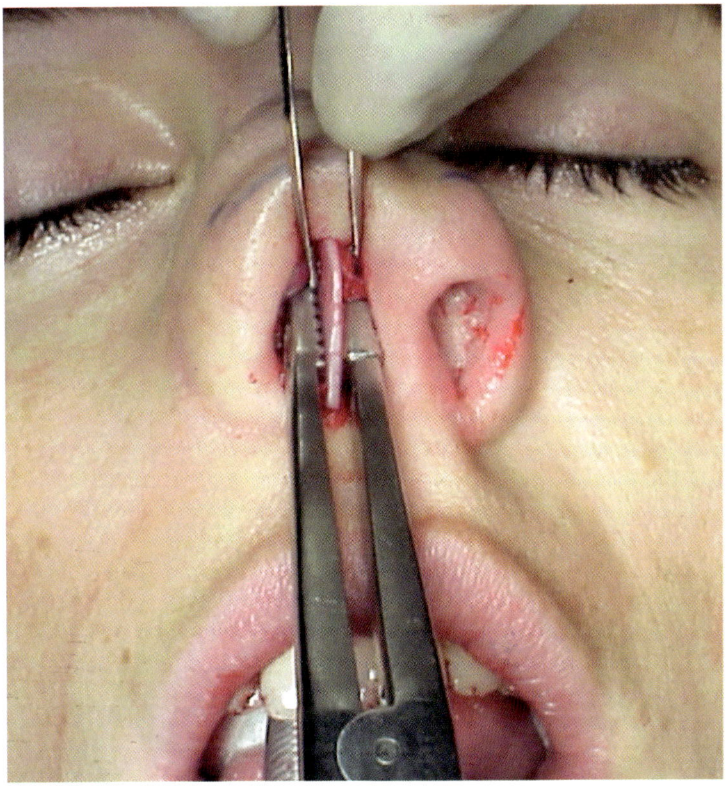

Figure 12b: Rubin's morselizer forceps inserted with the checkered branch on the right, with the aim of weakening the concave surface of the septal cartilage, and on the left the smooth branch, which has only the aim of opposing the opposite branch thrust

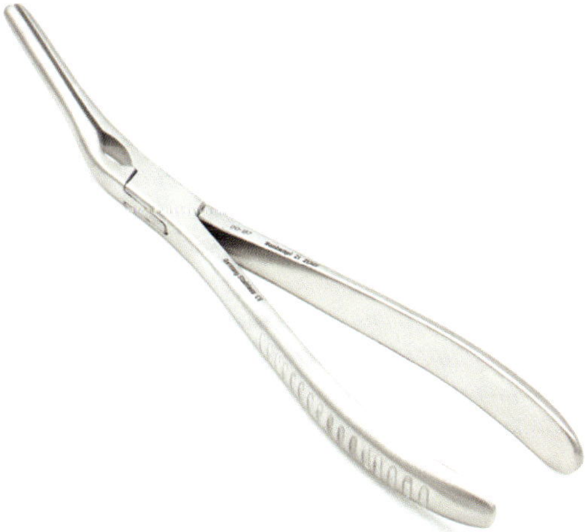

Figure 13a: Asch forceps

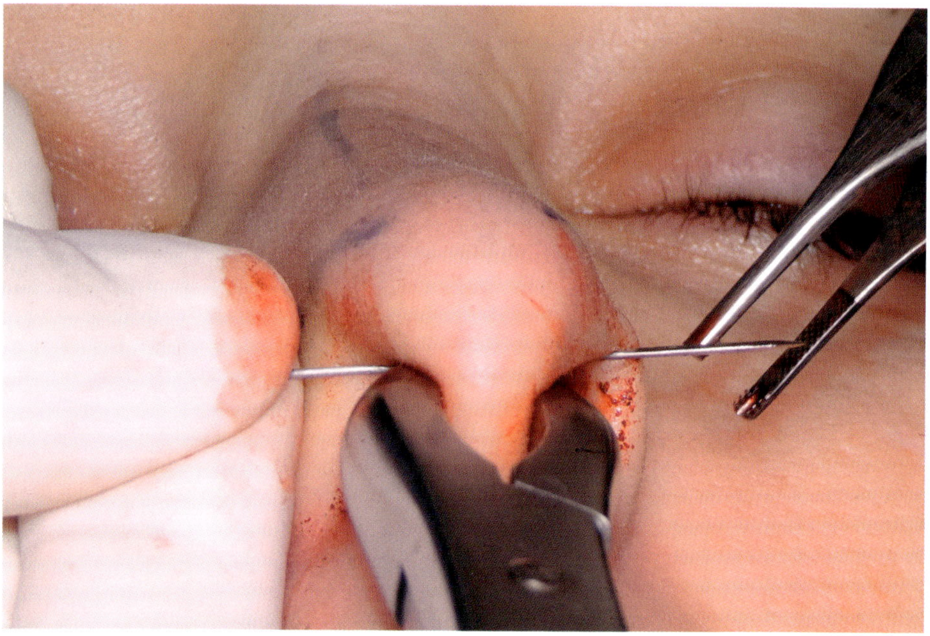

Figure 13b: holding an Asch forceps inserted in the nostrils,
a transfix stitch is placed superiorly to guide healing on the midline

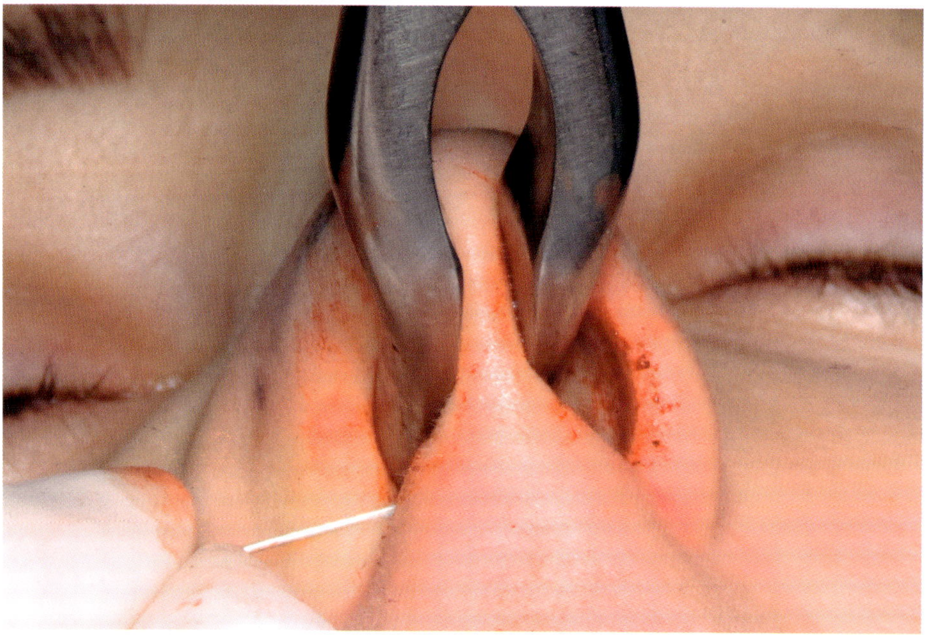

Figure 13c: a stitch in the lower part near the anterior nasal spine stabilizes the base of the septum

Then the chondromucosa acts as a hinge ensuring that the cartilage does not collapse into the nasal fossa when is repositioned on the midline. Two or three transfix stitches of vicryl rapid 3-0 are eventually applied to stabilize the septum. The nasal packing will be carried out at the end of the surgery.

References

1. Fuchs J. A rapid approach to the deviated septum in Rhinoplasty , Plast Recostr Surg 1956; 18:133.

CHAPTER 9

Treatment of the turbinates

The turbinates, as mentioned above, are regulators of the flow of air necessary for proper breathing. They should therefore never be removed but, if necessary, they can only be reduced, so that they may continue to perform their function. As breathing side changes many times during the day (see chapter 4), you should not rely on the response of a CT scan or other radiological examinations describing a hypertrophy of this or that turbinate, because its volume may depend on the time of the examination and not on a true hypertrophy. This obviously also applies to the inspection at the time of the examination.

I have already described the physiology of the turbinate (chapter 4), and it is necessary to remember that its volume increases with the typical mechanism of a corpus cavernosum, being it a cavernous body, until it touches the septum, and then withdraws a little. It follows that, if the septum is deviated, the turbinate of the part where there is more space will always be more voluminous than the contralateral one where the nasal fossa is more restricted. This condition is called compensatory hypertrophy because the increased volume of the turbinate is due to a need to the need to compensate the overly large space. When the septum is straightened by surgery, the turbinate that was on the side where the space was smaller will be able to perform its function well, while the one that was forced by the anatomical situation to be hypertrophic will find itself squeezed into a smaller space and therefore will adapt to the new and normalized anatomical situation in a long time. In the majority of cases this happens, but it is also possible that this adaptation does not totally happen, and therefore it is better to help it to shrink. To this end, an infiltration of 20-40 mg of Triamcinolone injected into the head of the turbinate can be decisive, especially if, in addition to the anatomical factor, there is an allergic factor contributing to the hypertrophy

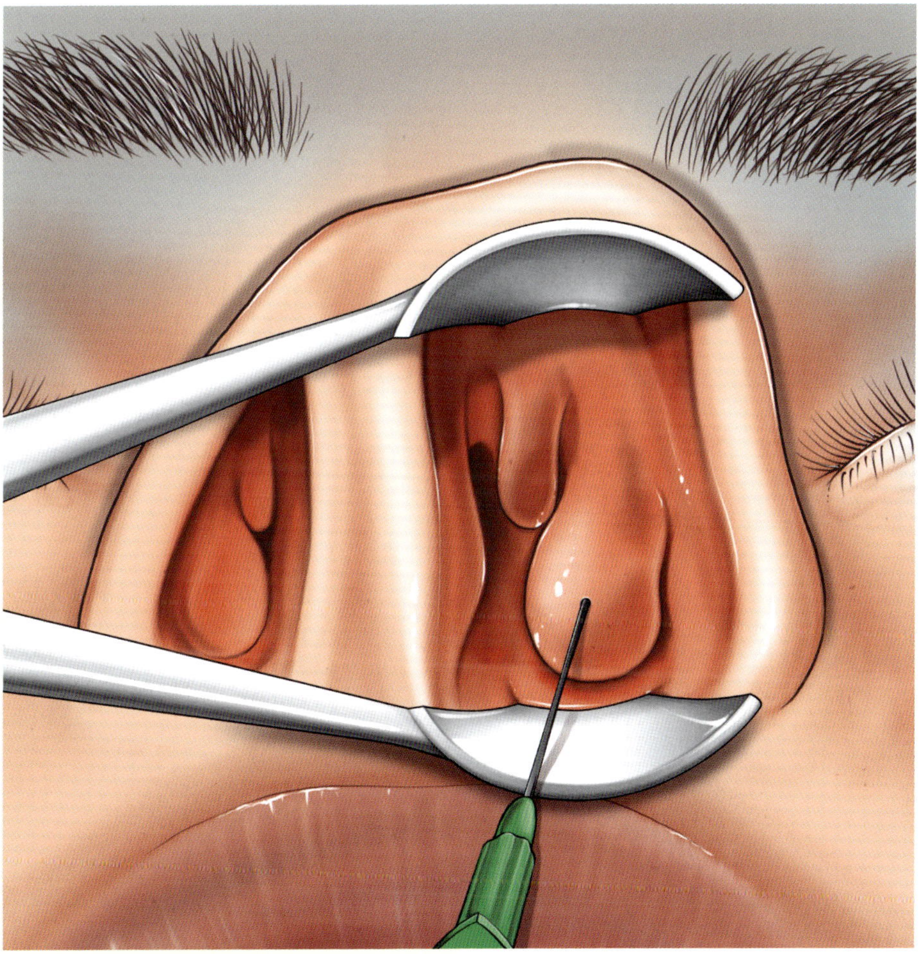

Figure 1: infiltration of triamcinolone in the head of the turbinate. This is effective when the allergic component is predominant, but dangerous because the substance injected can cause blindness via the bloodstream. If you decide to proceed, you must remain very superficial, aspirating before injecting, to be sure that you have not penetrated a blood vesse

(fig. 1). Infiltration must be carried out with extreme caution, making sure that the drug is not being injected into a vessel, as cases of blindness due to its passage through a vascular system connected to the ocular one have been reported. It is therefore necessary to infiltrate with the needle staying superficial, in the submucosa, to make a wheal that does not communicate with the vascular circle. If you are not sure of mastering this infiltration technique, it is better to give up and look for a valid alternative.

Alternatively, the turbinate must be reduced with diathermocoagulation in several places like the buttons on a mattress, or preferably with a tip that produces a plasma as in devices such as the coblator (Smith&Nephew) or the meghan (www.meghan-europe.com), which reduces the volume of the turbinate acting from within it without a significant increase in temperature. These devices work with radiofrequency technology, which induces ionic agitation in the tissues surrounding the electrode, generating heat, so it is not the electrode that heats up but the two to four millimeters of adjacent tissue. The energy used has a low power level so the temperature is maintained between 65° and 90° avoiding carbonization phenomena that occur instead in diathermocoagulation (1). The diathermocoagulation of the turbinates are carried out with an electrocautery on the turbinates' surface. They are small burns that are effective in reducing the turbinate but if they come into contact with the septum, they can stick to it causing adhesions called synechiae. Bipolar forceps can also be used, but again the repair process can induce turbinate-septal synechiae. The use of plasma-generating devices does not cause burns on the turbinates' surface and therefore there is no risk of causing synechiae (see also chapter 4). The shaft of the radiofrequency device has three marks to help you know how deep it is inserted (fig. 2). Hypertrophies may be bilateral or even left but as in most cases the septal deviation is left-convex, the turbinate on the opposite side has a compensatory hypertrophy which must be treated (fig. 3). The tip of the radiofrequency device is inserted starting from the head of the turbi-

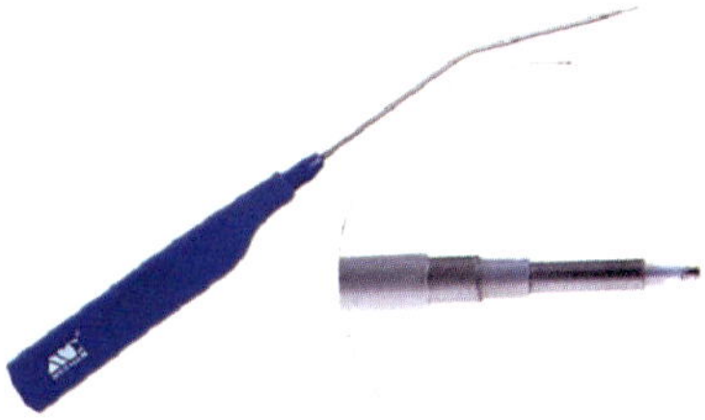

Figure 2: the radiofrequency device for treatment of the turbinates has a shaft with three marks to allow to check how deep it has been inserted

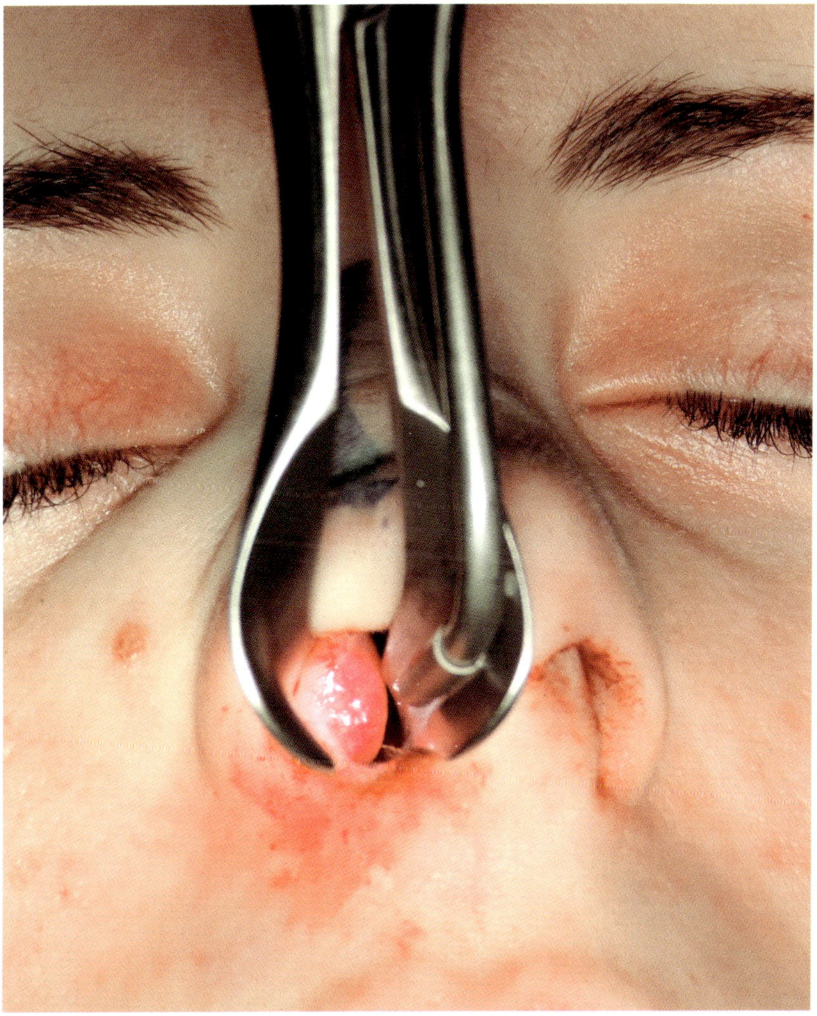

Figure 3: right lower turbinate with compensatory hypertrophy

nate until the third mark, and proceeding backwards the radiofrequency is activated (fig. 4). An application of a few seconds is sufficient, taking into account the characteristics of the device.

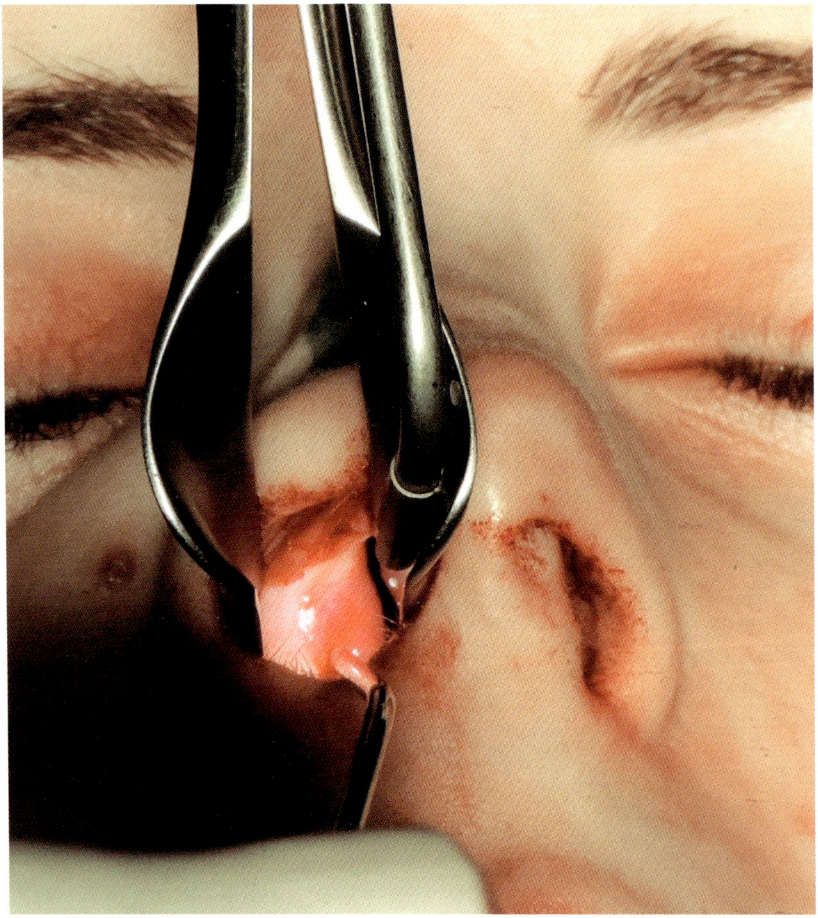

Figure 4: the tip is inserted into the turbinate, starting at its head, up to the third mark and then is gradually retracted to the second and eventually to the first one

References

1. Ferrario F Reductive surgery of the inferior turbinates: classification, analytical review and selection criteria for interventions. Proceedings of the AOOI conference Update in turbinate pathology-Verona 2010 p. 243. Torgraf, Galatina (Lecce)

CHAPTER 10

Osteotomies

Once the hump has been removed (see chapter 7), that is almost always the case when a rhinoplasty is performed on caucasians, the osteocartilaginous pyramid becomes a truncated pyramid. So it is necessary to narrow the lateral walls to return to a pyramidal shape.

If the lateral walls are not approximated the nasal mucosa comes in contact with the skin (figs. 1a, b). This condition can give rise to the open roof syndrome, described by Cottle, which involves pain and headache at low temperatures.

The two lateral bone walls of the nose are made up of the frontal process of the maxilla and the nasal bones. In order to tighten these walls, osteotomies must be performed. In some cases the bones have a considerable thickness, so the nose can have a wide aspect even if osteotomies have been perfectly done.

Let's now come to the technique to be performed: since the nasal pyramid has its apex at the nasion, i.e. a little more cranially than the intercantal line, the upper limit of the osteotomies will also be above this line, just where the nose ends and the nasal process of the frontal bone begins (fig. 2a). The mobilization of the lateral walls, that will bring the nose back to its pyramidal shape, must be carefully prepared so that the bony walls may move as a single block and no irregularities are produced at the point where the nasal bones articulate with the frontal bone.

Osteotomies must be precise otherwise asymmetries and deviations of the pyramid may occur. Therefore, before proceeding to the mobilization of the nasal bone walls, a careful preparation must be made with medial and lateral osteotomies. Only as a final step the fracture will be completed with a tran-

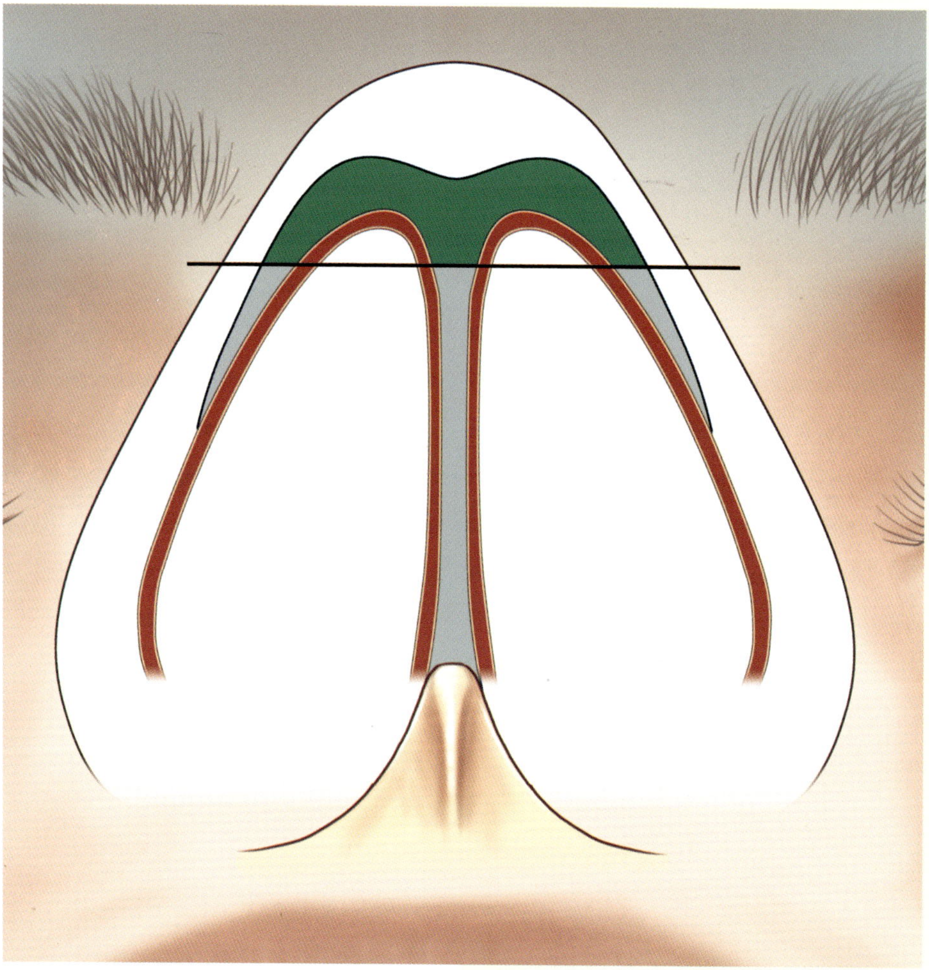

Figure 1a: the hump is removed, the nasal walls are spaced apart leaving a gap at the osteocartilaginous vault. The nasal pyramid has thus become a truncated pyramid, so the two walls need to be brought closer together to regain a pyramidal shape, otherwise the nose would remain wide and the internal mucosa would come into contact with the skin. At low temperatures, this condition gives rise to open roof syndrome

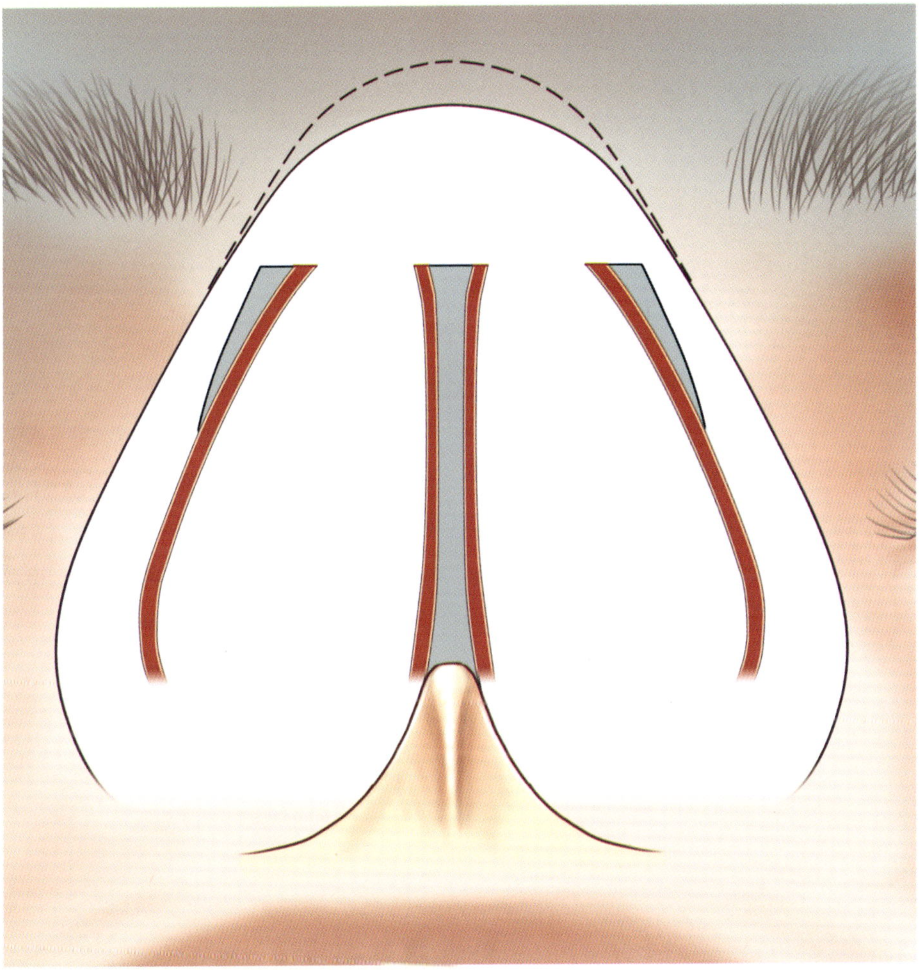

Figure 1b: open roof

sversal osteotomy done with a curved osteotome permitting the eventual approach of the lateral walls towards the midline. The suture between the nose bones and the frontal one has a very variable conformation but though osteotomies we must give a symmetrical result. For this reason, empirical methods such as hearing the different noise the osteotome makes when it reaches the frontal bone (1) must give way to something more certain, such as the method described below.

Fracturing the nasal bones is done in three stages.

- First stage of the osteotomies (medial osteotomy): to be sure that the fracture is performed exactly at the upper apex of the nasal pyramid, a straight osteotome is inserted on either side of the septum and a notch is made until the root of the nose, i.e. until the line have been drawn that corresponds to the beginning of the nasal pyramid (fig. 2a) To be sure of arriving exactly to the previously drawn line indicating the root of the nose, the thumb is put across it (fig. 2b). and with the osteotome the thumb is reached from the inside (video 1).(figs 2c, d).
- Second stage of the osteotomies (lateral osteotomy): a small incision is made in the eyelid skin (fig. 3a) in order to introduce a 4mm osteotome (video 2) (figs. 3b, c). This is used to make notches at the base of the lateral bony walls of the nose. Normally between three and four notches are needed to produce a fracture line. We start caudally, close to the anterior surface of the upper maxillary bone. Then we go up, towards the root of the nose following a slightly curved line until above the intercanthal line, reaching the point where the nasal pyramid ends and the frontal bone begins. (fig. 3d).

Why is the line of the lateral osteotomy a bit curved, starting low and with a slight tendency to go up? If the osteotomy follows a straight path starting low and remaining low, the two bony walls tighten completely, resulting in

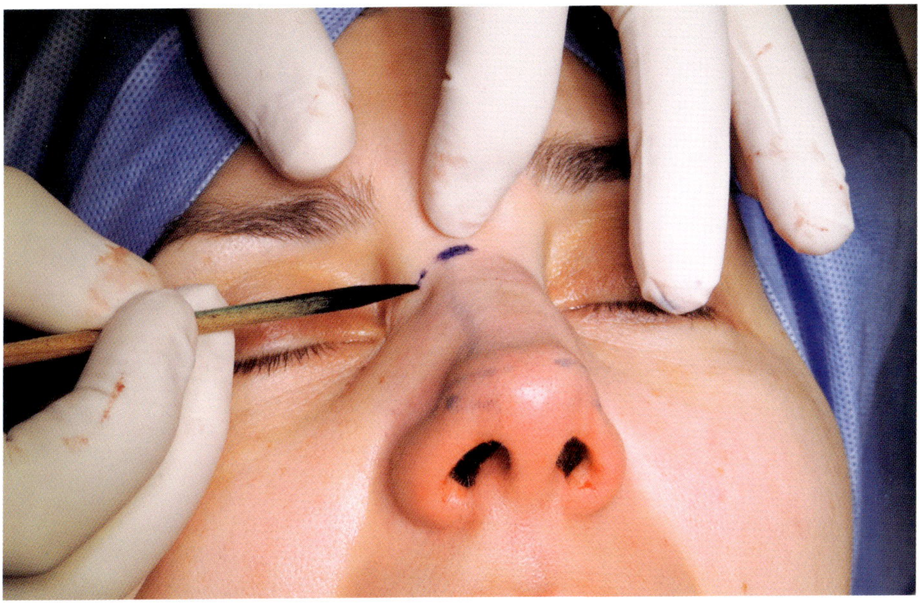

Figure 2a: the line drawn with methylene blue indicates the root of the nose that is the point where the nasal pyramid begins. This is the exact height at which the transverse osteotomies should be made, and with a hinge movement the nasal walls may to come together towards the midline

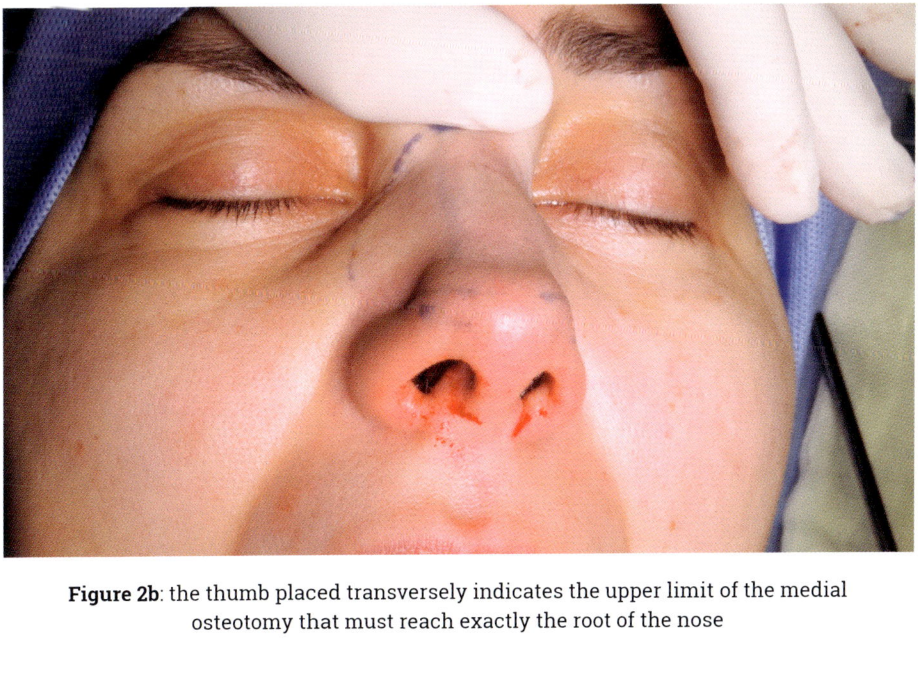

Figure 2b: the thumb placed transversely indicates the upper limit of the medial osteotomy that must reach exactly the root of the nose

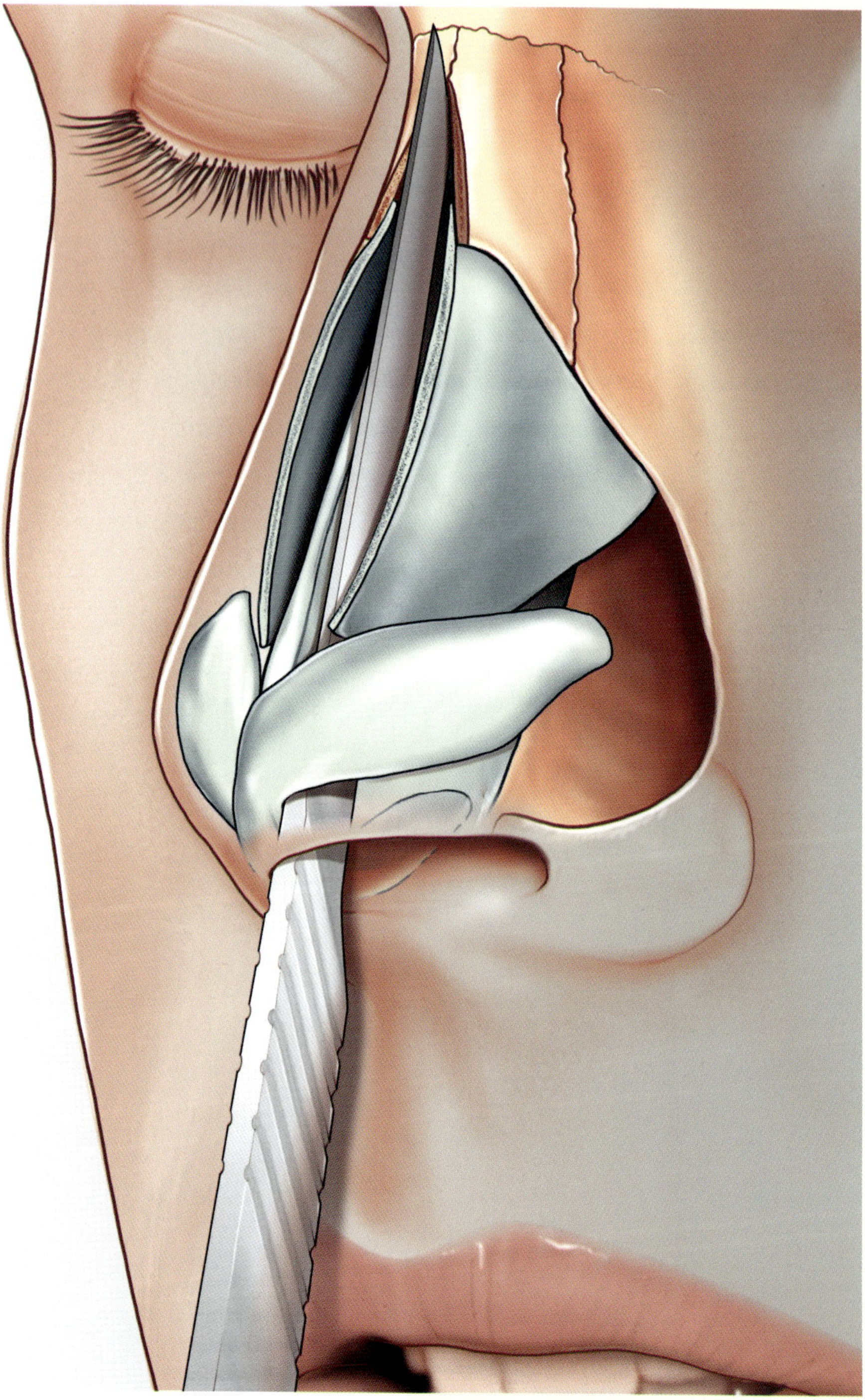

Figure 2c: diagram of medial osteotomies

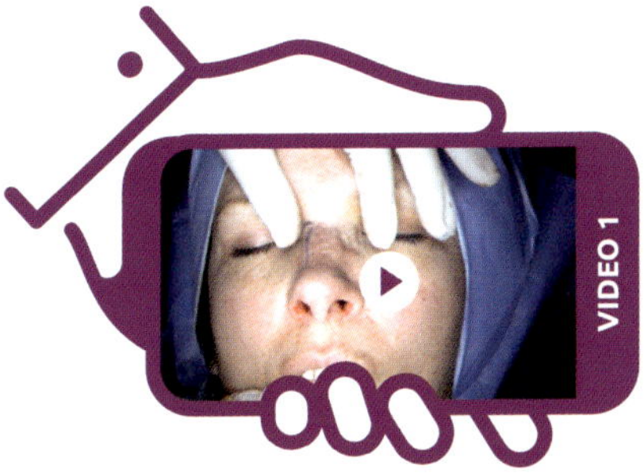

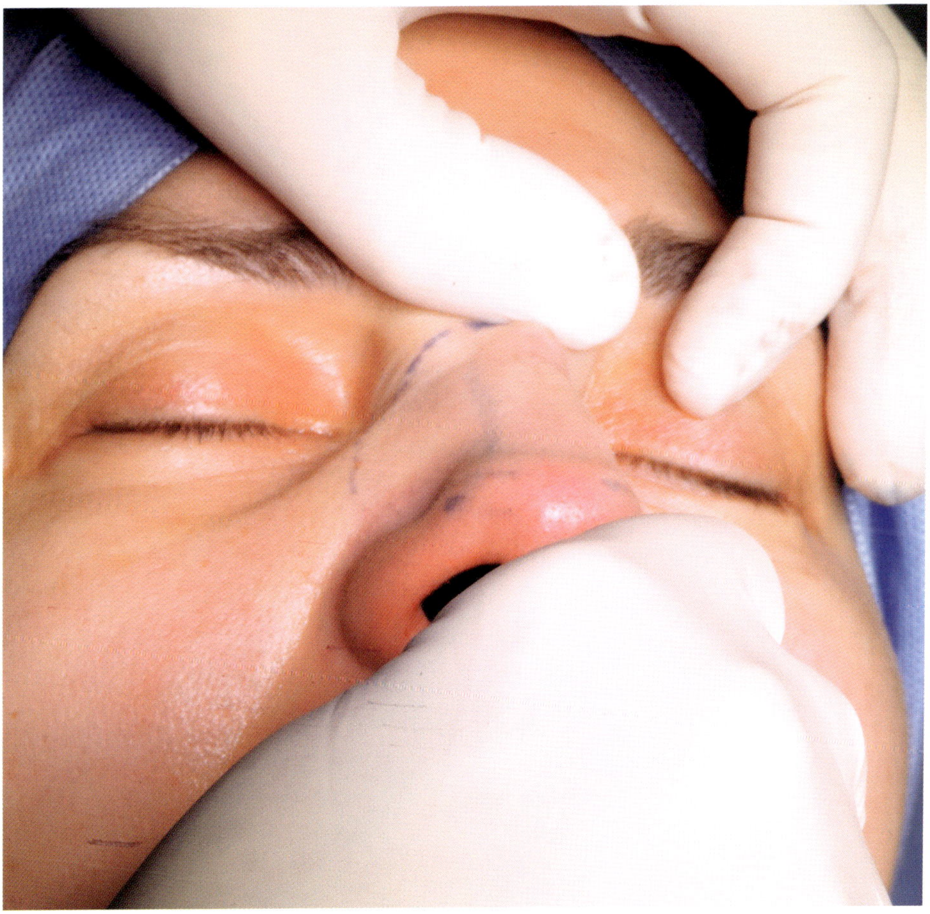

Figure 2d: a wide osteotome makes it possible to locate the exact position of its tip and therefore to check when it has arrived exactly at the predetermined point, i.e. where the thumb is placed transversely

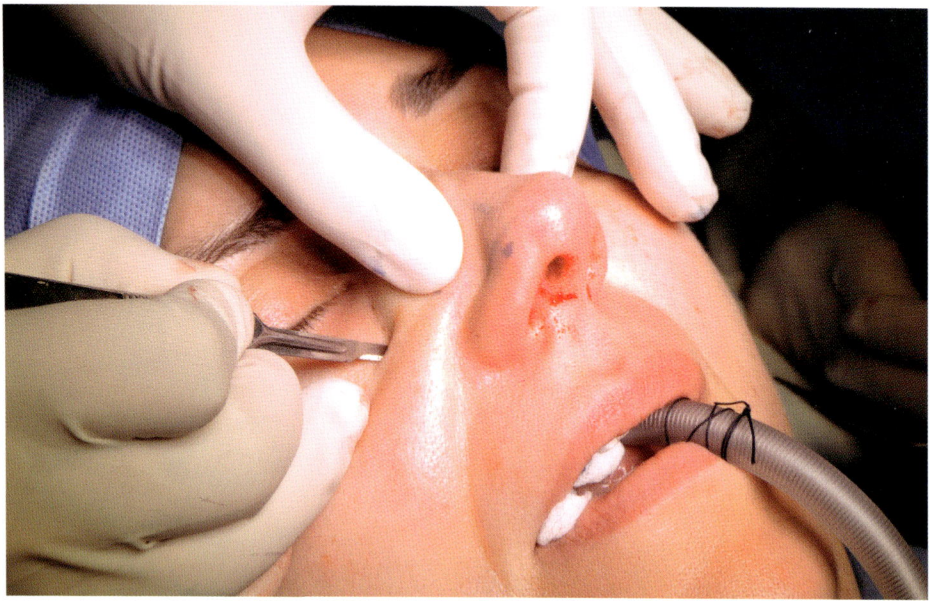

Figure 3a: the lateral osteotomy made by an incision in the eyelid skin leaves no visible traces

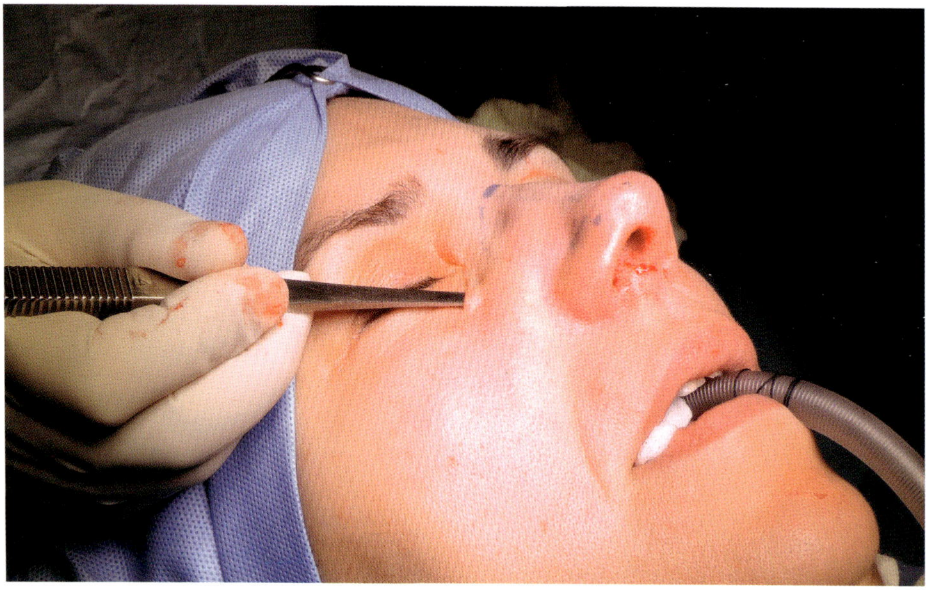

Figure 3b: a 4mm osteotome is introduced through the eyelid incision and with three or four notches the bone is fractured, leaving intact numerous soft tissues connections that have the important task of preventing the collapse of the bony walls of the nose into the nasal cavity

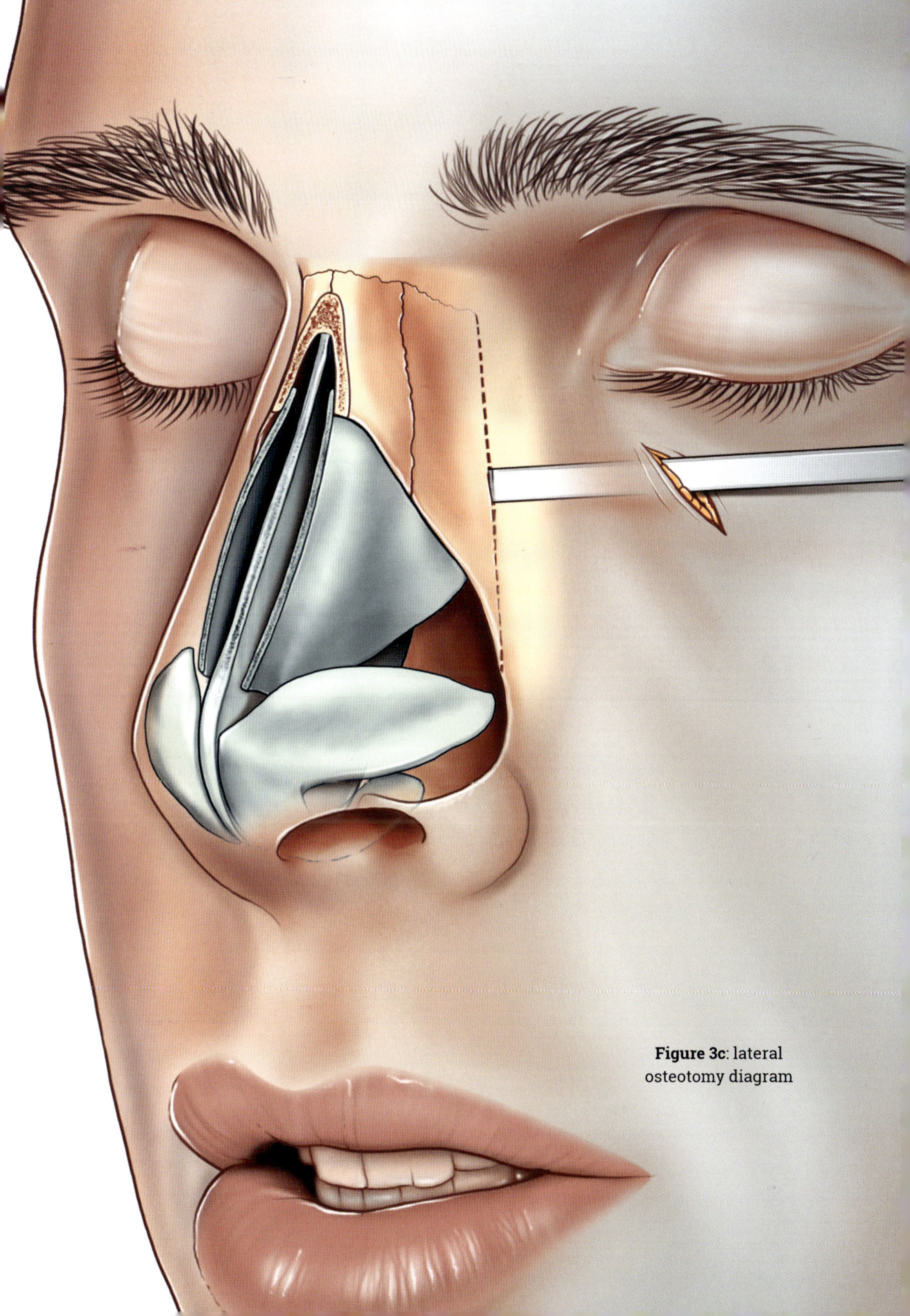

Figure 3c: lateral osteotomy diagram

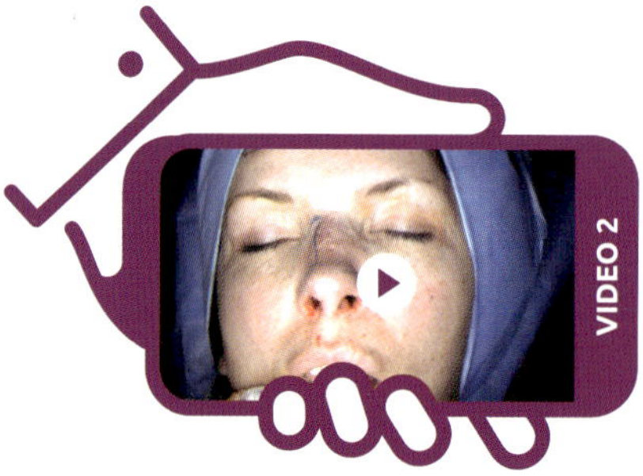

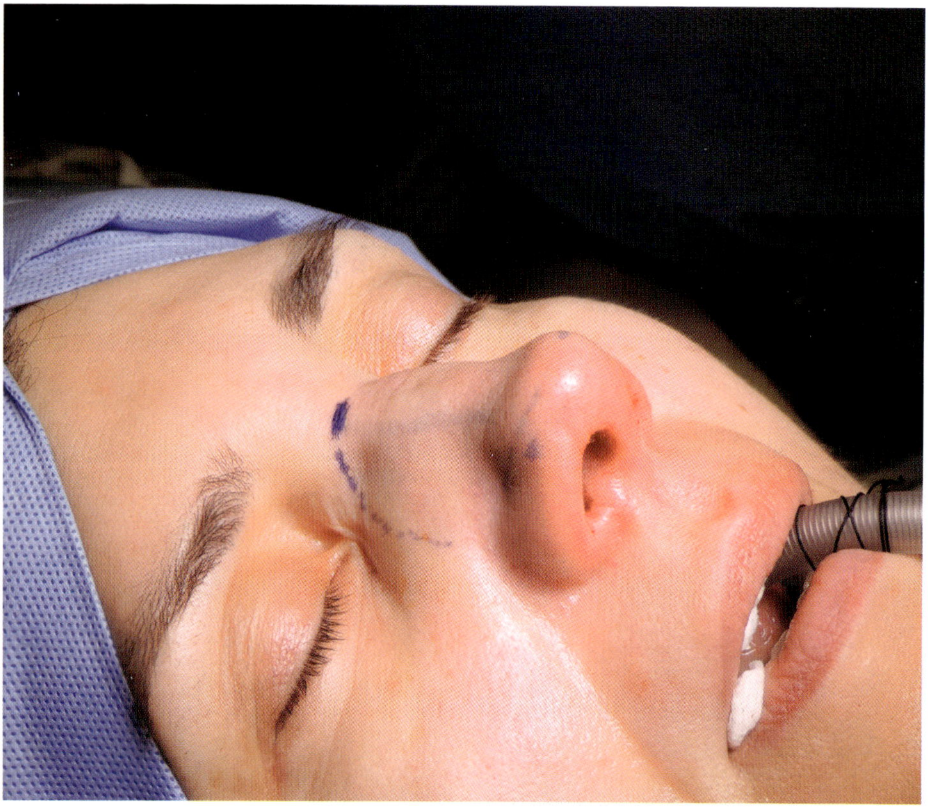

Figure 3d: the fracture line to be followed starts low and ends by curving upwards. In this way the apparent distance between the eyes does not change because the width of the nose at its root remains the same. If, however, the fracture is directed downwards even in the most cephalic part, the apparent distance changes and the patient's self-image may change

a sharp nose, very narrow even at the root. If, on the other hand, the line starts low and goes up, the apex of the pyramid remains wide. If, on the other hand, the line starts low and rises a little, as is recommended in most cases, it tightens in a more harmonious way.

- Third stage of osteotomies (transverse osteotomy): a curved osteotome is introduced into the nasal cavity, first on one side and then on the other, with the curvature facing laterally. It is pushed down to the bottom of the notch that was produced by the medial osteotomy performed at the first stage, and a fracture of the bony bridge still existing between the medial and lateral osteotomies is made (fig. 4a). By exerting pressure on the nasal bone with a finger while proceeding with the transverse osteotomy,

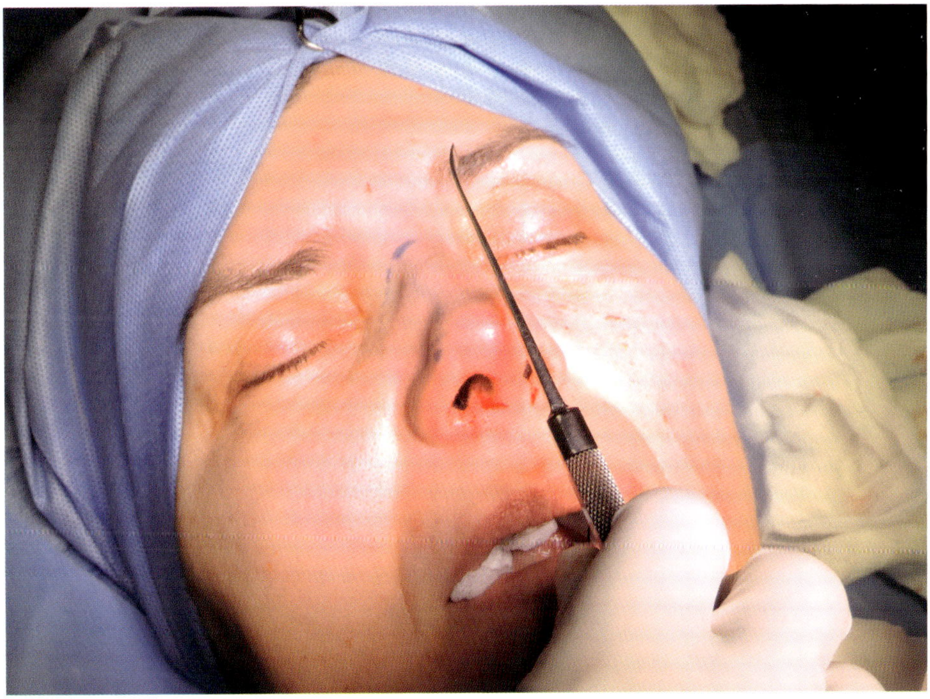

Figure 4a: a curved chisel is introduced till the bottom of the notch made with the medial osteotomies, in order to fracture from inside out the residual bone bridge at the root of the nose

as soon as the fracture is complete, it's possible to feel the bone collapse and come close to the septum (fig. 4b). The lateral bone walls of the nose are then fully mobilized inwards where they will rest against the septum giving back the nose its pyramidal shape (video 3). The access from the eyelid permits to do the osteotomies leaving soft tissues bridges that prevent the collapse of the nasal bones inside the nasal cavity. Therefore it is more reliable than continuous linear osteotomies which instead are more likely to not be able to prevent this movement.

As an alternative to the external route, an incision can be made in the nasal vestibule at the base of the piriform aperture. An osteotome is introduced, and the lateral osteotomy, which from this position must necessarily

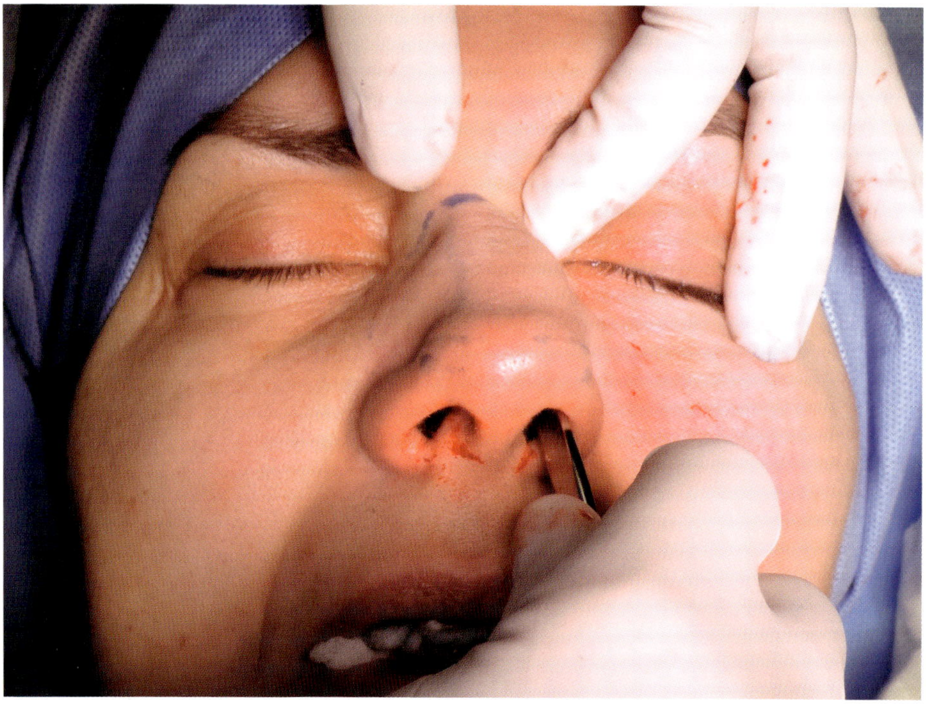

Figure 4b: the lateral wall is pushed with the finger, and as soon as the fracture is complete the bone collapses and approaches the septum

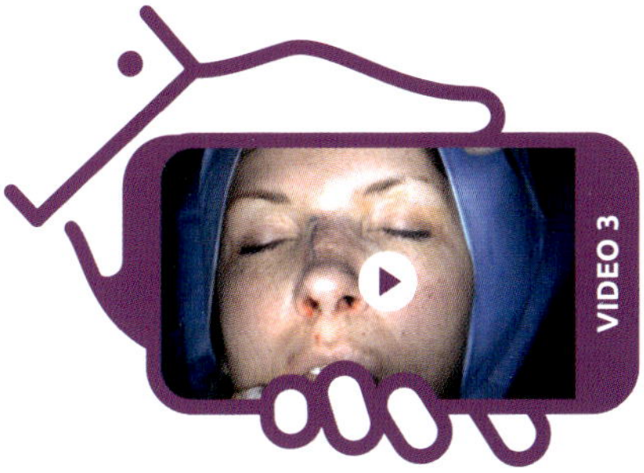

be continuous, is done along the same fracture line described in the external osteotomy. With this osteotomy technique the connections between bones and soft tissues are disjointed linearly, so bones are more likely to slide into the nasal fossa. This movement is called telescoping because of the similarity with the invagination characteristic of telescopes among its elements. The consequence of telescoping is that on the nasal dorsum, on the sides of the septum, a step is formed by the void left by the bones that have sunk a few millimeters into the nasal cavity. The nasal dorsum will therefore be non-regular with an imperfect dorsum due to the presence of a groove along the septum on the side where the bone has sunk into the nasal cavity. Therefore, the choice of proceeding with the lateral osteotomy by an external route is preferable because if the access is made from the vestibule it must be taken into account the possibility of causing this imperfection.

References

1. Gualdi A. Rhinoplasty, Illustrated Manual. Acta Medica SEE Florence 2014; p. 105.

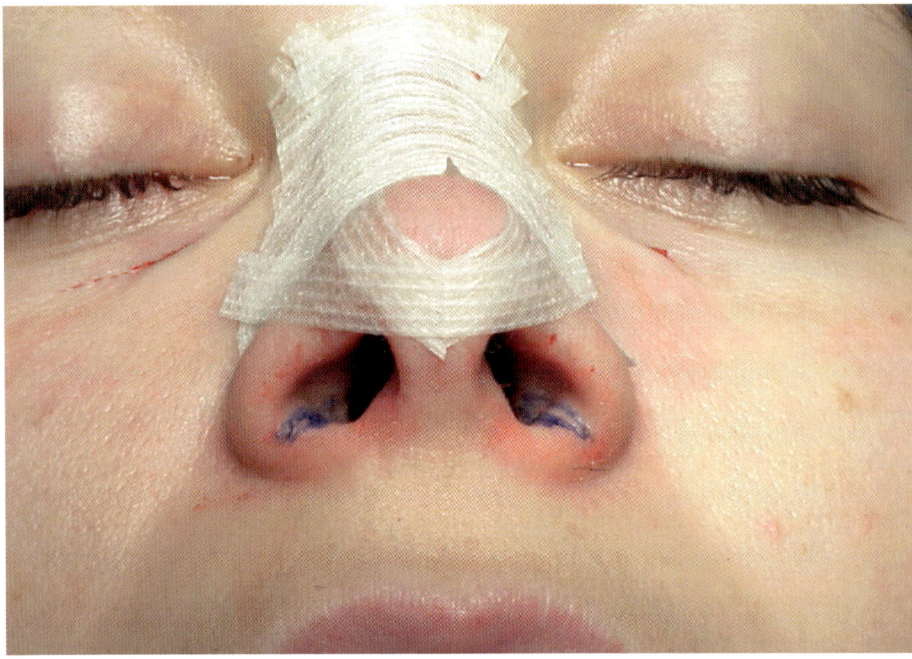

Figure 2: to round the nostrils, a wedge of skin to be removed is drawn reducing the horizontal part (Sheehan technique)

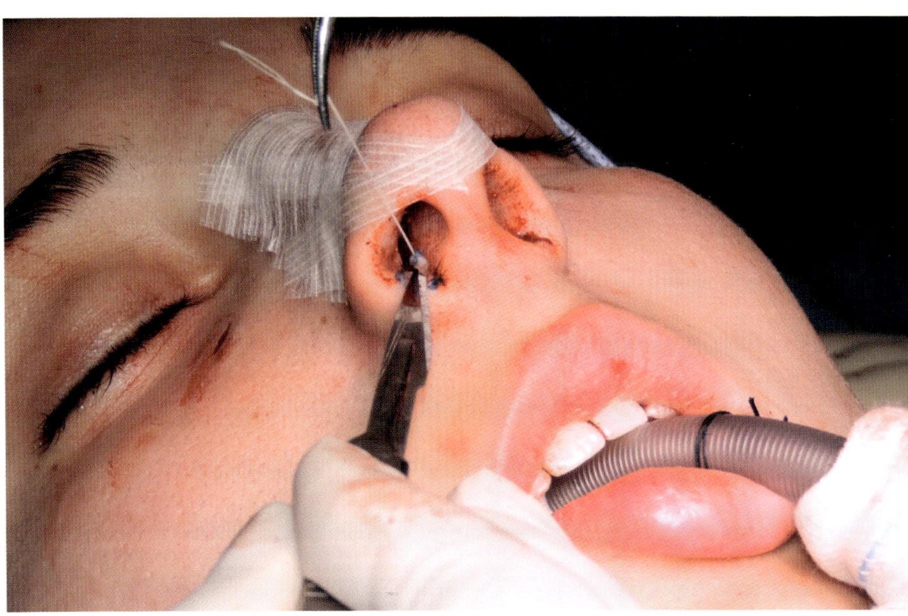

Figure 3: a suture thread is passed in the middle of the drawn wedge, and exerting traction on it, the incision with a blade 11 scalpel is made easily

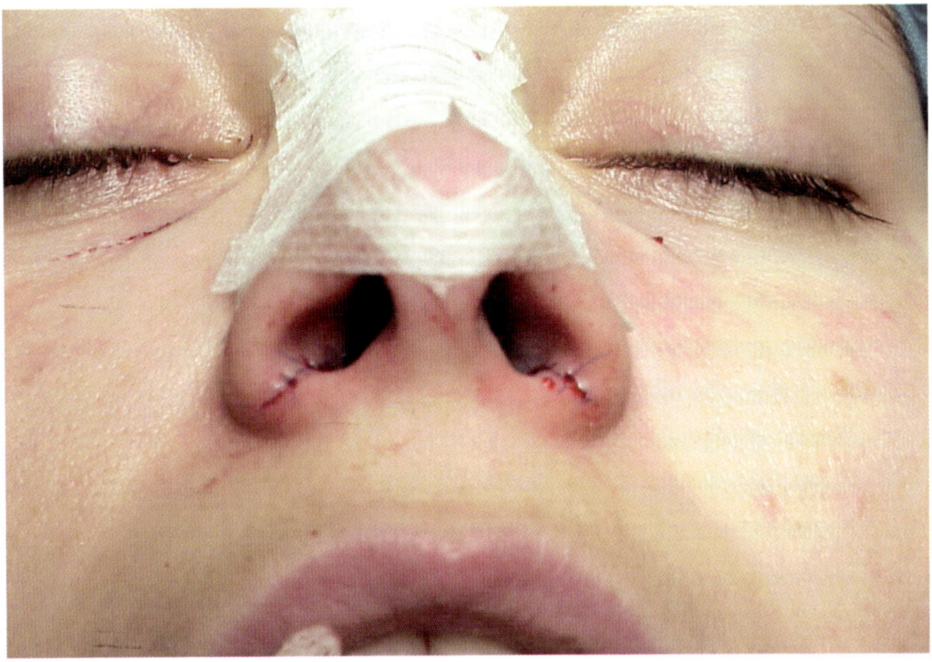

Figure 4: result of the nostril rounding maneuver

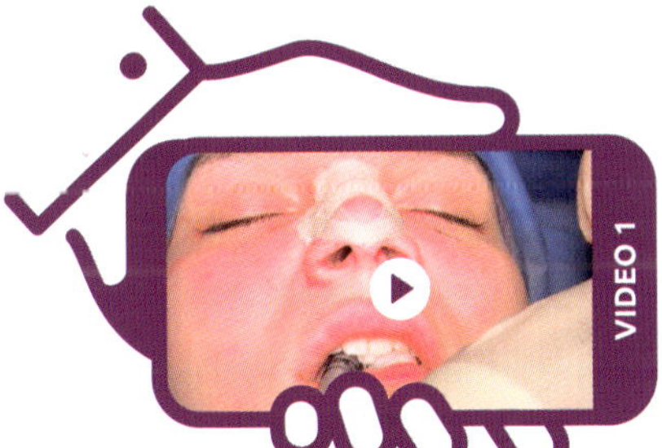

Sometimes the removal of such a wedge may only be necessary on one side. This happens when the nose has grown deviated under the growth thrust from one side of the septum, thus one nostril has grown longer than the other. When rhinoseptoplasty is performed to bring the nose back to the midline, the nostrils need to be symmetrized by reducing the larger one with the procedure described above.

CHAPTER 12

Dressings

At the end of the operation the nose is covered with steristrips. Their application immobilize the supporting structures of the nose, i.e. the bones and cartilage, limits oedema, and does not to leave dead spaces where some blood could collect. Over time any blood collection in the supra tip area can organize itself becoming scar tissue that alters the shape of the nose. The steristrips are impregnated by the plaster put to immobilize the bones and therefore act as an adhesive for the plaster.

For an effective immobilization of the tip, two steristrips are first placed longitudinally, on either side of the nasal dorsum and joined in front of the nasal tip just above the columella. Then a steristrip is placed as a loop with one end along the edge of the methylene blue mark on the right ala and the other on the contralateral one. The loop is folded exactly in the middle, and with a needle holder the two parts of the steristrip are tightened compressing the skin no longer supported by cartilage so helping it to adapt to the new anatomic shape (fig. 1a). Further steristrips are placed between the supratip area and the root of the nose (fig 1b) (video 1).

The supratip consists in the presence of a bulge just above the nasal tip. It may be due to an insufficient lowering of the quadrangular cartilage, or even to a collection of blood between the quadrangular cartilage and the overlying skin that became scar tissue. Blood collection is more likely to form if the septum has been lowered too much as suggested by Sheen (1). However, if the dorsum of the septum is linear and the skin is kept adhered to it with a plaster using the technique just described, there is no longer any space for the blood to collect. The differential diagnosis between the two

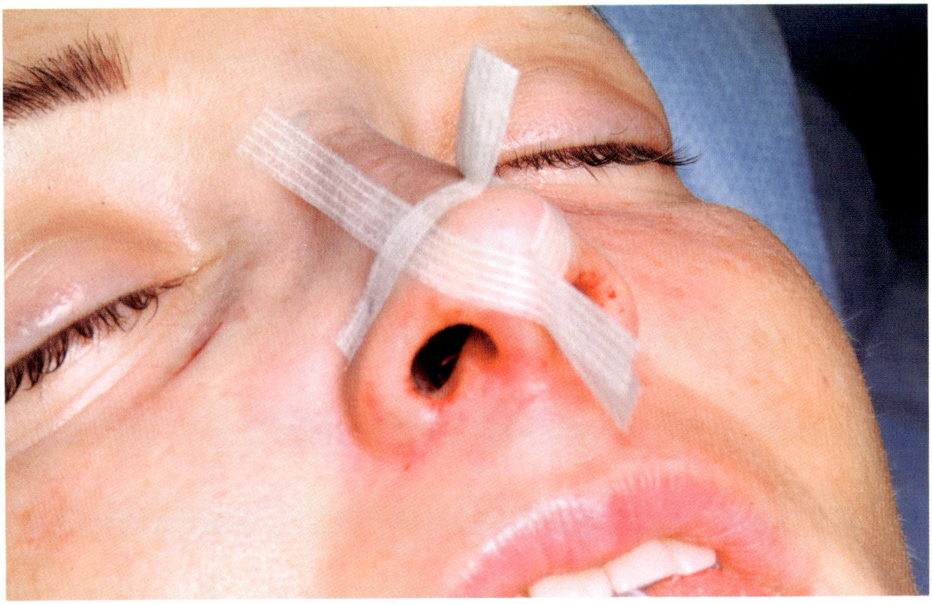

Figure 1a: two steristrips are placed on either side of the nose to tighten the tip. The third one has the task of compressing the skin corresponding to the area where the cephalic margin of the alar cartilage has been removed, helping the skin to retract

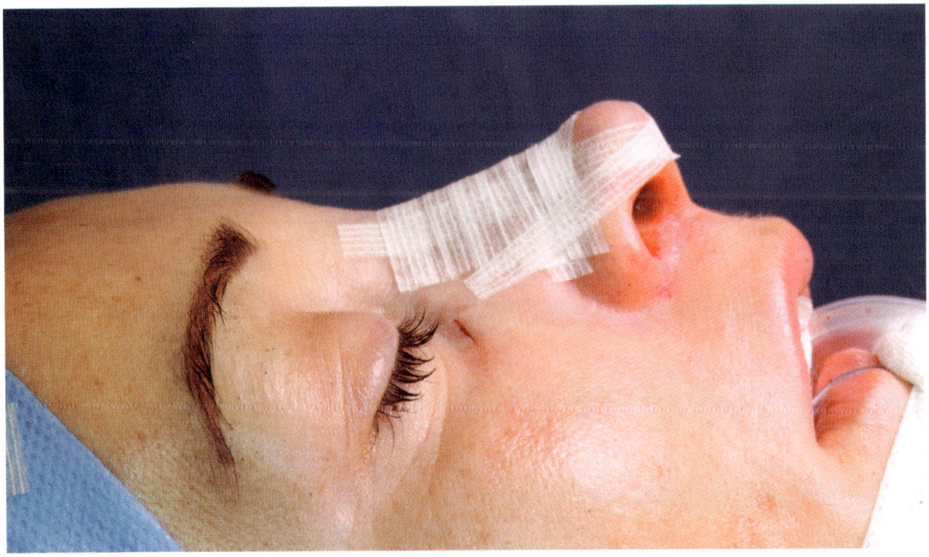

Figure 1b: the entire dorsum is covered with steristrips that limit the postoperative edema. The plaster which will be applied will adhere to the steristrips

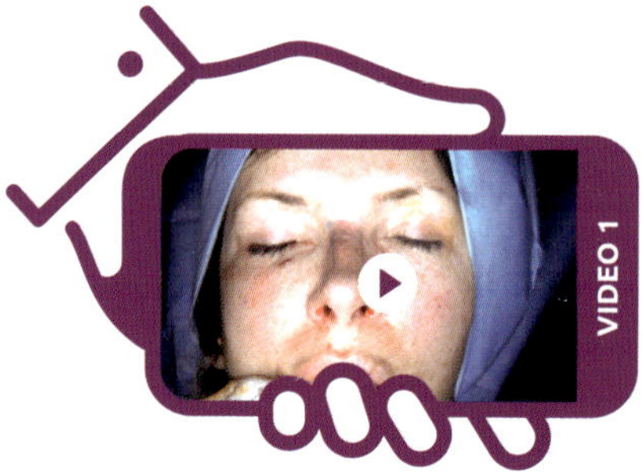

types of supratips is made by simple palpation: if the bulge is supported by a hard structure, this will be the upper part of the septum that has remained too high; if, on palpation, the structure supporting the swelling is softer, this is scar tissue due to an organized hematoma. These are the most likely causes of supratip, but it is also possible that the upper lateral cartilages overlap the septal cartilage, or that it might be due to mispositioned grafts, or mucosa left between the septum and the overlying skin (I have also had one case due to an incipient rhinophyma!). The secondary treatment of these two different conditions consists in the first case in lowering of the septum, and in the second case in a careful undermining of the skin just below the dermis (fig 2a), leaving the scar tissue adherent to the septum, and hence easily removable with Pellegrini Scissors or a blade 11 scalpel (fig. 2b).

Once the dressings have been placed, the nasal packs are inserted into the nasal cavities (figs. 3a, b). If a septoplasty has been done, packing will consist in the introduction of a Merocel pack with an internal tube. If, on the other hand, a rhinoplasty without septoplasty has been performed, a small amount of paraffin gauze dressing is put to protect the incisions. Some space to allow the passage of air will be comfortable and can easily be made by introducing a closed forceps into the nasal cavity to press the gauze against the nasal walls. (video 2).

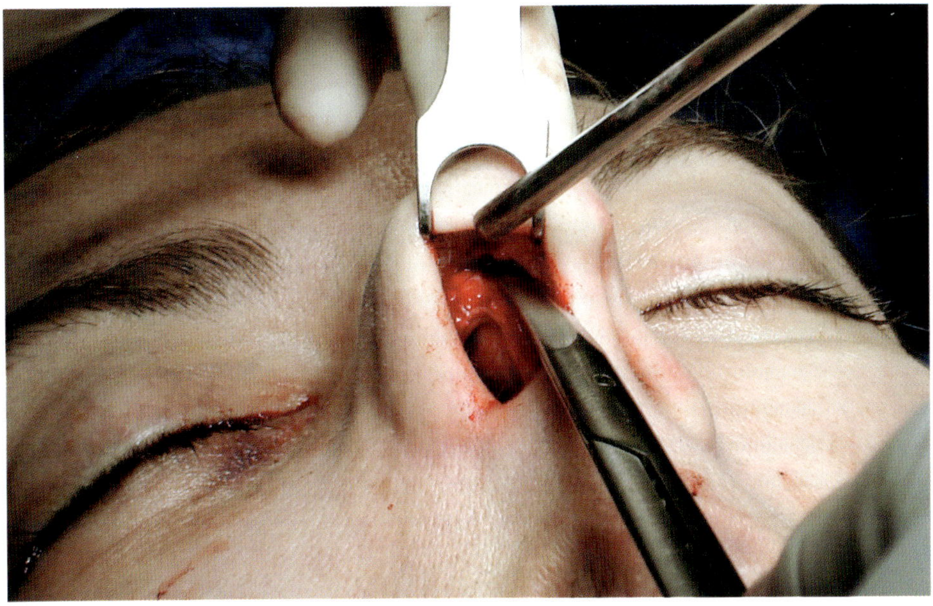

Figure 2a: treatment of supratip scarring: scissors are used to undermine the skin in correspondence of the supratip along a cleavage just below the deep dermis leaving the scar to be removed attached to the septum

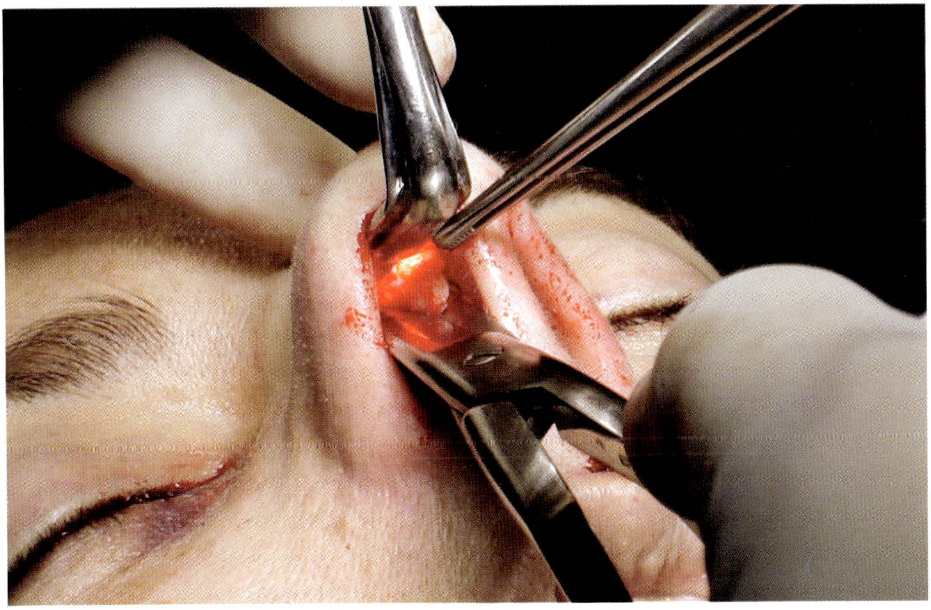

Figure 2b: easy removal of the scar tissue forming the supratip using Pellegrini scissors

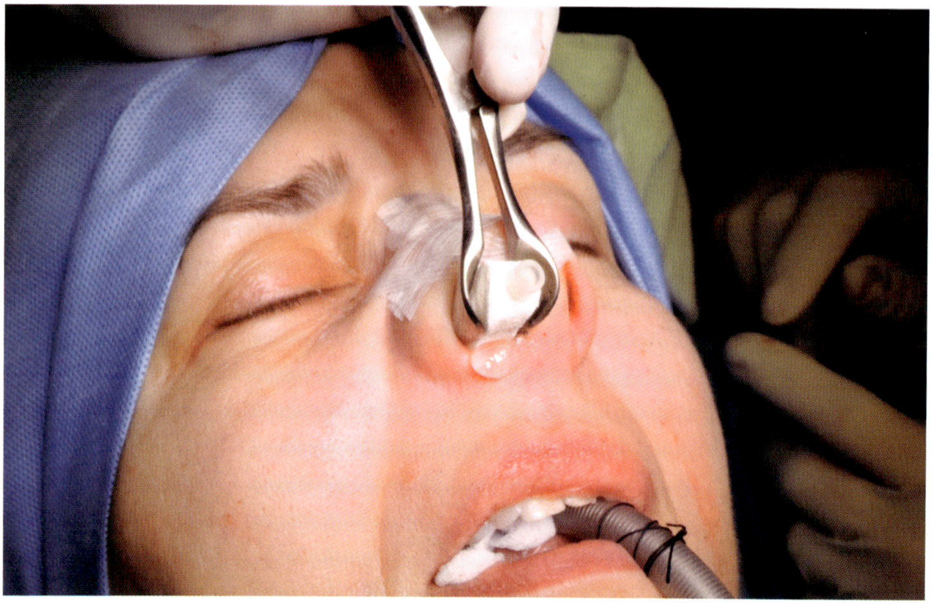

Figure 3a: insertion of Merocel packs containing a small tube that allows a little air to pass through. A long Killian is inserted first and the pack is slid along it

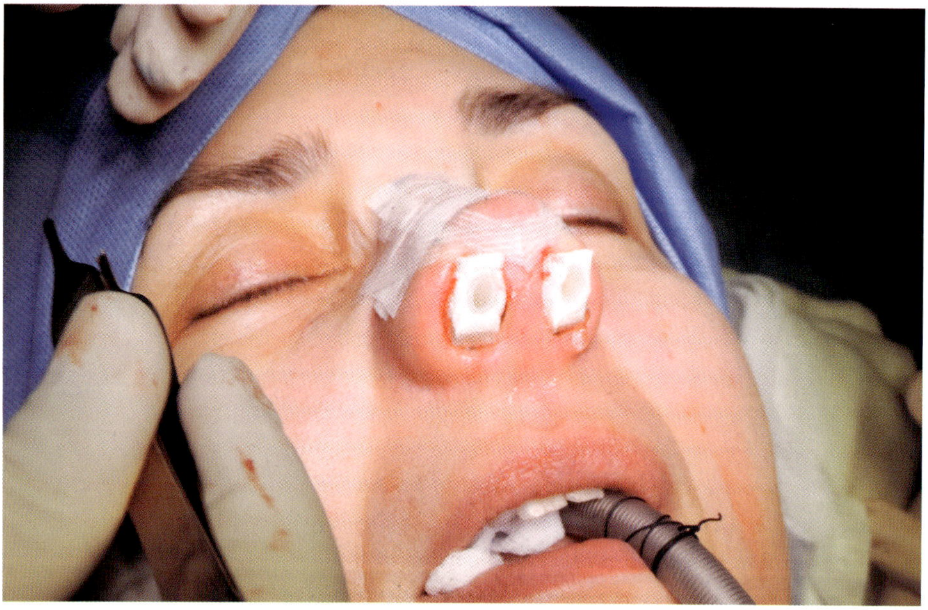

Figure 3b: pack inserted bilaterally in case of septoplasty. If the septoplasty is not performed, a paraffin gauze dressing is sufficient

After packing, the plaster cast is applied. The plaster should be placed staying on the patient's head and held between the fingers until it hardens. (fig. 4) (video 3)

The position at the patient's head avoids a parallax error that would lead to a crooked plaster position. The operator's sight from the patient's side leads to an altered optical perception, which is misleading when assessing whether the observed structures are on axis or not.

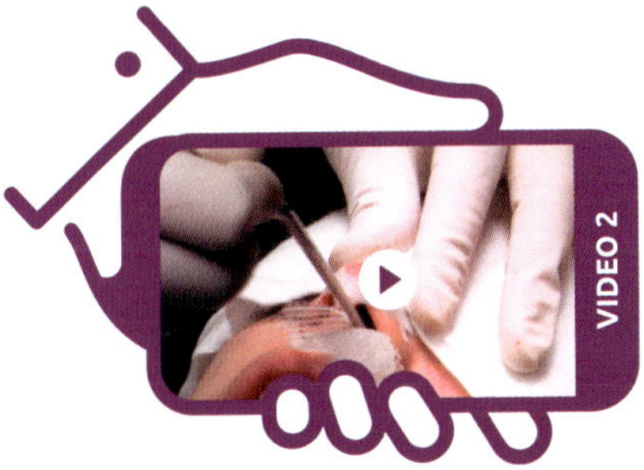

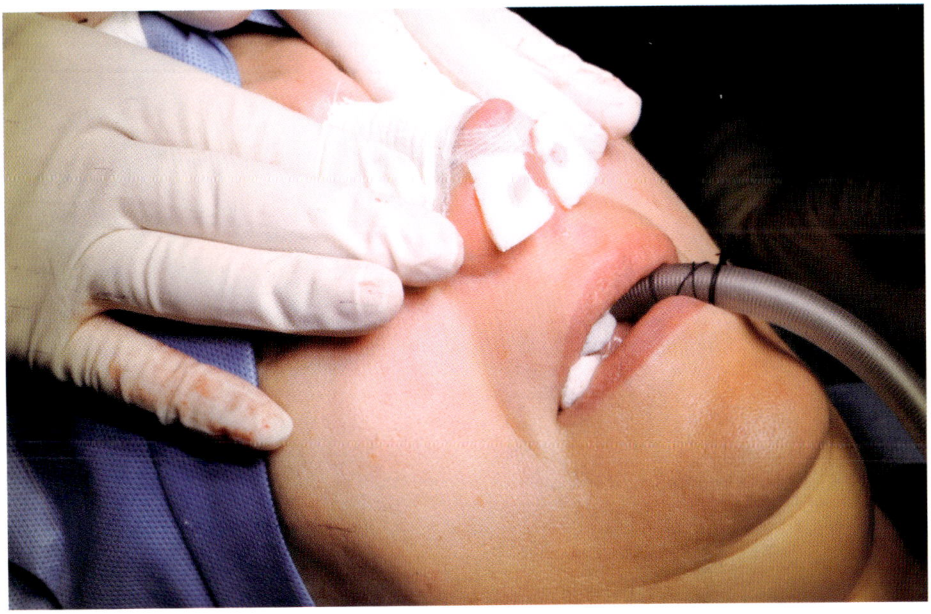

Figure 4: the plaster should be placed from the patient's head so as not to incur in a parallax error that would lead to put it not straight

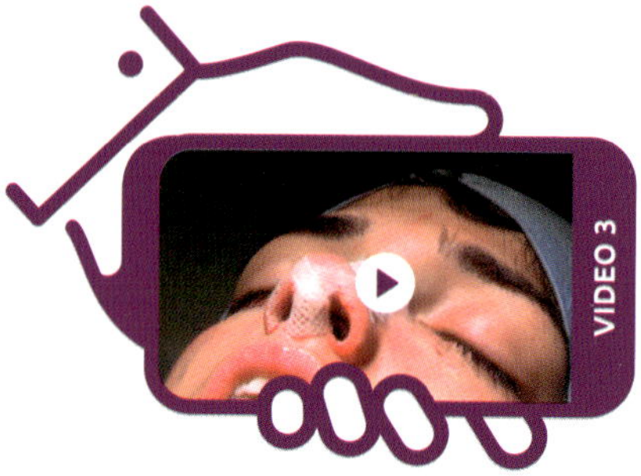

The plaster must contain only the pyramidal structures and therefore must extend from the root of the nose until the boundary with the nostrils.
Larger plaster casts, that also cover the glabella, should not be used. Putting a plaster that covers the glabella is a mistake and should not be done. The glabella in fact normally swells, leading to an elevation of the plaster which, due to its adhesion to the underlying steristrips, lifts the skin from the underlying skeletal framework. This movement favours accumulation of blood between the skin and underlying structures that may give rise to an irregularity of the dorsum, consisting of a convexity overlying the final part of the septum, which is called supratip (see previous paragraphs). The application of stristrips on the forehead to block plasters that extend till there, worsens the situation because the swelling of the glabella becomes the fulcrum of a lever that will produce a real suction in the area of the supratip.
Other splint devices may be used, but none has the cheapness, functionality and practicality of plaster, which requires no special equipment to be used, but just water.

Reference

1. Sheen J. Aesthetic Rhinoplasty. The C.V. Mosby Company, Saint Luis Missoury, 1978.

CHAPTER 13

Nasal packing

If the nasal septum has not been operated on, nasal packing is not necessary (chapter 12). However, paraffin gauze dressing should be placed in the nasal cavities to prevent the blood, which inevitably runs down in the first few hours, from clotting inside the nostrils with consequent obstruction of the air passage. Removal of blood clots may cause further bleeding and it is therefore not appropriate. The paraffin gauze dressing can be removed the first day, once bleeding stops. Softening the clots with hydrogen peroxide helps not to detach crusts when the gauze is removed. The patient should remain calm, without exerting any effort, and should breathe through the nose during the next half hour to allow the cavities to dry out reducing the possibility of subsequent nosebleeds.

What to do in case of epistaxis

Small nosebleeds are often stopped by placing a gauze pad soaked in hydrogen peroxide. For cases that are more difficult to control, tabotamp or similar products such as surgicel can be used, limiting the use of nasal specula as much as possible so as not to deform the structures and therefore not to disturb the healing process.

If nose surgery extends to the septum, it is necessary to guide its healing in the midline with straight packs to avoid the formation of angles and curves. Nasal packs must be soft enough not to cause ischemia of the chondromucosa of the septum. A small tube placed inside the pack will allow some air to pass through, thus alleviating the discomfort of having a completely closed nose. Packing is necessary when undermining the septum a lacera-

CHAPTER 17

Spreader grafts

Spreader graft is by definition a cartilage graft whose function is to spread. Spreader grafts are used to keep the triangular cartilage away from the septum, because when it is too close to it, its valvular function is impaired (chapter 6). In fact, when the triangular cartilage gets too near the septum, the space between them is reduced as well as the movement necessary to perform its valvular function. Respiratory disturbances are inevitable also if the septum presents a convexity in the area adjacent to the triangular cartilage.

In primary rhinoplasty it doesn't make sense using a spreader graft unless the septum at the level of the valve has a deviation that cannot be adequately corrected. If the deviation of the septum is such that cannot be straightened safely, the cartilage can be weakened so that it retains no memory of its curvature, and two cartilage splints can be placed on both sides of the septum to keep it straight (fig. 1). Clearly, this can maintain the septum in axis, but will cause widening of the nose at the level of where it was placed (fig. 2)

The spreader graft is therefore intended to prevent respiratory problems caused by malfunction of the Mink valve, but also to prevent an imperfection consisting of dimpling of the lateral wall of the nasal pyramid immediately below the nasal bones, which occurs if the triangular cartilages are collapsed against the septum (fig. 3).

The cartilage graft, that has the function of pushing the triangular cartilage away from the septum, must be about one centimeter long, i.e. about the same length of the side of the Triangular cartilage that approaches

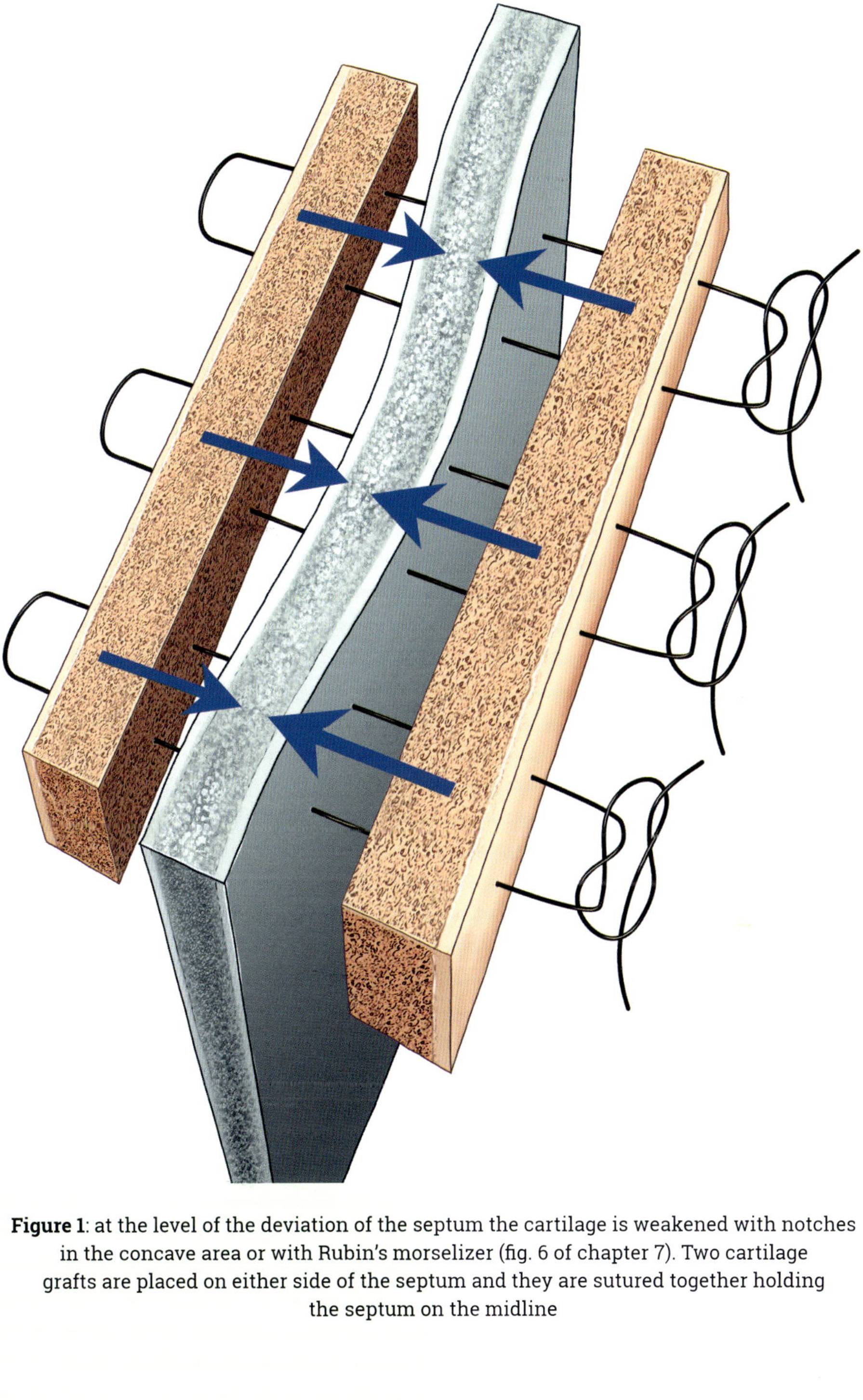

Figure 1: at the level of the deviation of the septum the cartilage is weakened with notches in the concave area or with Rubin's morselizer (fig. 6 of chapter 7). Two cartilage grafts are placed on either side of the septum and they are sutured together holding the septum on the midline

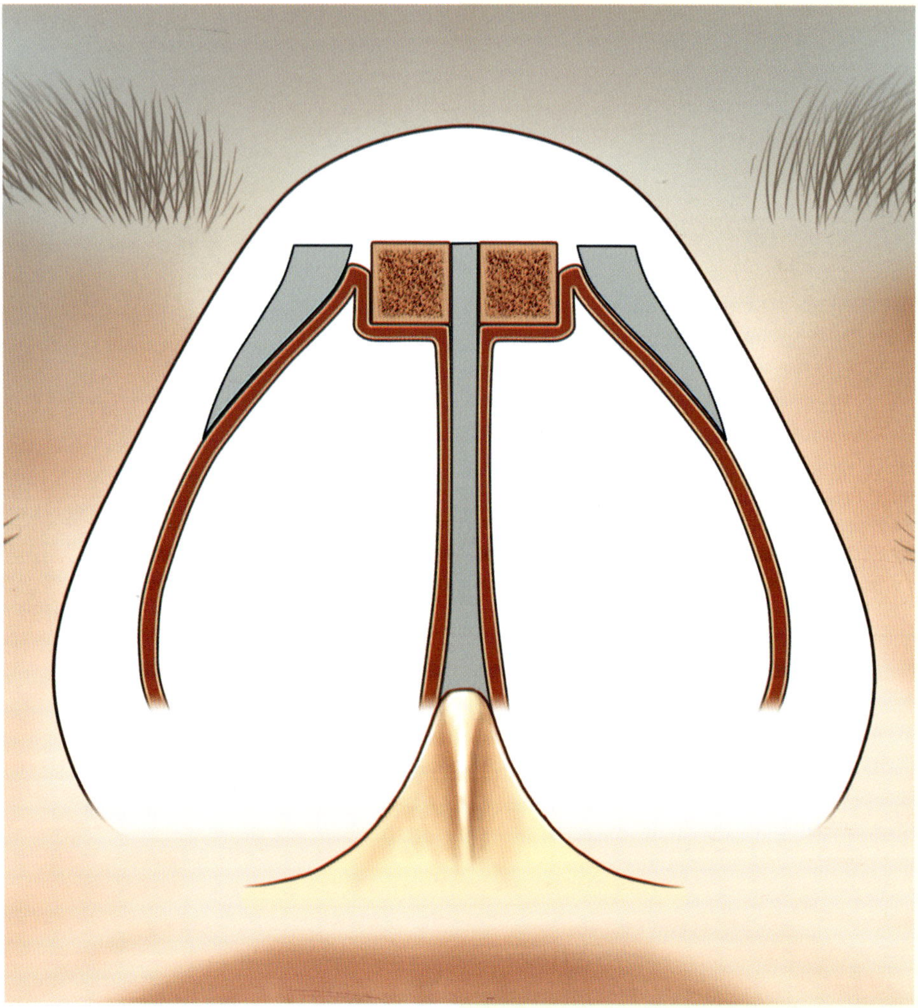

Figure 2: spreader grafts placed on either side of the septum displace laterally the triangular cartilage and therefore the nose will have a wider appearance

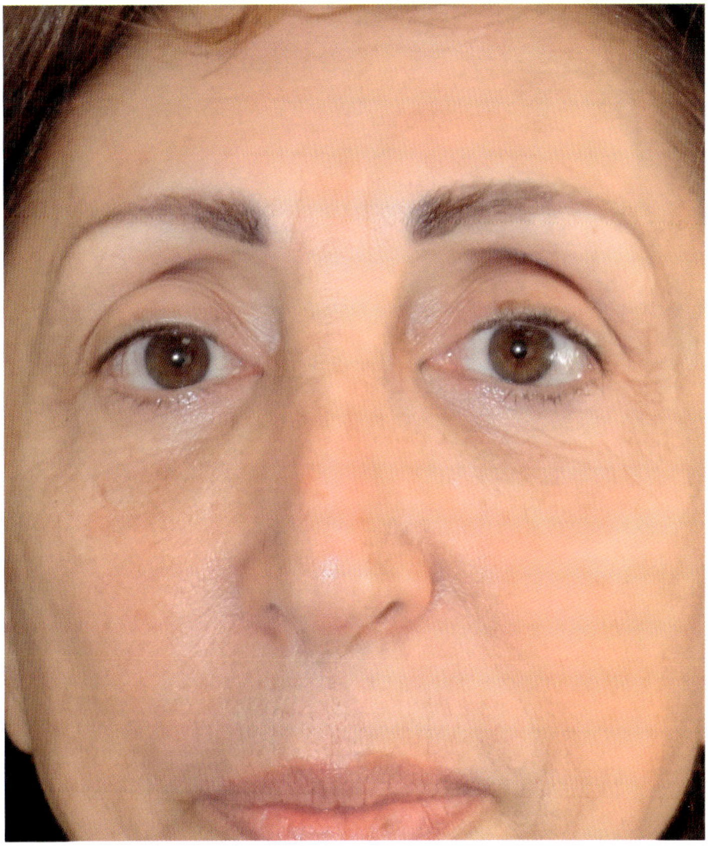

Figure 3: typical dimpling of the lateral walls of the nose due to the collapsed triangular cartilages

the septum. Its thickness should be adequate to spread the cartilage out effectively (approximatly 2 mm), and a couple of millimeters high, so as not to obstruct the nasal cavity. The preferred cartilage for the spreader graft function is the one of the septum, but other donor areas can also be used. The placement of this graft is easy when the septum has not been undermined, as it is sufficient to create a pocket under the perichondrium with an elevator. This manoeuvre is done starting from the anterior margin of the septum and sliding the elevator along the upper edge of the quadrangular cartilage which forms the cartilaginous dorsum (fig. 4). The pocket made this way is precise, so that the graft introduced cannot move. It is more difficult to place spreader grafts if the perichondrium of the quadrangular cartilage has been completely elevated, or in primary cases where the dorsal border of the quadrangular cartilage has been lowered. In these cases the graft must be immobilized with stitches, because there is no precise pocket to rely on. If a spreader graft is to be used during primary rhinoplasty, the submucosal technique should be used (fig. 5).

In the submucosal technique the mucoperichondrium is elevated along the upper portion of the septum and below the triangular cartilages and further up, below the periosteum of the nasal bones. The reduction of the hump is done in the same way as described previously (chapter 7). A possible spreader graft can then be placed because it will be protected by an intact chondromucosa.

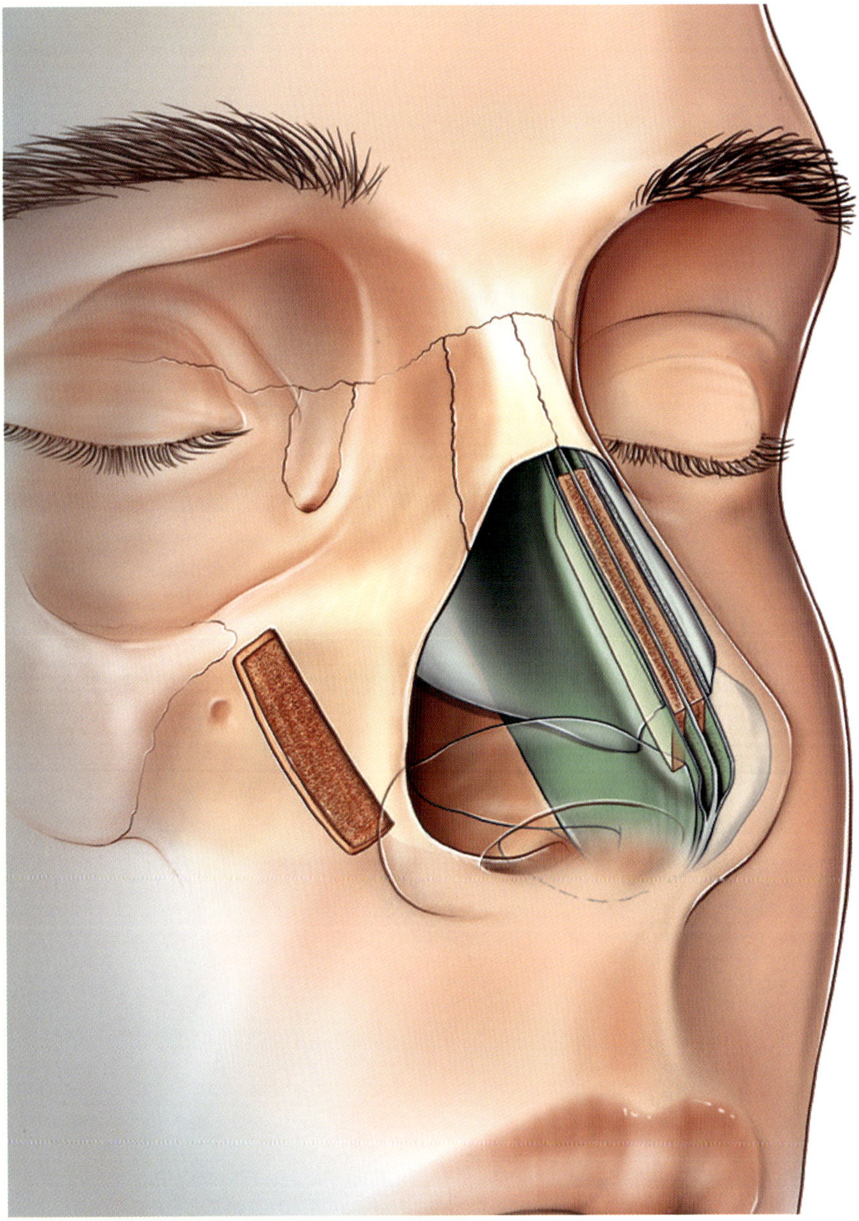

Figure 4: in the picture, on the left, the graft taken from the septum is seen.
The Spreader Graft pocket is made by tunnelling along the septum from the caudal margin of the quadrangular cartilage to the lower edge of the nasal bones. Its function is to keep the triangular cartilage away from the septum

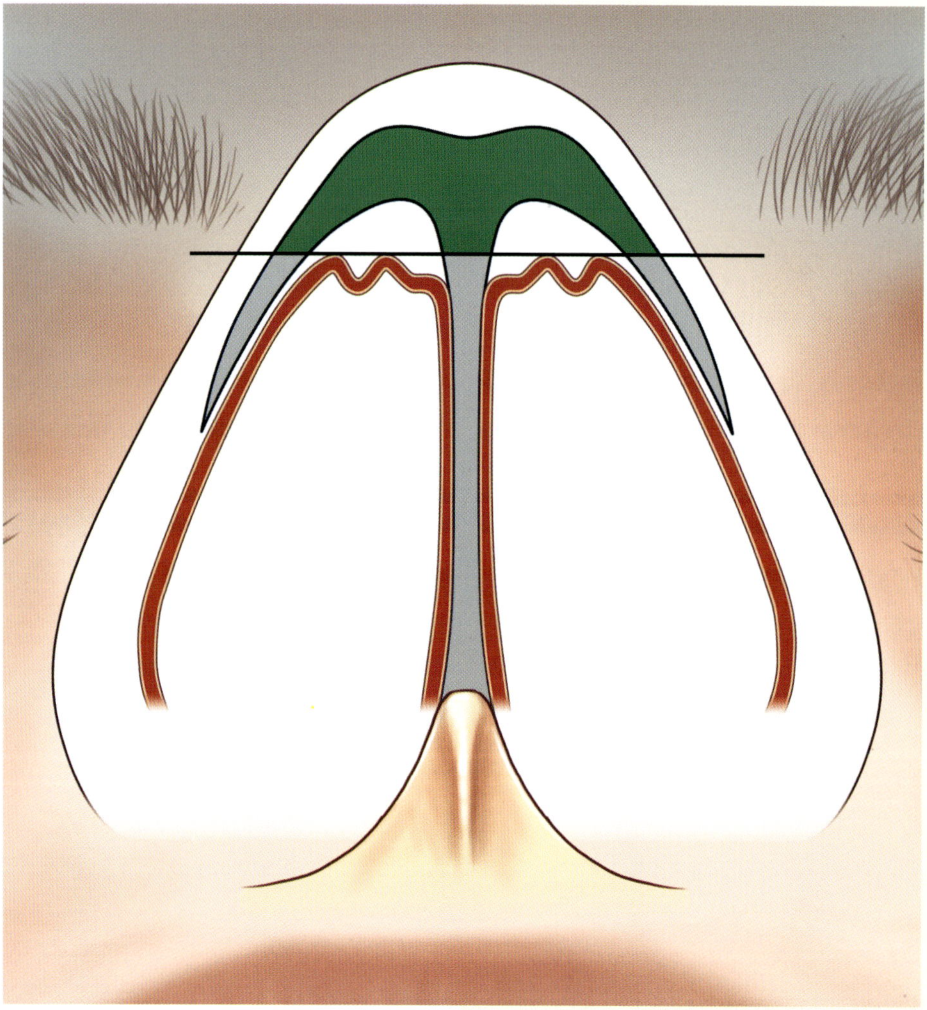

Figure 5: if grafts are going to be used on the sides of the septum it is necessary to be sure that they are covered with chondromucosa. Therefore the submucosal technique will be used, whereby the chondromucosa is elevated from the septum and from the inner surface of the nasal bones

CHAPTER 18

The use of cartilage grafts. How and why

Rhinoplasty is an artistic procedure, perhaps the one that best denotes the surgeon's taste and technical skills. A good execution of a basic technique usually gives excellent results, but sometimes the use of cartilage grafts may be necessary. Cartilage grafts are used with different aims: as a filler, to better define the tip, to widen the nasolabial angle, and as a spreader graft to improve the breathing performance (chapter 17), or as a support of collapsed parts.

In deviated noses, the causes of the deviation can be recent or remote. They are recent when the nose was straight, but due to trauma it became crooked. They are remote when during the development it has grown crooked. While in the first case we have a lot of normal components (as long as it was originally a straight nose) that have shifted so theoretically it is sufficient to put them back straight, in the second case bones and cartilages have grown asymmetrically, with different sizes and curvatures. Of course it is more difficult to make symmetrical a nose in which, for example, one alar cartilage is larger than the other, perhaps even with different curvatures. Often the deviated septum has grown pushing the tip to one side, and under this thrust the cartilages have grown differently. Also the nostrils can be one larger and the other smaller for this same reason. With a good grasp of the anatomy and with a clear vision about what you want to achieve, it's possible get to a successful correction. Sometimes, however, it is necessary to use cartilage grafts to fill gaps or mask uncorrectable curvatures (figs. 1a, b). The graft insertion technique involves drawing the site where the graft

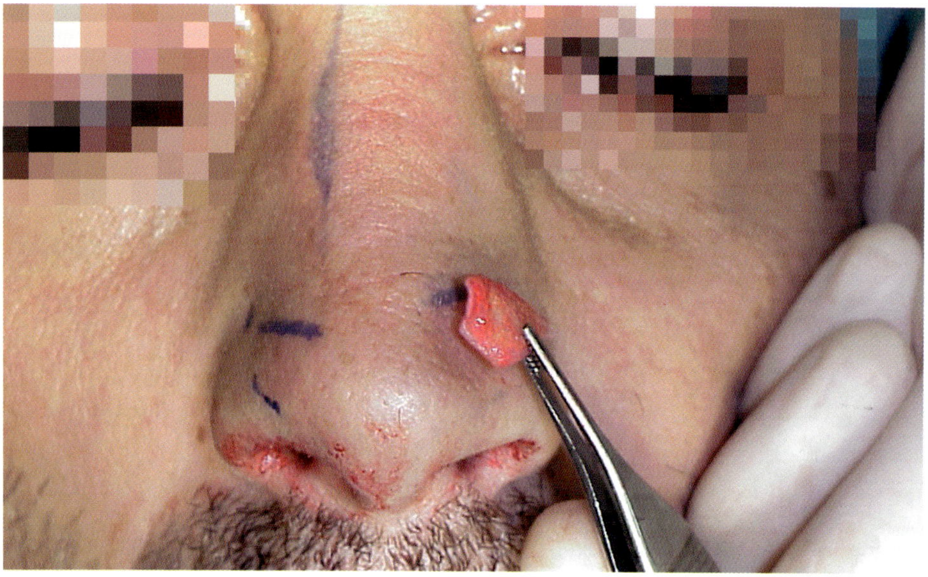

Figure 1a: the curvature of the left lateral crus presents a concavity which can be filled inserting a graft to fill the visible depression, so as to optically symmetrize the nasal tip

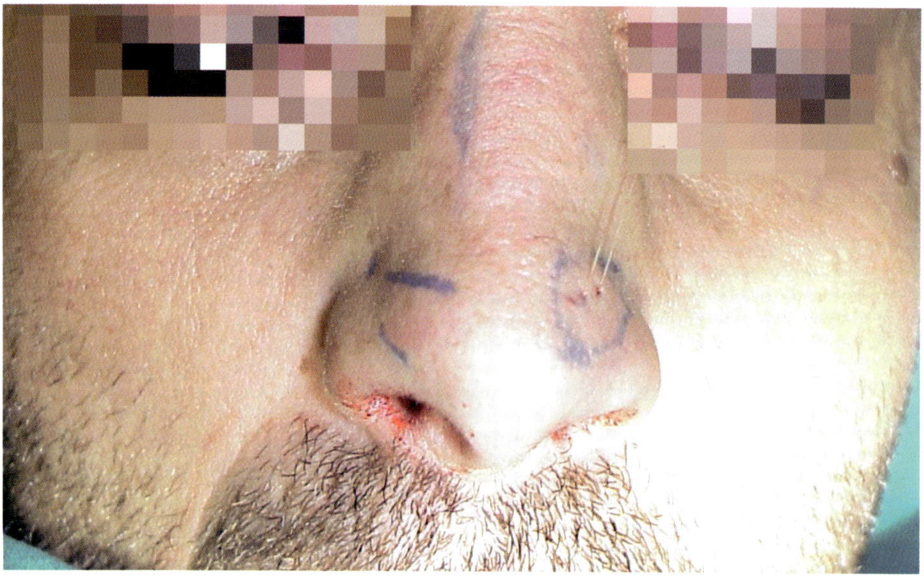

Figure 1b: the depression area, delineated with methylene blue, was filled with an Alar cartilage graft inserted through a short marginal incision. A transcutaneous stitch makes safe its position without fear of displacement

will have to be inserted, the creation of a pocket, and the insertion of the graft. A suture stitch is passed into the graft and with the help of a syringe needle is passed into the pocket cavity. The two ends of the suture thread are passed through the syringe needle so that the graft is positioned with the correct orientation (figs. 2a, b, c, d, e, f) (video 1). The same procedure can be used for the nasolabial angle (figs. 3a, b).
Cartilage grafts can be taken from different sites depending on the purpose

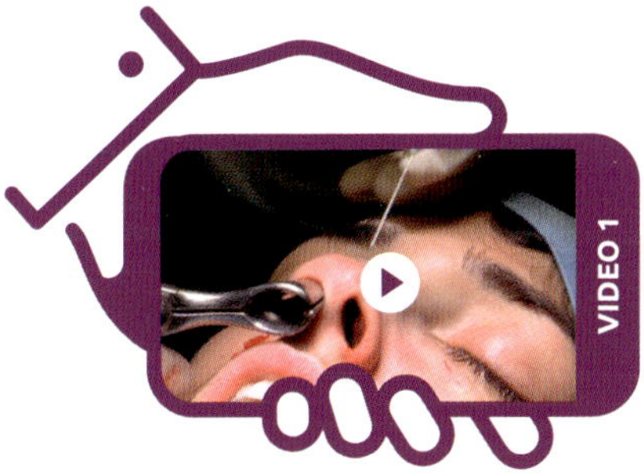

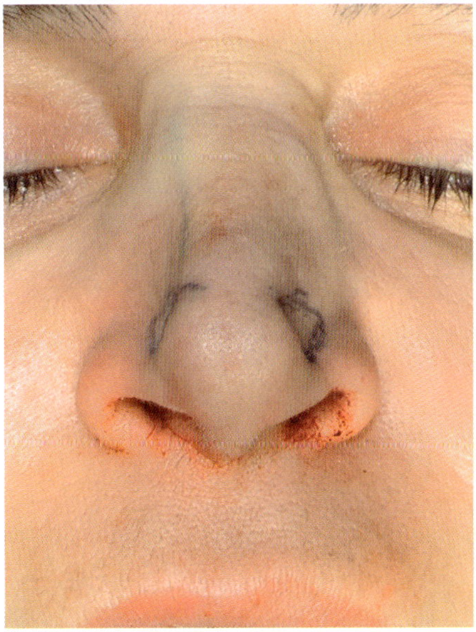

Figure 2a: drawing of the area to be filled with a cartilage graft

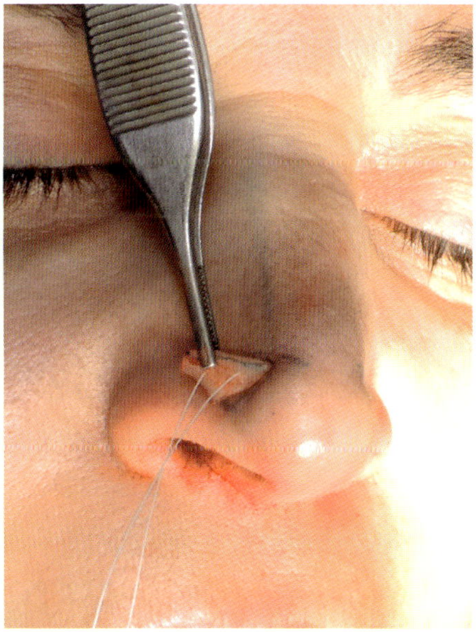

Figure 2b: checking the orientation to be given to the graft

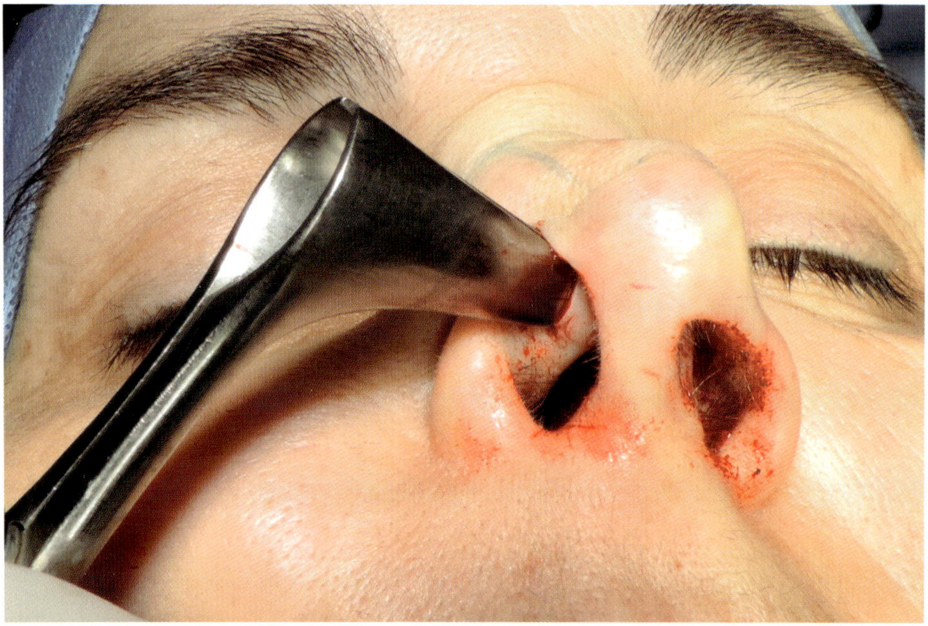

Figure 2c: a Killian is introduced from a small marginal incision once the graft pocket has been created

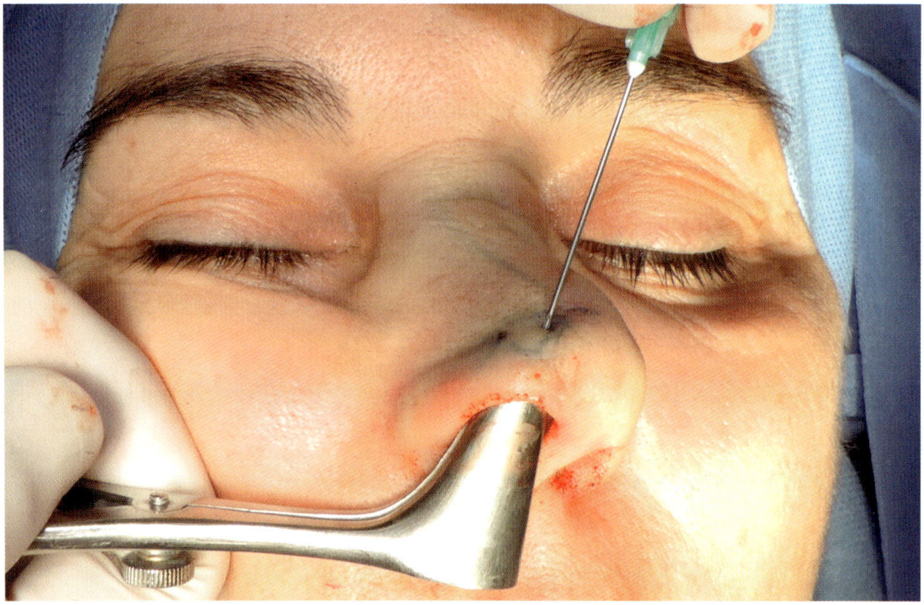

Figure 2d: a syringe needle is introduced by passing it between the Killian branches so that it does not take false paths

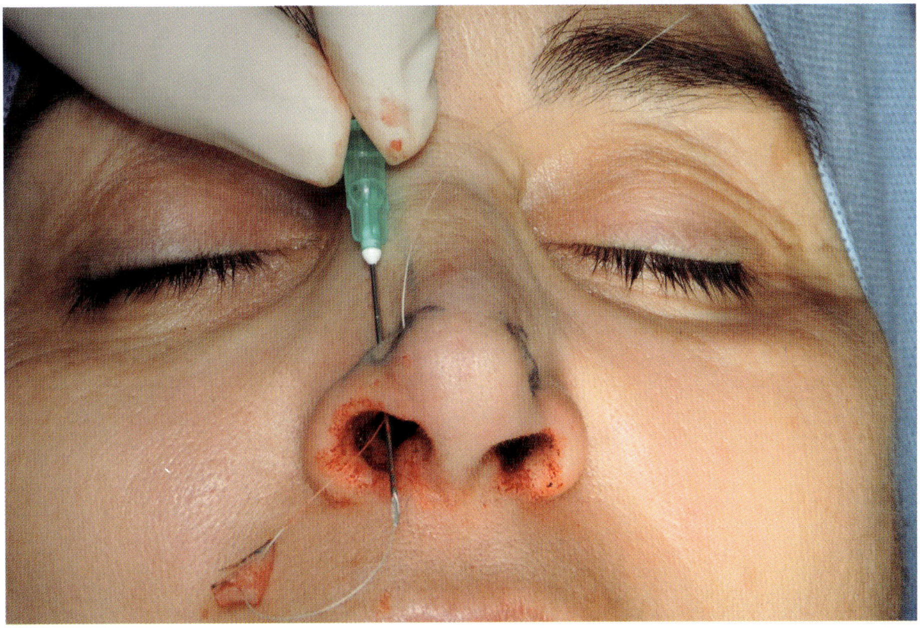

Figure 2e: the stitch thread is passed through the needle that is then withdrawn. Pulling the thread, the graft is locked in the desired position

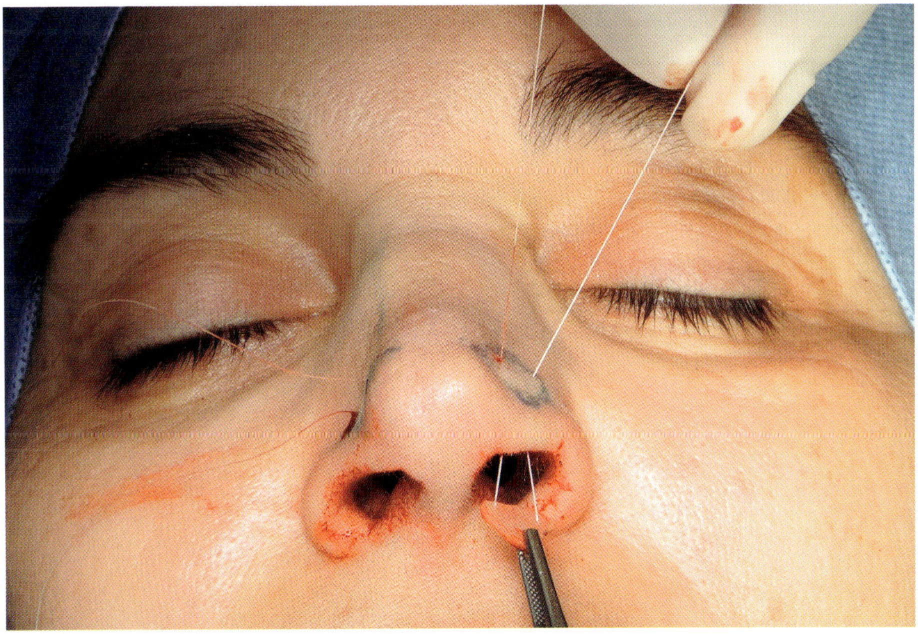

Figure 2f: positioning the graft into the left nostril

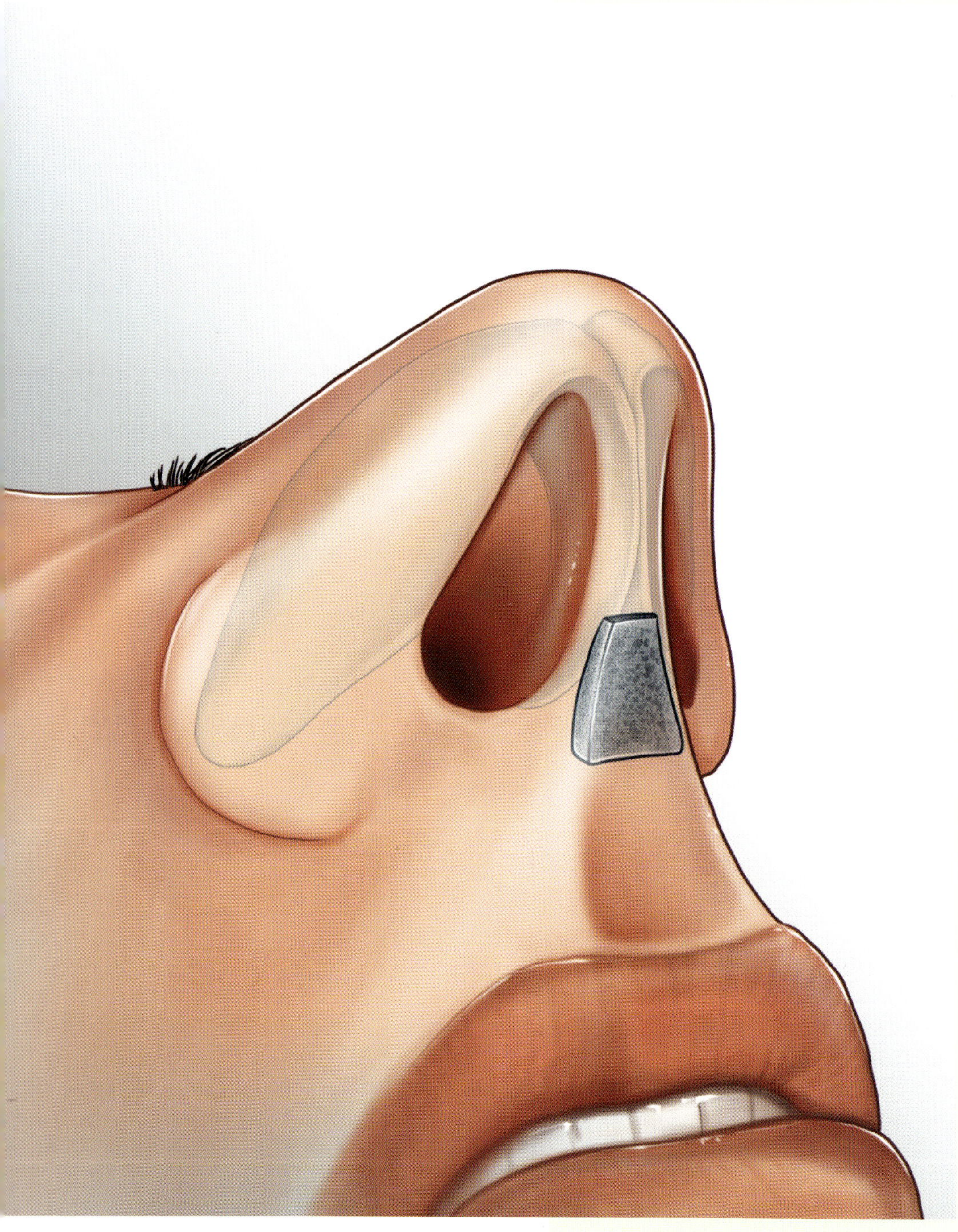

Figure 3a: increasing of the nasolabial angle with cartilage graft

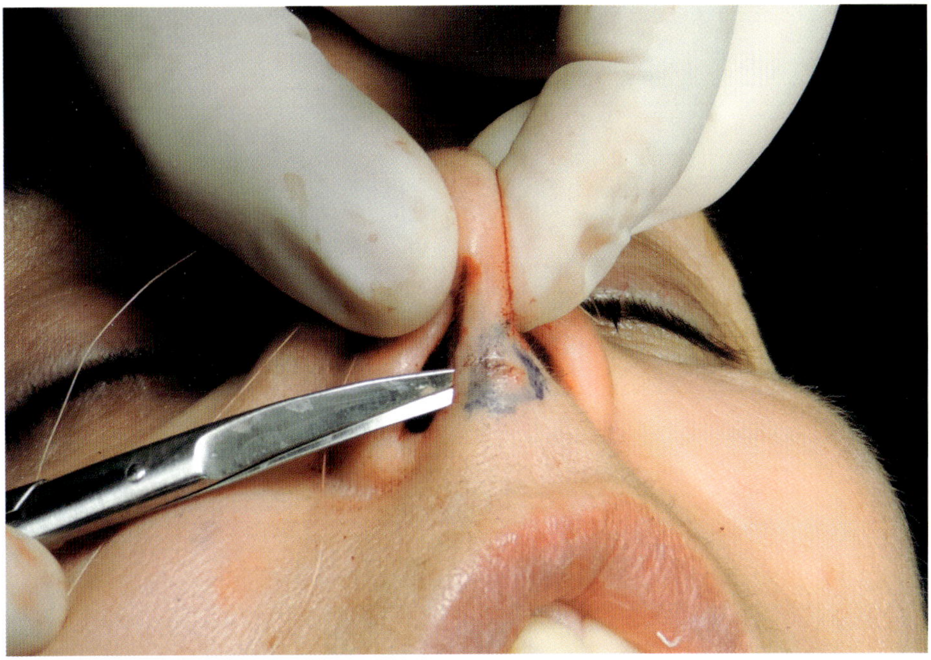

Figure 3b: preparation of a pocket for the graft used to widen the nasolabial angle

they are to serve. Non-septal cartilage is used bearing in mind their tendency to bend over time. This phenomenon occurs due to their being placed in a different context and for functions other than their primitive role. If a straight and rigid cartilage is needed, it must be taken from the septum. These two characteristics make it suitable to act as a support and to fill volumes without curving over time. The alar cartilages are less stiff and are curved. Their shape are such because they are in a certain context of forces. When the forces affecting the cartilages change, their curvature will necessarily change. The same problem applies to cartilages taken from the ribs or the auricular pavilion, i.e. they curve over time. The removal of cartilage from the auricular pavilion is done through a retro-auricular incision at the concha, thus leaving no appreciable trace (fig. 4). The graft can be used individually or be combined with other pieces to serve our purpose. To hold

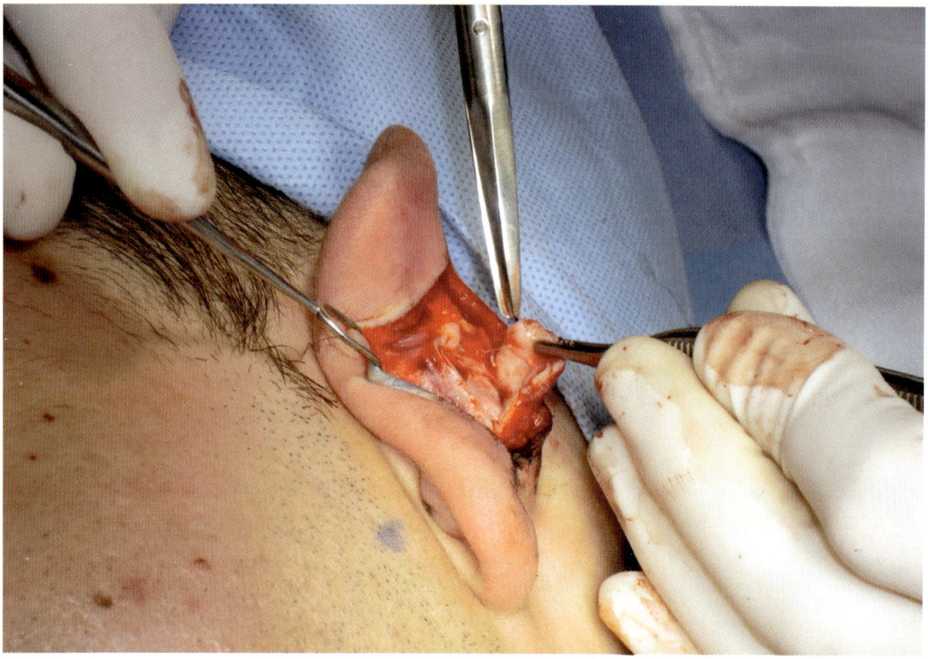

Figure 4: collection of cartilage from the auricular concha with access from the posterior surface of the auricle

the fragments in place and facilitate their mating, they can be transfixed with needles so that the suture stitches may pass through without them moving (figs. 5a, b).

Finally, as a source of cartilage, costal cartilage can also be considered. This is the most difficult to obtain and the one that changes the most over time. It can be cut into tiny cubes and rolled in a muscular fascia to augment the nasal dorsum.

The alar cartilage can be weakened to break up the forces that might cause it to bend. Various techniques exist for this purpose, from the use of Cottle's cartilage crusher (fig. 7) to Rubin's morselizer (fig. 6). The alar cartilage is suitable for re-insertion into the ala where it can also act as a support against an ala collapse, or even as a filler, in which case it should be crushed to prevent bending that may occur over time.

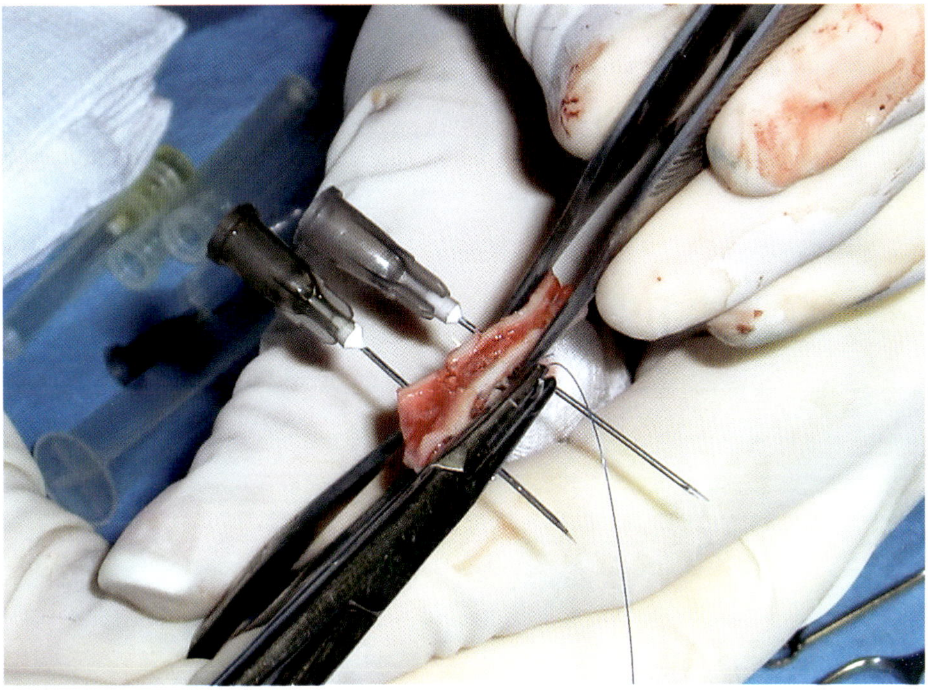

Figure 5a: two fragments of cartilage united with stitches. Needles are used to hold the grafts while stitches are applied

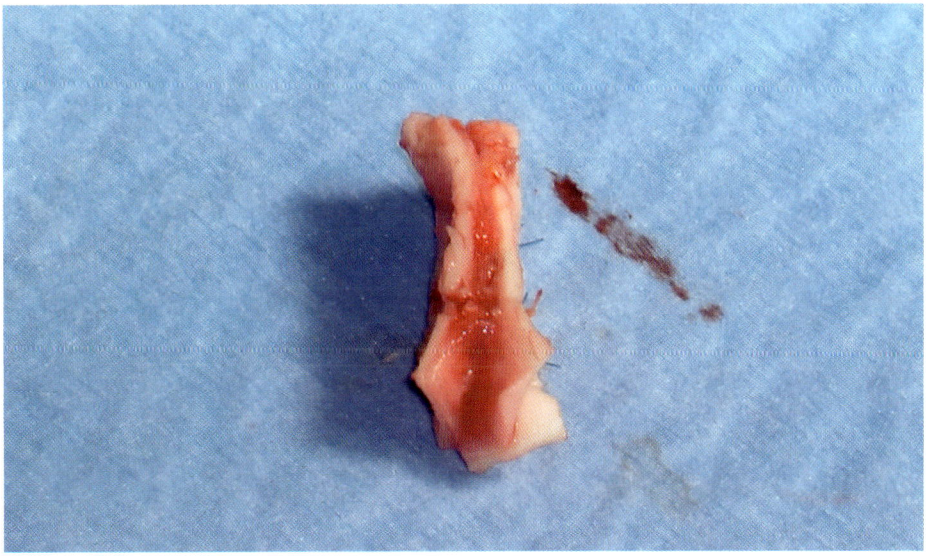

Figure 5b: prepared graft

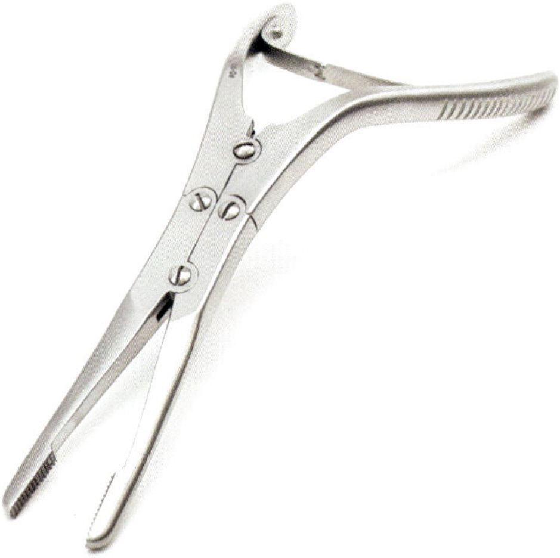

Figure 6: Rubin's morselizer, used to weaken the cartilage and make it loose its memory in order to prevent subsequent curling

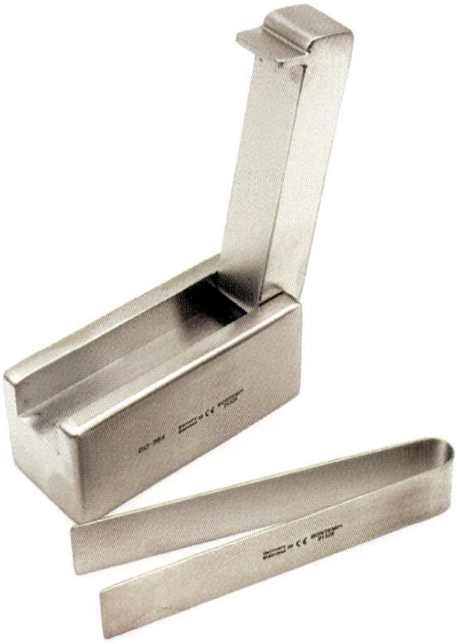

Figure 7: Cottle's cartilage crusher, which serves the same purpose as Rubin's morselizer, but crushes a lot the fragment to be used

The auricular cartilage breaks easily and over time becomes curved, so it should be used for small fillings such as the nasolabial angle, or if there are no viable alternatives.

Since in aesthetic surgery it is necessary to give good results, and these must be stable over time, the less we rely on luck, the better. The septum can be used avoiding using it to raise the dorsum. When the nasal dorsum is raised using the cartilage of the septum, some problems are likely to occur. The first one is mobility. The cartilage does not bind to the bones nor to the cartilages of the dorsum resulting in unnatural mobility. The second problem is visibility. Edges and margins may become apparent once the edema following rhinoplasty has been reabsorbed. It is therefore necessary, if dorsal increasing is needed, to consider the possibility of wrapping small fragments of cartilage in tabotamp or surgicel, or in a strip temporalis muscle fascia, to be inserted on the nasal dorsum. The fascia is stable over time, while the tabotamp reabsorbs, but leaves a little fibrosis which softens the irregularities due to the lack of uniformity of the cartilage fragments wrapped in it. As an alternative to cartilage grafts, alloplastic materials can be used (in my experience PTFE or goretex) which fill very well, are soft, do not move and I have never seen them becoming infected, although it can happen. Since they are soft, they cannot have a supporting function but only a filling function.

CHAPTER 19

Alloplastic materials

If the volume needs to be increased and autologous grafts cannot be used, the use of alloplastic materials may be indicated. There are various types of material, both rigid and soft.

Personally, the only alloplastic material I use is PTFE (polytetrafluoroethylene or goretex). The decision to use only this material derives from the consistently positive experience with its use: no extrusion, no resorption no cases of infection. Once, when a part of the implant had been badly placed and protruded into the nasal cavity, it remained there for a long time without becoming infected; it was sufficient to trim the exposed part so that healing with complete epithelialization of the nasal mucosa could take place without infection. Of course, infections can always occur, but in my experience it never happened.

PTFE is not rigid and therefore not suitable for supporting stresses, e.g. projecting the tip, but is suitable for filling where volume is required (figs. 1a, b, c, d).

The best indication of PTFE is an augmentation of the nasal dorsum. In order to proceed with the precise positioning of the graft, the extent of the graft to be used is outlined with methylene blue (fig. 2a) and a graft of suitable size is prepared (fig. 2b).

It is prudent to wet the graft with an antibiotic solution (fig. 2c), prior to its definitive insertion (fig. 2d).

To increase the width of the nasolabial angle, a subcutaneous pocket is made and PTFE of the desired shape is inserted. (figs. 3a, b). At the glabella mimic movements are present and therefore PTFE grafts are not suitable to fill it because tend to curl.

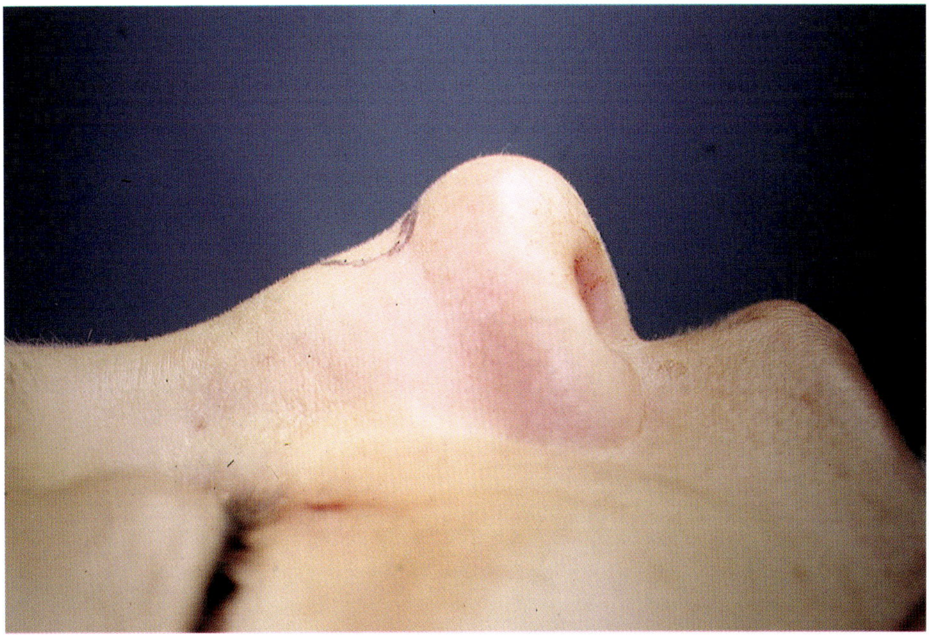

Figure 1a: depression of the dorsum at the supratip

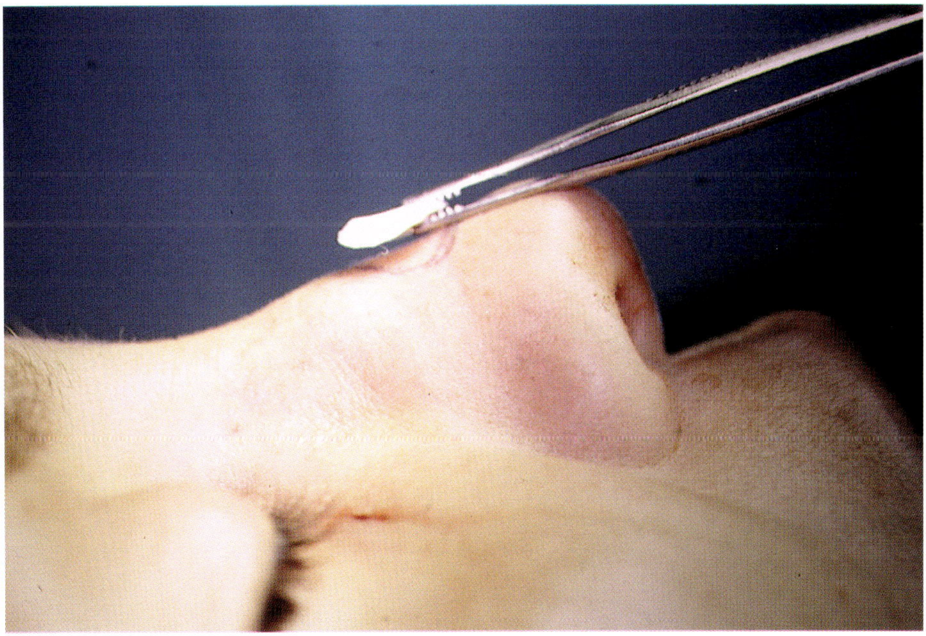

Figure 1b: alloplastic PTFE graft to be inserted to fill the depression

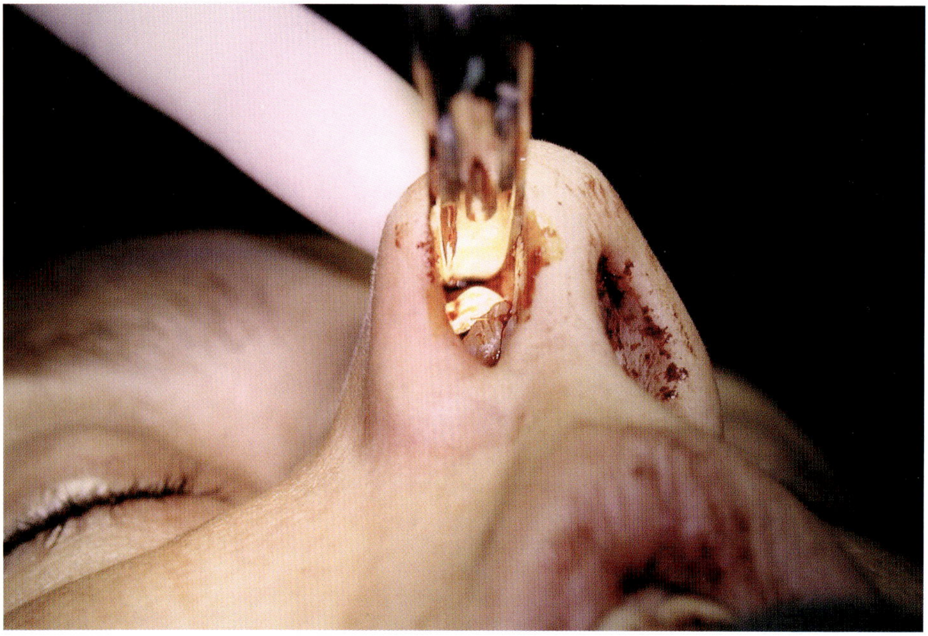

Figure 1c: graft inserted

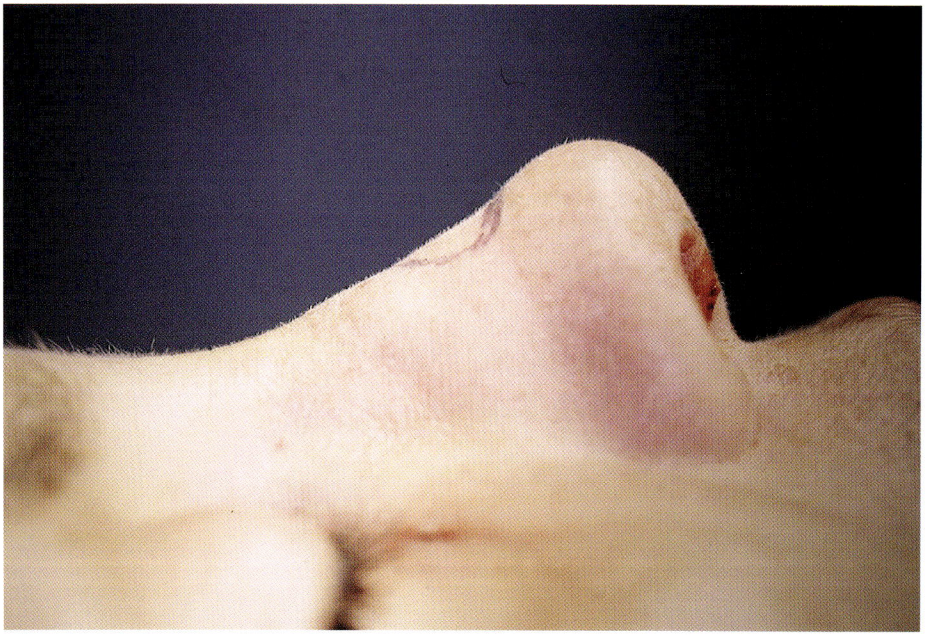

Figure 1d: correction achieved

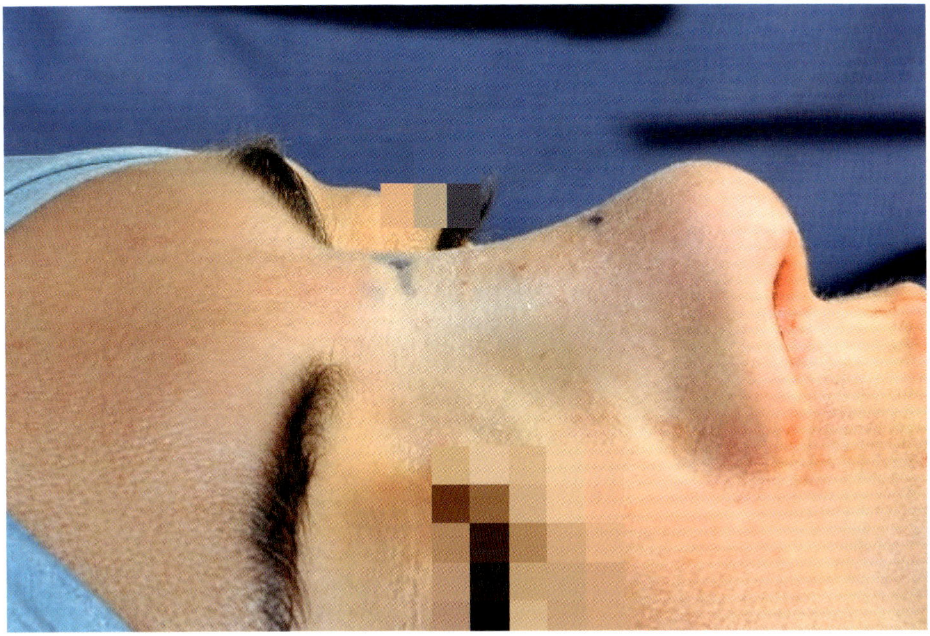

Figure 2a: the dorsum to be filled is marked with two methylene blue dots

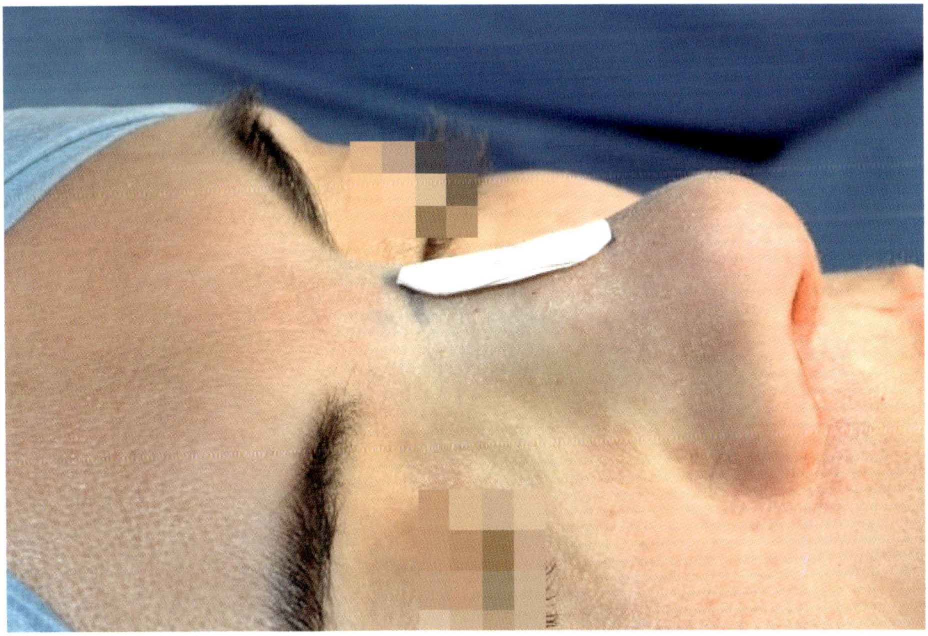

Figure 2b: PTFE graft prepared in thin overlapping layers

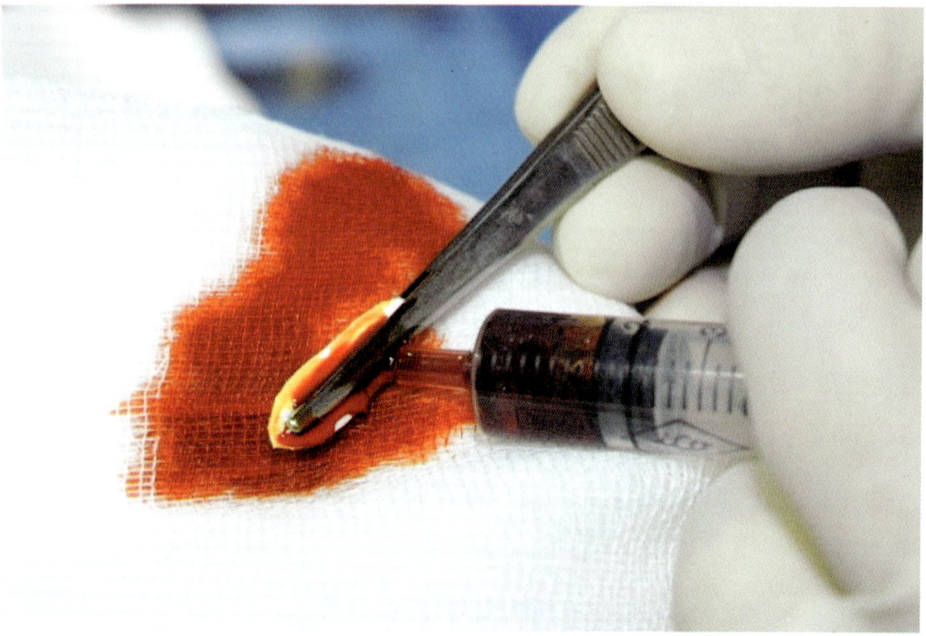

Figure 2c: graft being wet with rifampicin

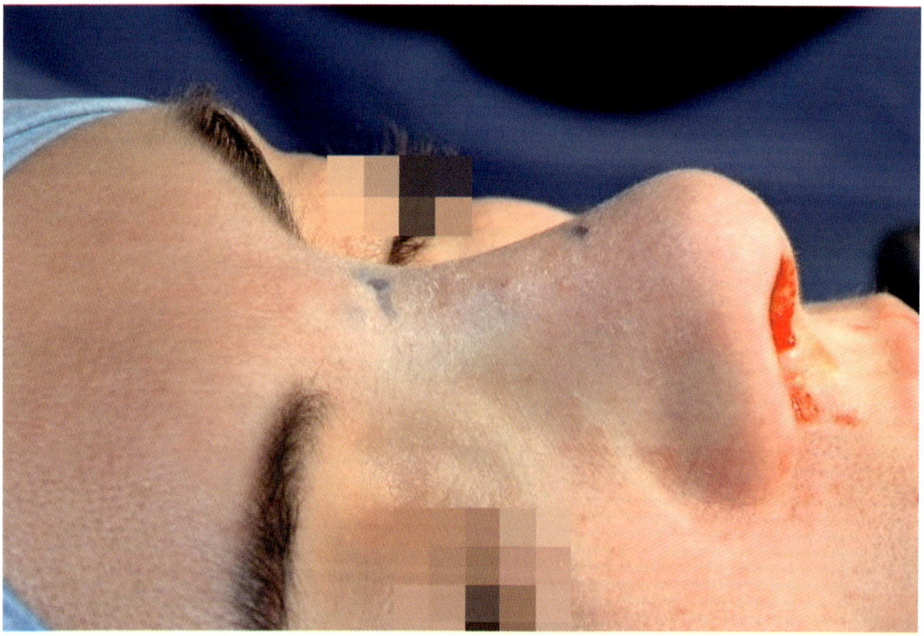

Figure 2d: view of the filling obtained

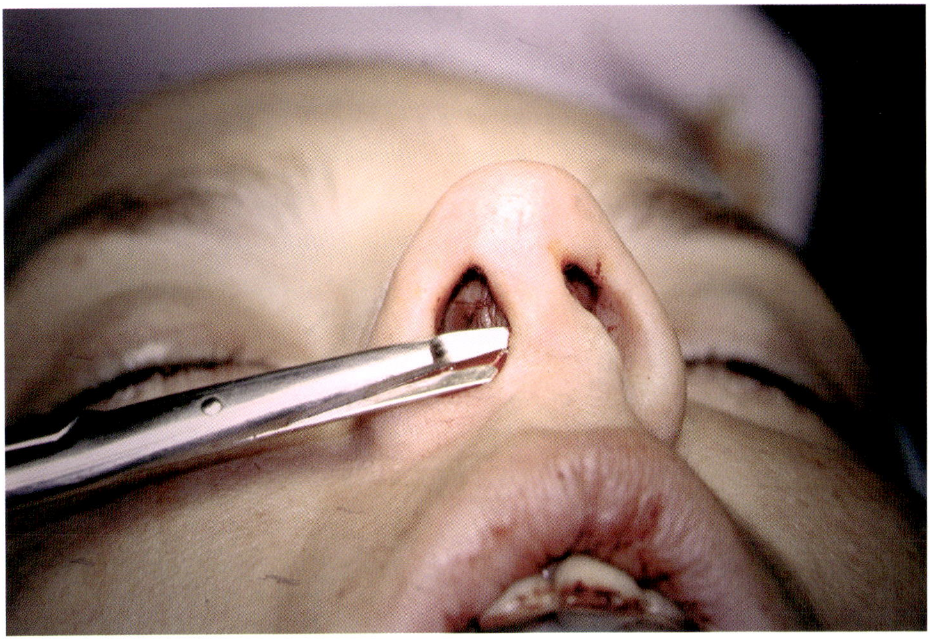

Figure 3a: preparation of the subcutaneous pocket

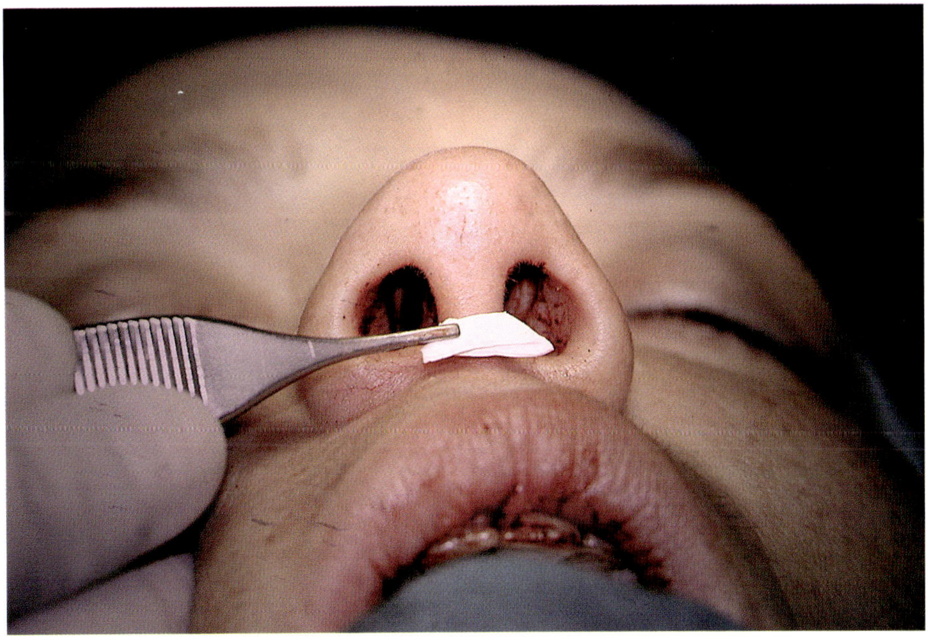

Figure 3b: prepared PTFE graft

PTFE is soft, exists in various thicknesses, can be placed in overlapping layers kept together with a stitch of vicryl rapid 5-0 (fig. 4).
If the margins of the graft cause a visible step under the skin, the edges can be smoothed out using a scalpel. While the malleability of the material is an advantage in that it adapts well to the structure on which it is placed, it can also be a disadvantage since it can bend in an undesirable way during insertion, leading to irregularities that may be visible. In order to avoid this, it may be advisable to place the graft on an instrument such as a chisel which acts as an introducer, such as the baker's pizza shovel (fig. 5a) . Stitches passed through the skin help securing of the graft in the desired location (fig. 5b). Also Asch forceps may be used to deposit the PTFE in the desired point (fig. 5c). A check with direct view is appropriate to see if the graft is in the position desired.
I have no experience of other alloplastic materials. Once I removed from the

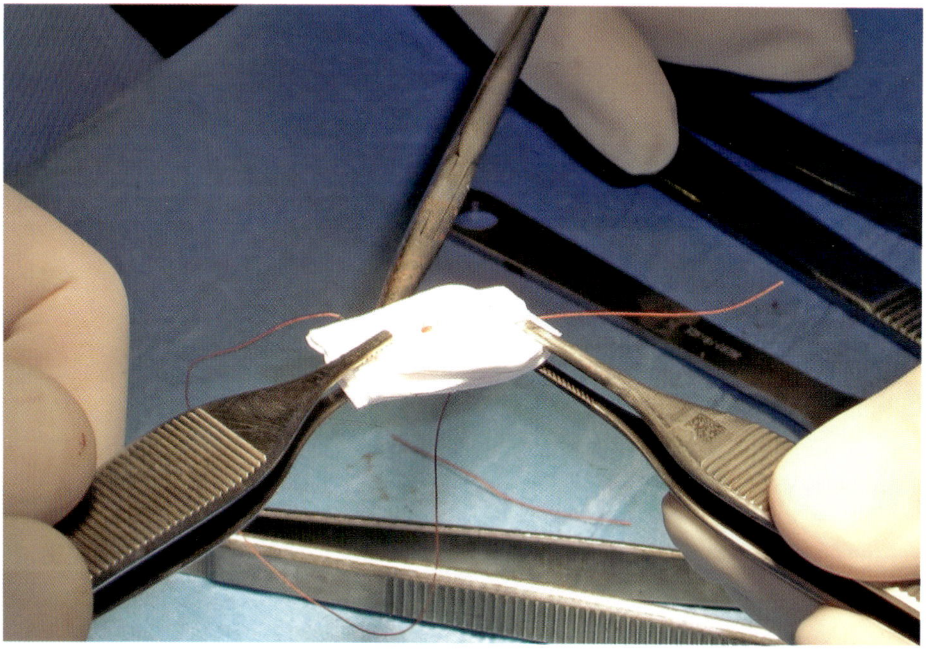

Figure 4: overlapping PTFE layers are held together by absorbable sutures

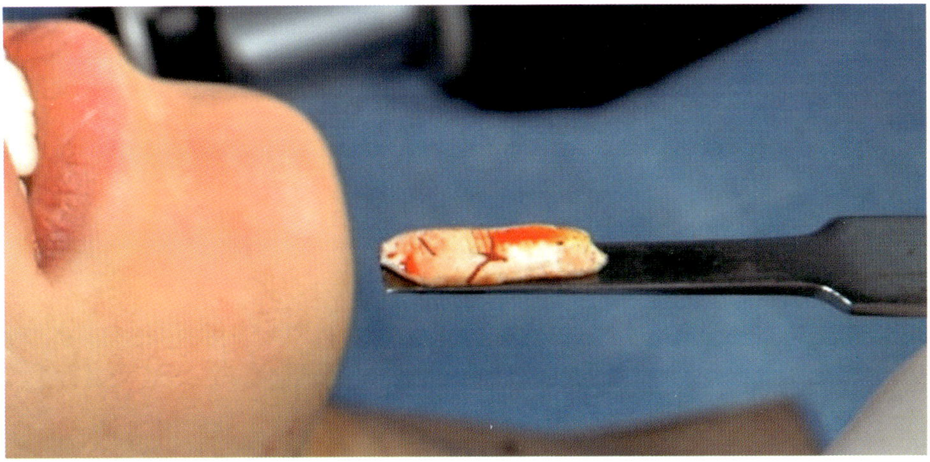

Figure 5a: a chisel on which the graft is laid may be used to introduce the graft

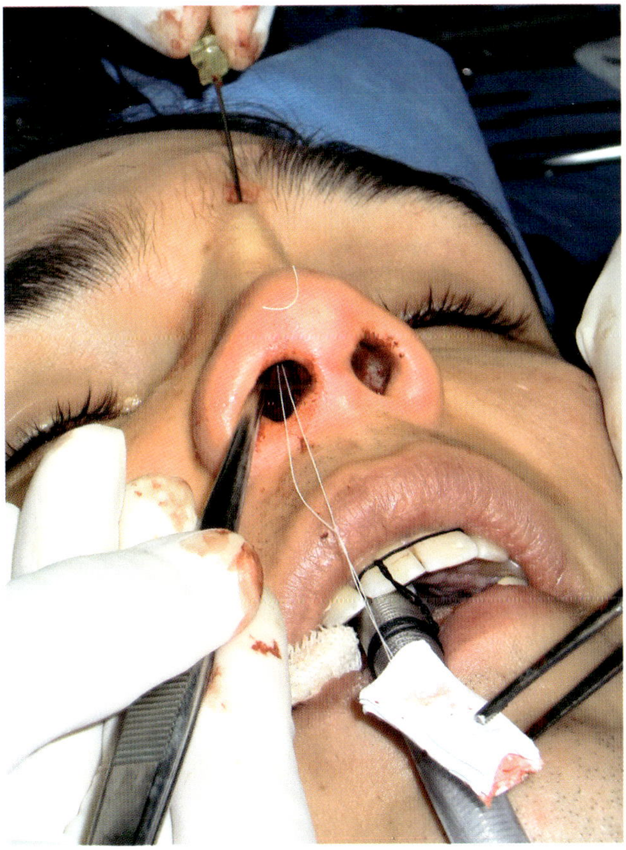

Figure 5b: a stitch can be placed to pull the graft to the desired location

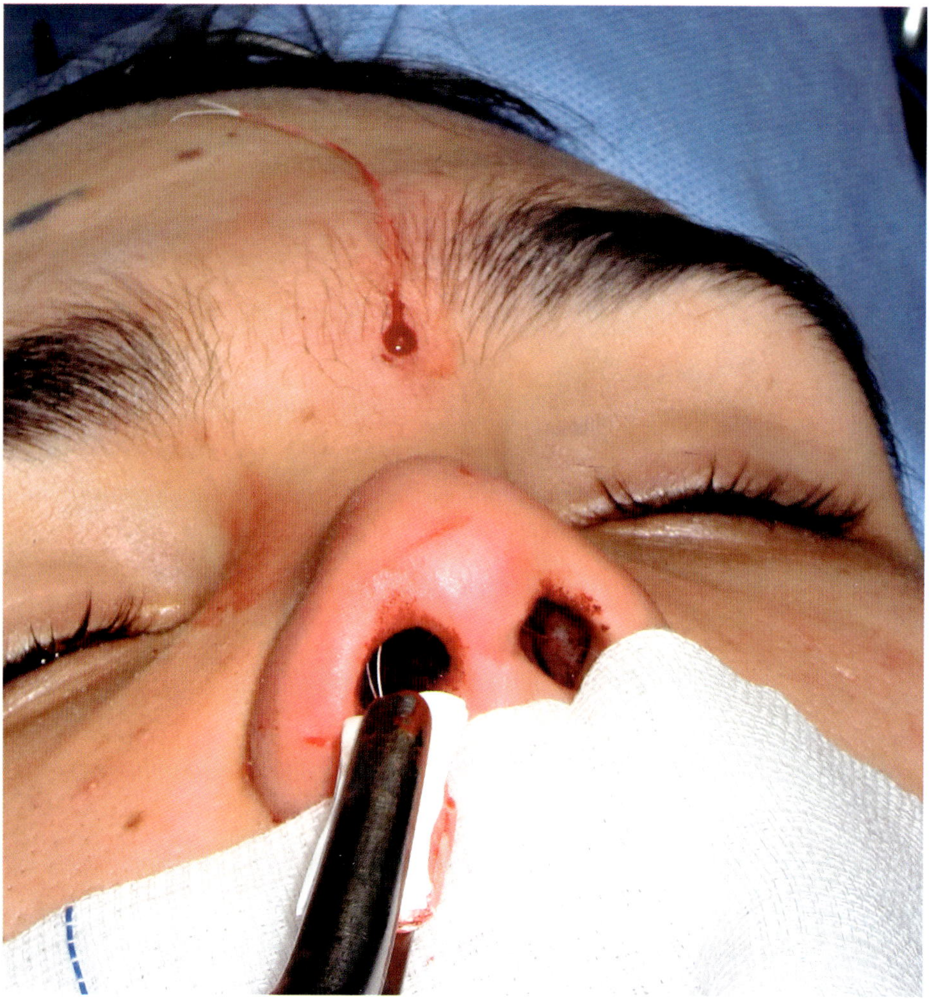

Figure 5c: the graft can be accompanied with an Asch forceps

dorsum of the patient's nose, an ivory graft that had been there for many years but had the disadvantage of being mobile, and replaced it with PTFE. Non-biological hard materials, i.e. not made of bone or cartilage, like silicone, can cause a decubitus and should therefore not be used.

CHAPTER 20

The humpless or saddle-nose

Many passages of this chapter have been covered in other chapters. In this one they will be briefly summarized to recapitulate the techniques that can be used in saddle-noses.

If the nasal dorsum is not to-be reduced, it must be evaluated whether the nose should be narrowed or not. If it needs to be narrowed, medial and lateral osteotomies and subsequent immobilization with a plaster are necessary (chapter 10). If it does not need to be narrowed, this is a rare case where the pyramid does not need to be modified.

The tip (chapter 7) may need an increase in projection or simply a reduction. In the latter case Diamond or hockey stick techniques are applicable. When an increase in projection is required, the first option is to expose the alar cartilages through a rim Incision, locating the Deneb point, stabilizing it with a 5-0 vicryl rapid stitch, and bringing both lateral crus of the alar cartilages closer to the midline and suturing them together, one against the other, thus extending the medial crus and obtaining a more projected tip (Berson's technique, chapter 7).

As an alternative to this technique, a graft can be taken from the septum, opened into a Y shape so that the two oblique branches of the Y reproduce the shape of the tip as in the butterfly technique of Ponti. The vertical branch of the Y is inserted between the medial crus. The depth of insertion of the vertical branch of the Y between the medial crura determines the greater or lesser projection of the tip (fleur de lys technique by Tessier, chapter

7). Other types of grafts can be used to increase the projection of the tip but with slightly different effects. Onlay grafts and Sheen's shield project less, but change the shape of the tip, making it more defined.

Onlay grafts are placed at the tip above the Intermediate crura to further project the tip and make it more defined. Cartilage taken from the septum can be used for this purpose, but also the ones taken from the nasal alae are suitable because these grafts are very small and will deform very little over time. Onlay grafts can be introduced through a small incision made along the lower edge of the alar cartilage, or they can be fixed with stitches after exposing the alar cartilages with the so-called delivery technique and eventual stabilization of the Deneb point to be sure of symmetry.

For the Sheen shield graft the procedure is similar. However, the purpose for which it is used changes a little: the shape of the tip obtained is squarer, has a real facet, and better simulates the presence of two domus.

The projection of the tip can also be increased with grafts that make higher the support of the medial crus at the anterior nasal spine. For this purpose, one or more layers of cartilage (but also of PTFE or goretex) are placed in front of the anterior nasal spine. Very suitable for this purpose are grafts taken from the cartilage of the auricle, because they are thick and, given the small size of the fragments used, without the unpleasant side effect of curving over time.

How to increase the dorsum

When choosing which route to take for dorsum augmentation, various possibilities must be considered: bone, cartilage or alloplastic material grafts. Bone grafting should be reserved for special cases where rigidity and supportive strength are required, such as in boxers' noses, whose structures have lost the shape and rigidity is necessary.

The use of such grafts is therefore a rarity in Aesthetic Surgery and beyond the scope of this book.
The cartilage grafts (chapter 18) can be taken from the septum or from other nasal cartilages, from the auricle or from the costal cartilage. We have already drawn attention to the fact that the only cartilage that does not bend over time is that of the septum, but this advantage is accompanied by the disadvantage of being rather rigid, so when is laid on the dorsum gives rise to movements that can persist over time. Another disadvantage is that if the skin of the nose is thin, which is often the case in the upper half of the pyramid where the dermis is less thick, the graft may be visible. The other cartilages can be used in various ways as explained in chapter 18.
Also costal cartilage can be used as a filler, but once taken out from its context, where peculiar strengths that allow it to perform its function correctly are present, its shape changes, assuming curves that can be become evident over time, therefore it is not advisable to use it as it is. If it is cut into many little pieces it can be used as a filler. This diced cartilage can be wrapped inside a strip of superficial fascia of the temporal muscle so that it can be distributed evenly along the surface to be filled without visible irregularities on the surface of the nasal dorsum. As an alternative to the fascia of the temporal muscle, the cartilage fragments can be wrapped in surgicel or tabotamp. However, it should be borne in mind that these materials, currently used as hemostats, are reabsorbed, leaving a slight fibrousness that may not hide eventual irregularities in the distribution of the pieces of cartilage.
The alloplastic material i currently use to increase the dorsum is PTFE (chapter 19).

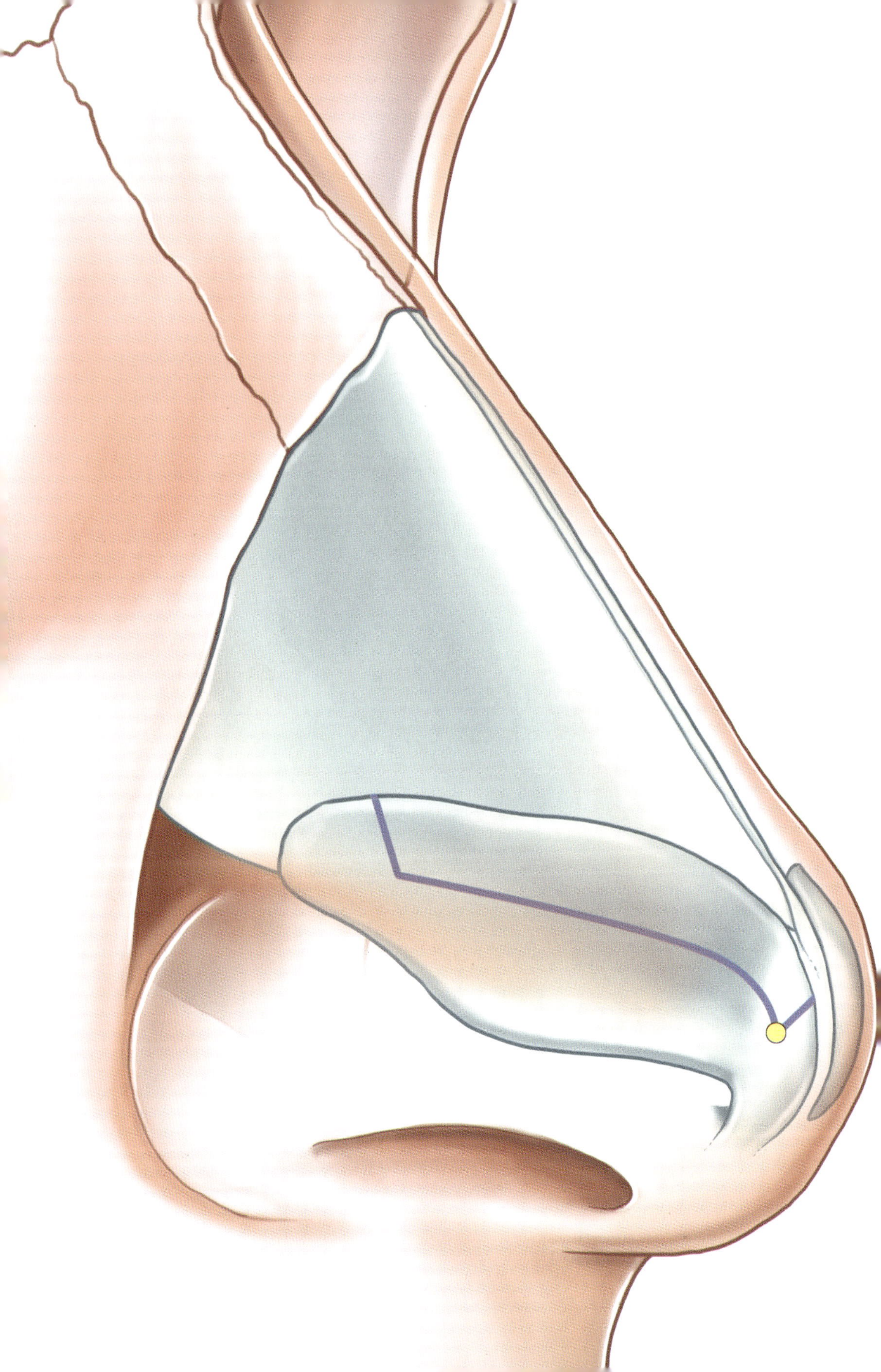

CLINICAL CASES

CASE 1

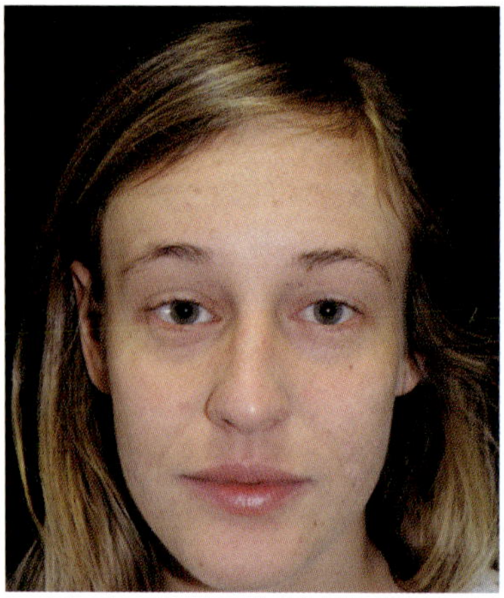
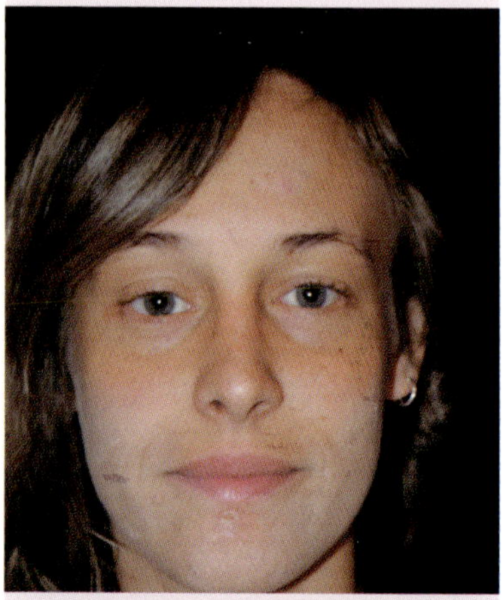
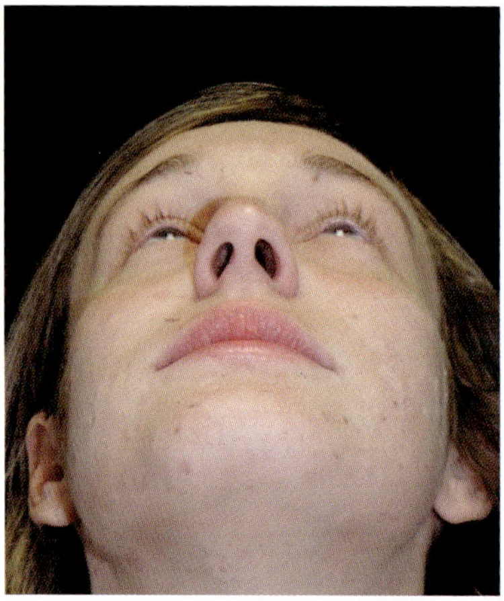
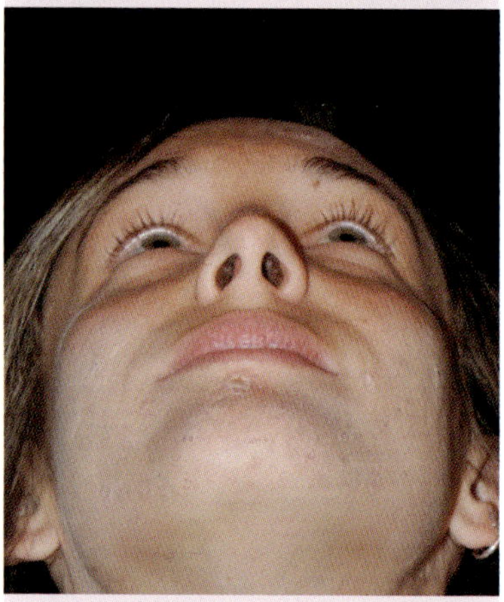
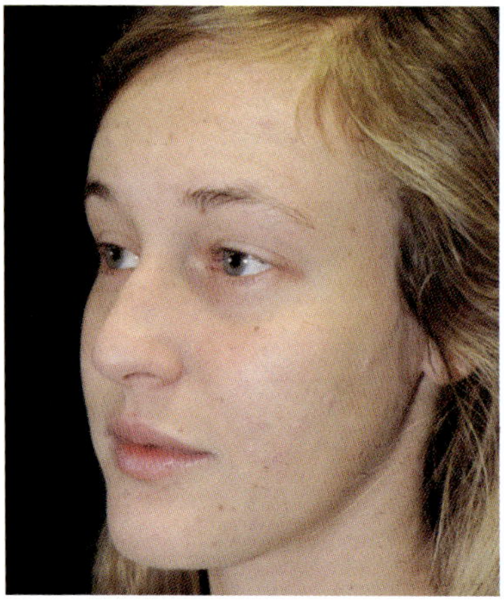
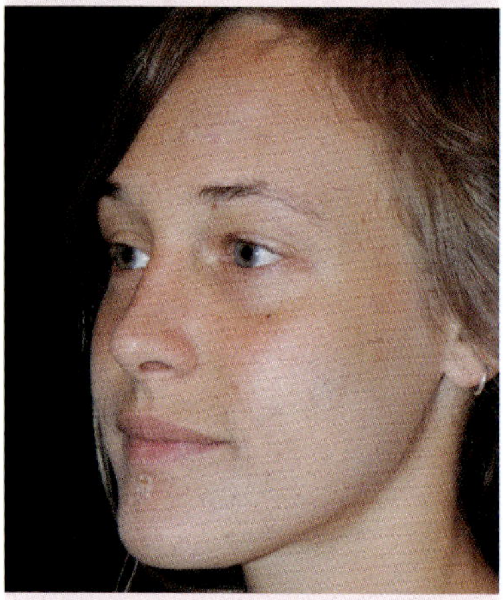

Patient with facial asymmetry appreciable in the photo from below in which it is noted that the right maxilla is in a posterior plane compared to the contralateral. The mandible is also asymmetric; the anterior septum is deviated and has caused the deviation of the pyramid to the right side, and obstruction of area 4 of Cottle.
Surgery performed: rhinoseptoplasty: lowered dorsum, shortened and tilted septum,

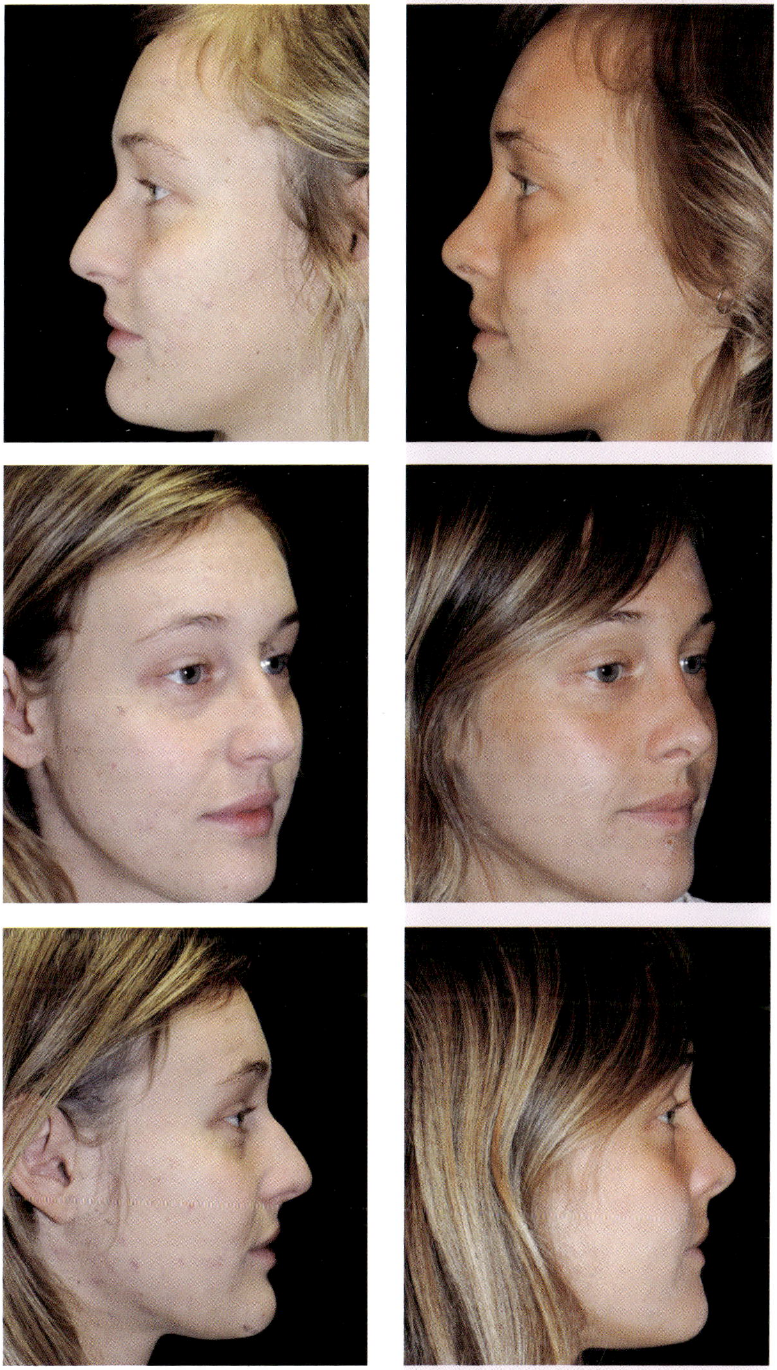

reduced tip using hockey stick technique. The triangular cartilages were shortened to accompany the shortening of the septum. The deviation was corrected with bilateral subperichondral access to the septum and removal of the deviated part at the level of area 4, and serial incisions on the right anterior surface. The hypertrophy of the turbinates was treated with radiofrequency equipment. Basal osteotomies to conclude.

CASE 2

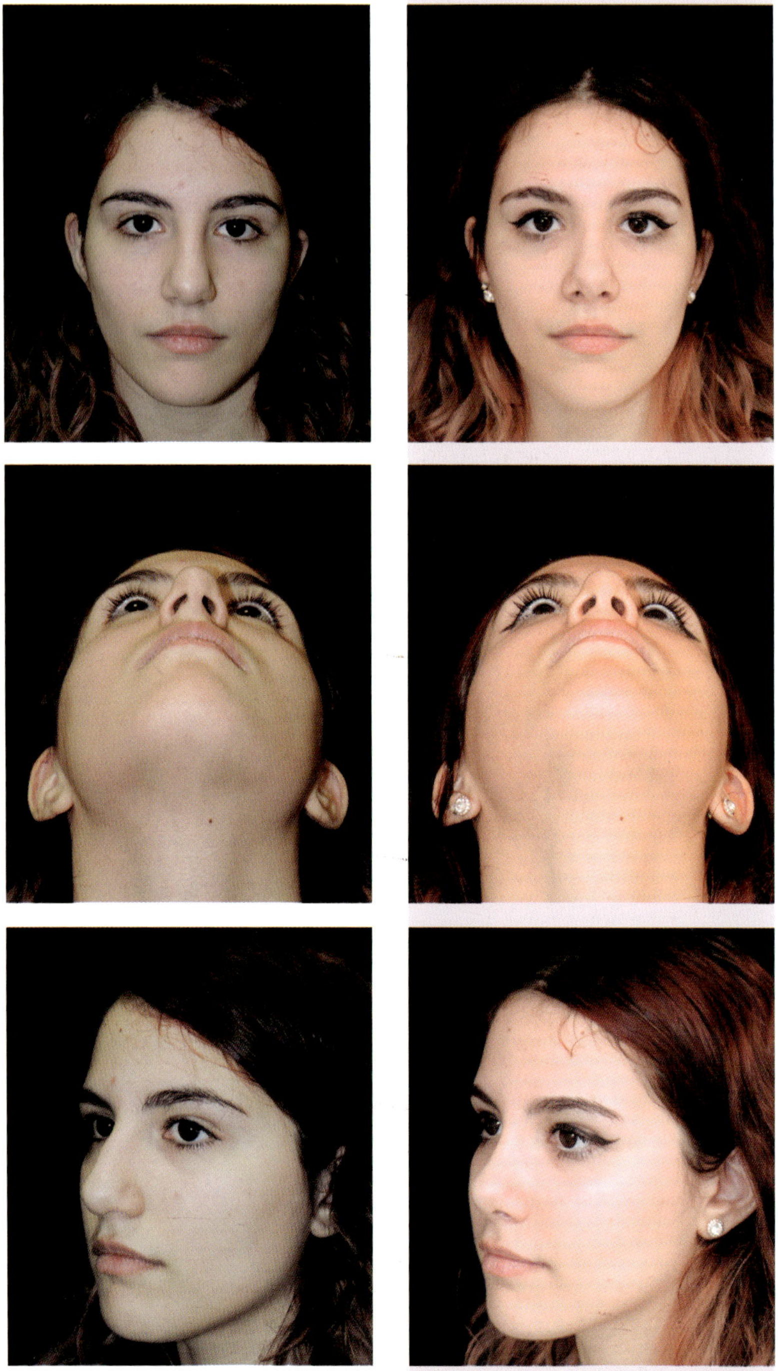

Asymmetry detectable by non-horizontal eye line and left maxilla in a posterior plane compared to the contralateral. Asymmetric alar cartilages, the right being larger and the left nostril larger. Deviation of the septum that protrudes slightly into the right nostril (Cottle's area 1). Left-convex deviation of Cottle's area 4.
Correction with rhinoseptoplasty: lowered dorsum, shortened and tilted septum,tip plasty

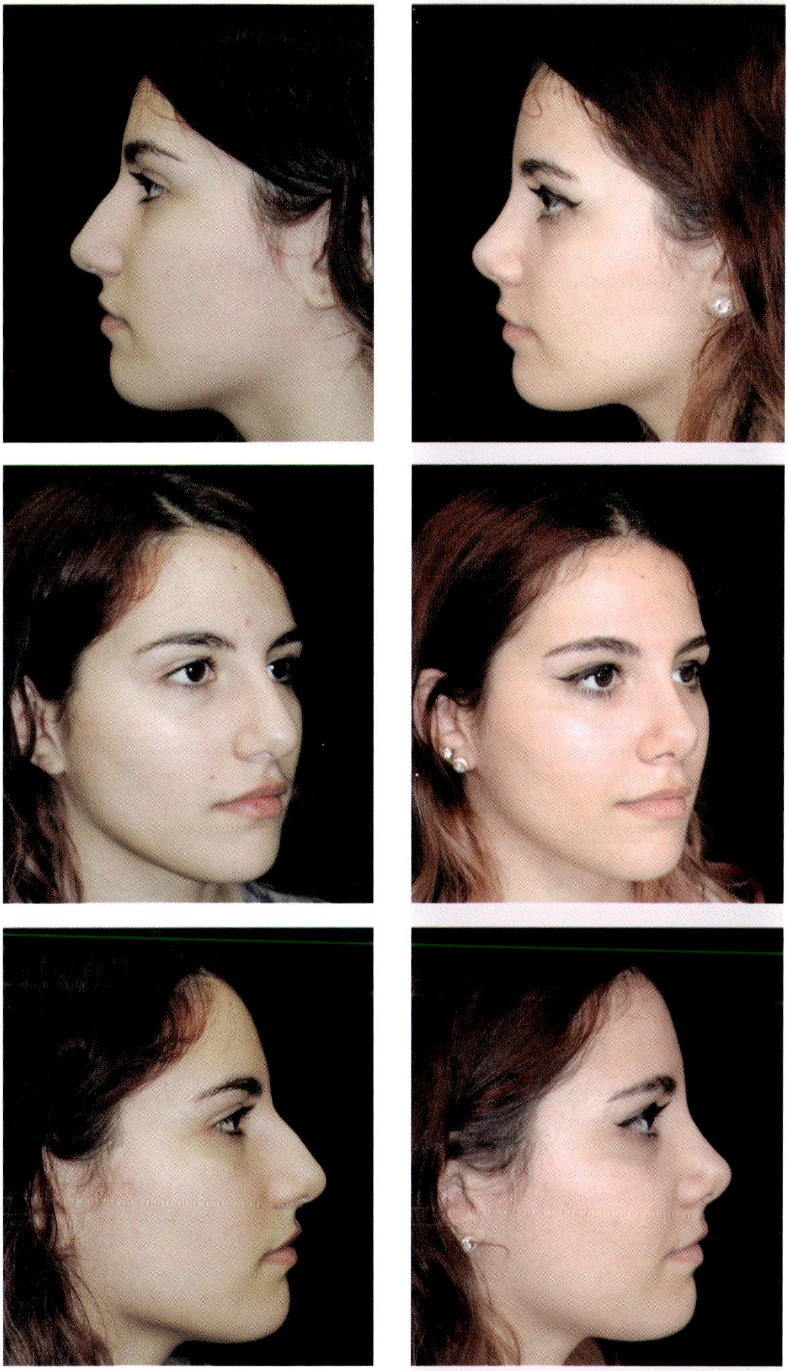

with hockey stick to the right and Diamond to the left; Killian septoplasty modified by bilateral chondromucosa and periostiomucosa elevation, removing of cartilage and bone spur of vomer and perpendicular lamina of ethmoid that was the obstructing left nasal cavity. Reduction of the turbinates with radiofrequency and reduction of the left nostril. Basal osteotomies.

CASE 3

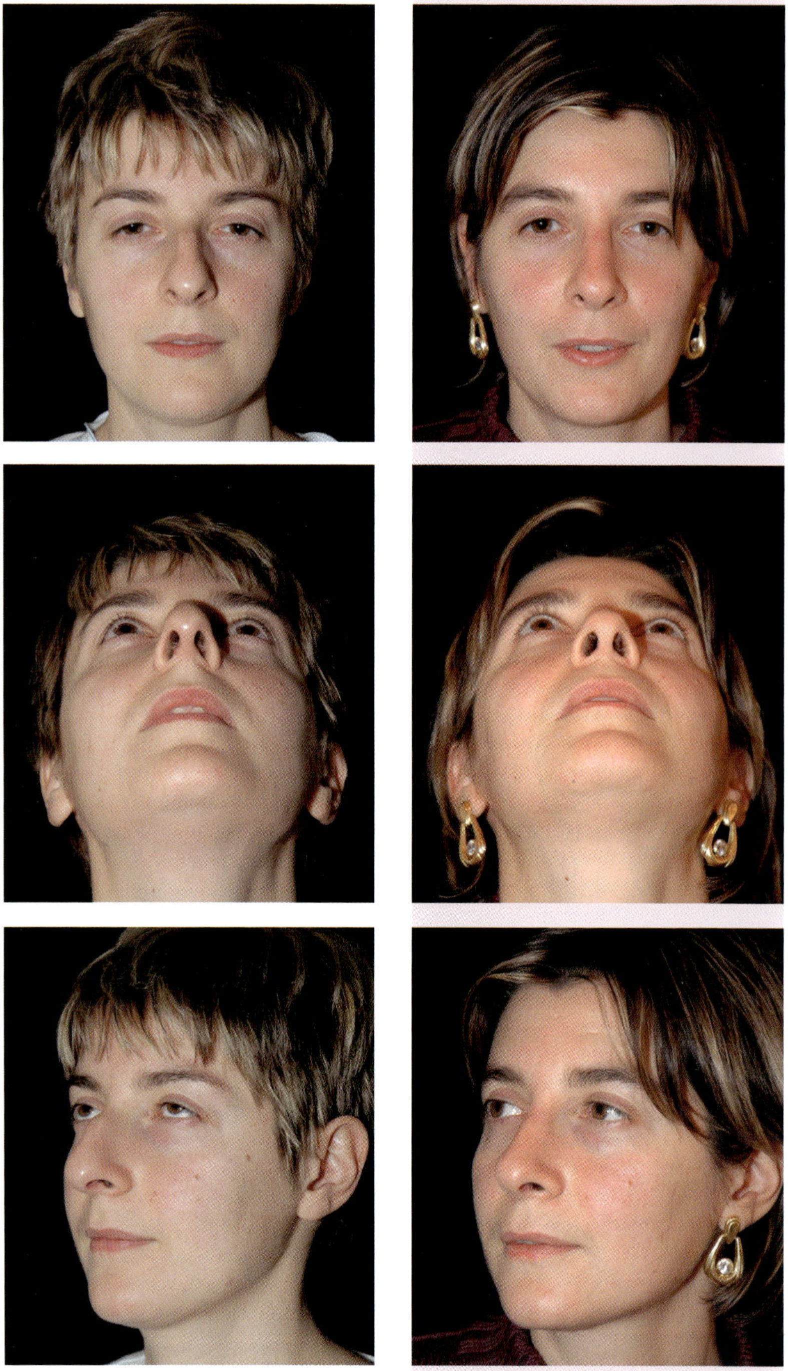

Correction: lowered dorsum, shortened and tilted septum, the lateral crus of the alar cartilages was repositioned closer to the edge of the nostril to permit their reduction leaving a lower margin of at least two millimeters to support the ala. The tip was reduced with hockey stick technique. Basal osteotomies.

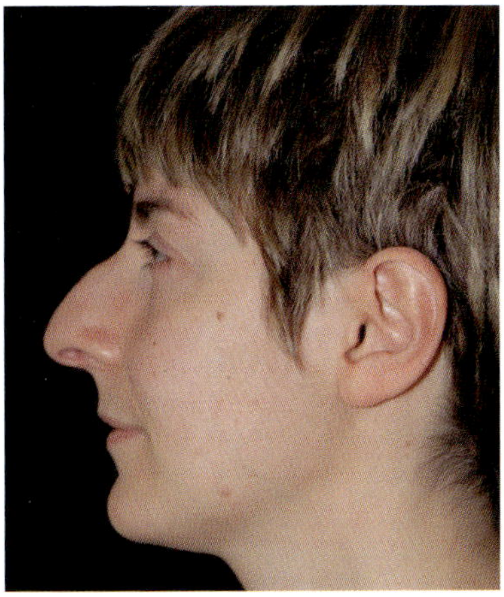
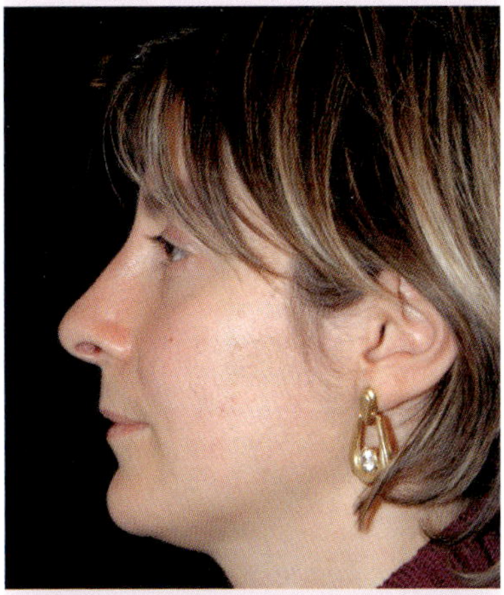
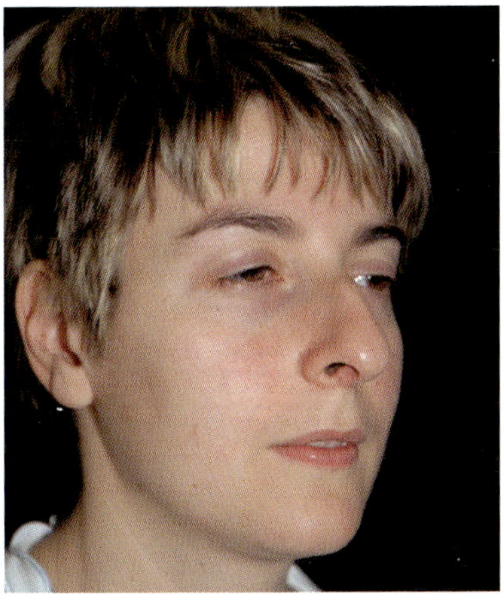
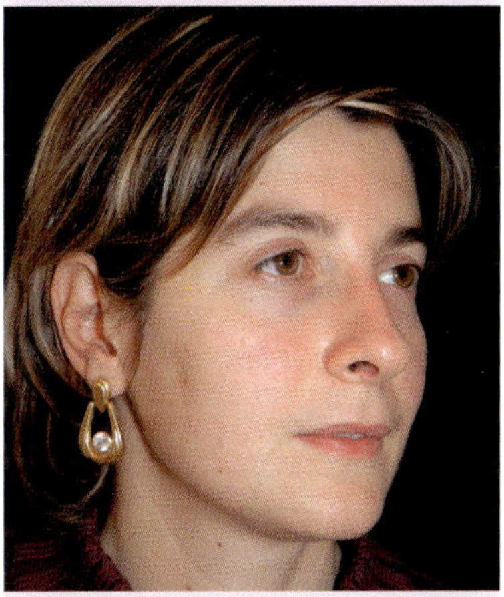
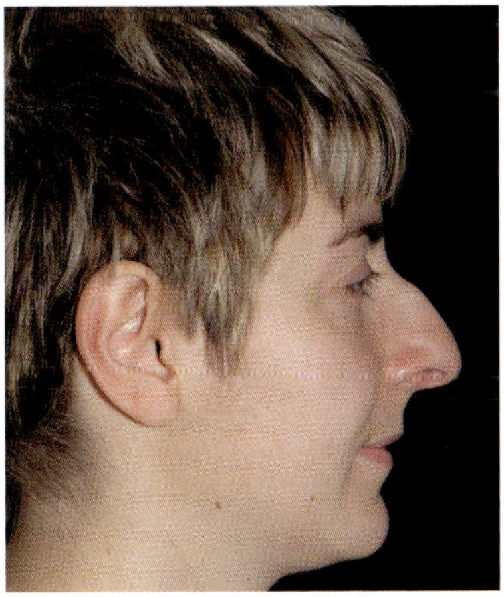
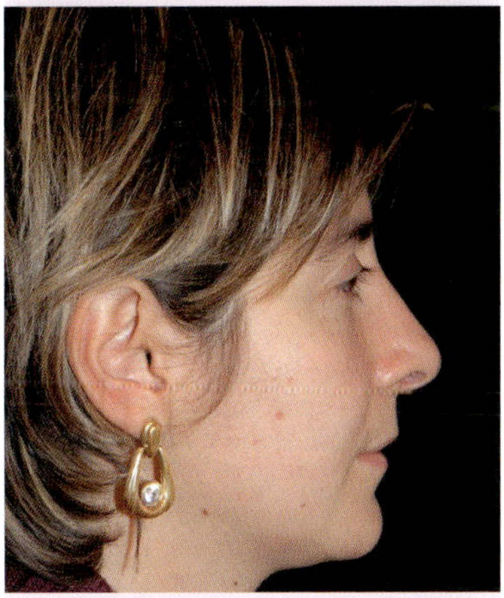

CASE 4

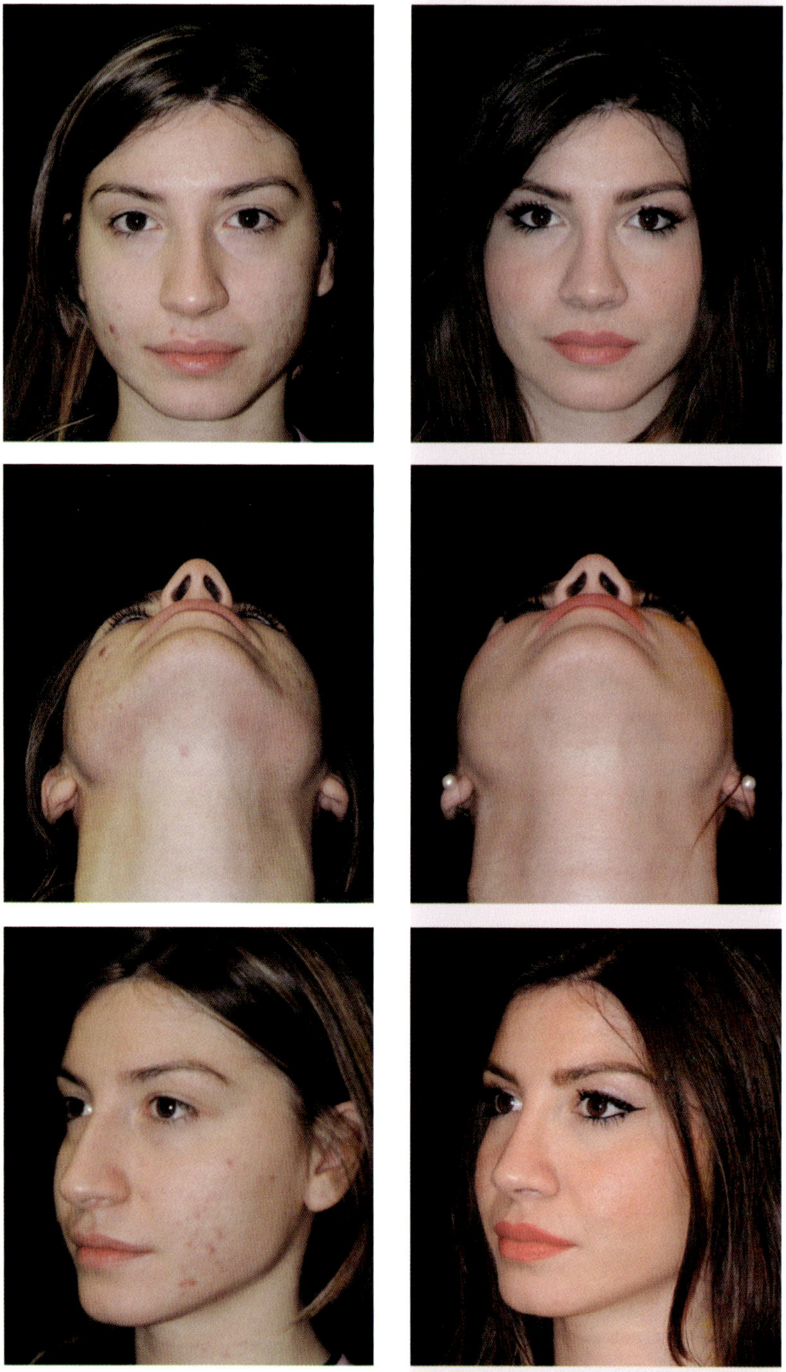

The patient had undergone a nose fracture and presents a bone spur in Cottle's area 4. Correction: rhinoseptoplasty. Lowered dorsum, alar cartilages treated with the Diamond technique. Access to the septum with bilateral mucoperichondrial elevation extended to the periosteum posteriorly, then removal of the left spur in Cottle's area 4. Reduction of the nostrils. Basal osteotomies.

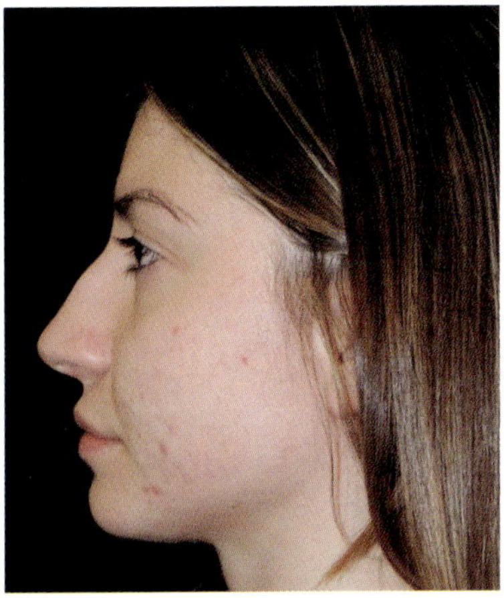

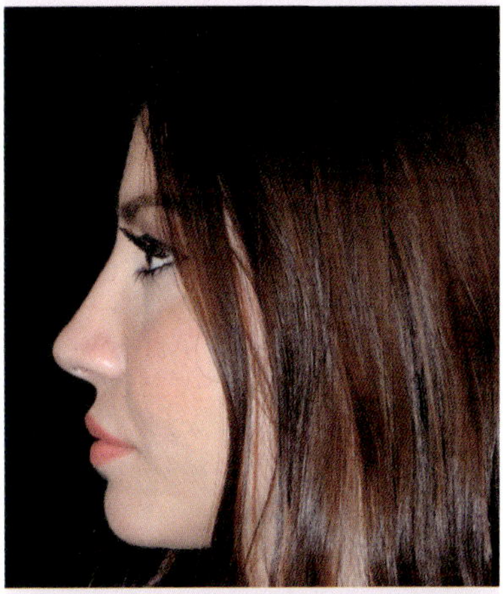

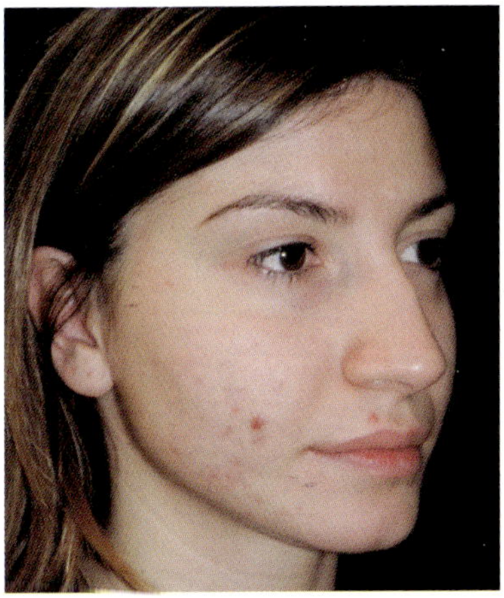

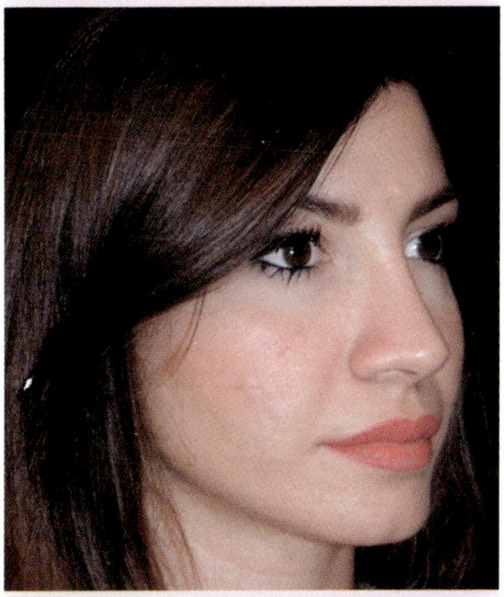

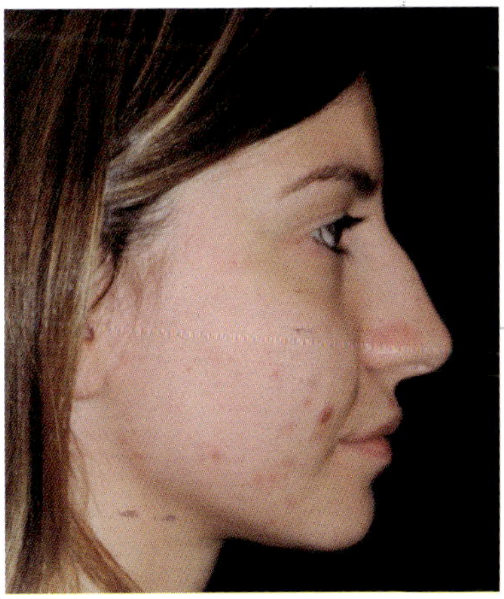

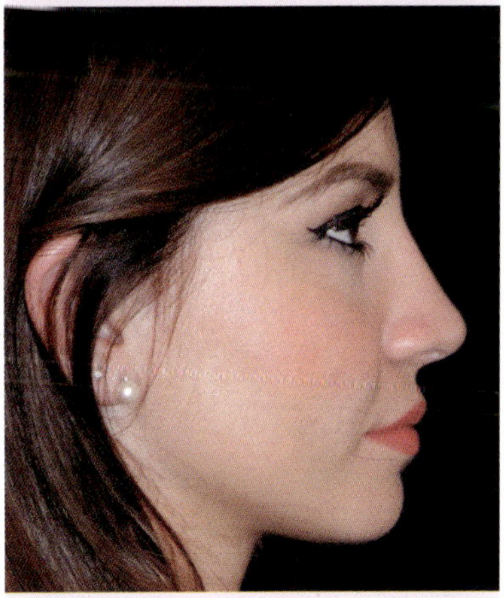

CASE 5

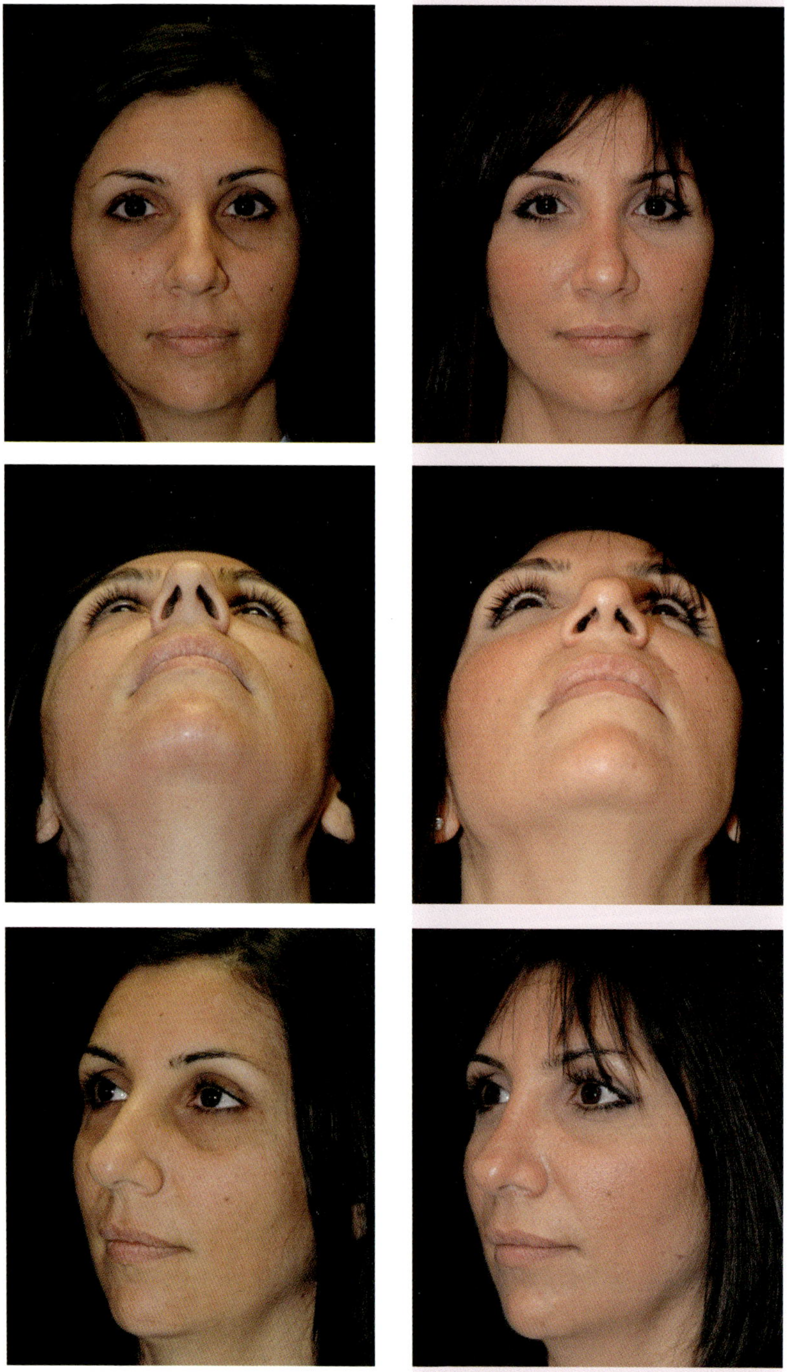

Correction: lowered dorsum, shortened and tilted septum, tip adjusted with hockey stick technique. Removal of a strip of cartilage from the lateral apex of the lateral crus to allow lateral sliding of the cartilage in relation to the skin of the ala. Triangular cartilages completely undermined from the overlying skin and shortened. Reduction of the turbinates with radiofrequency. Basal osteotomies.

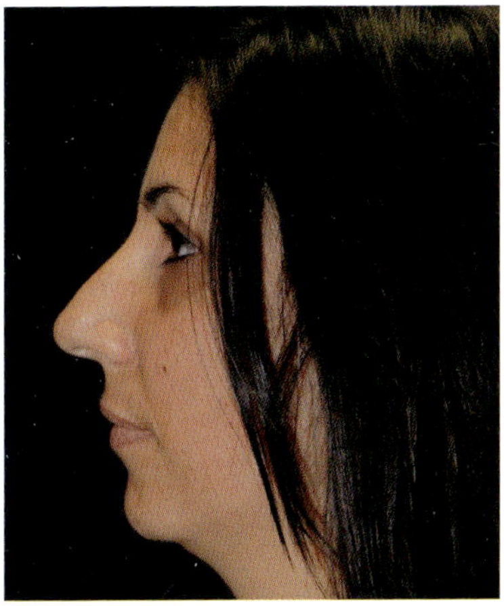

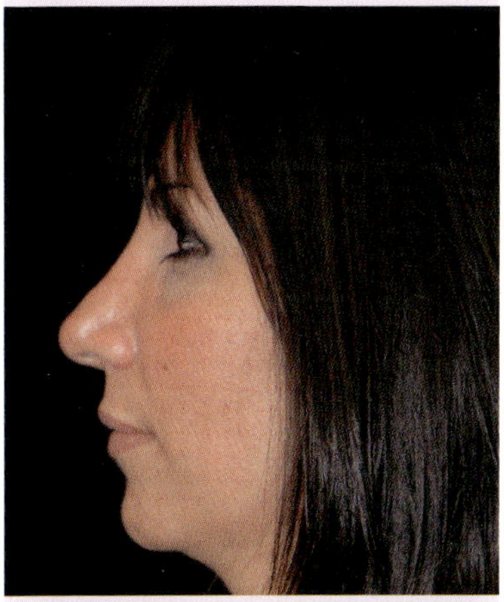

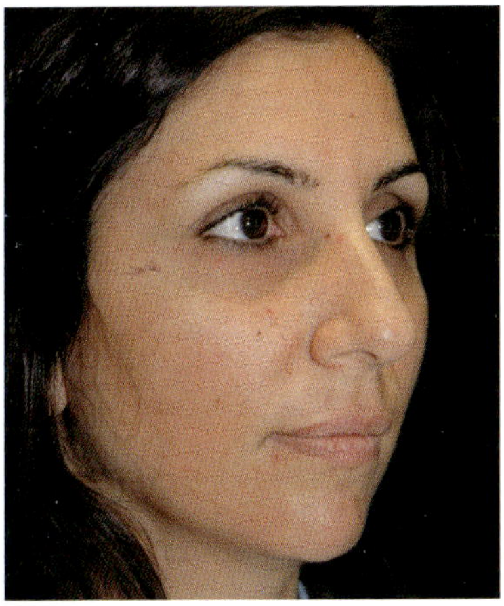

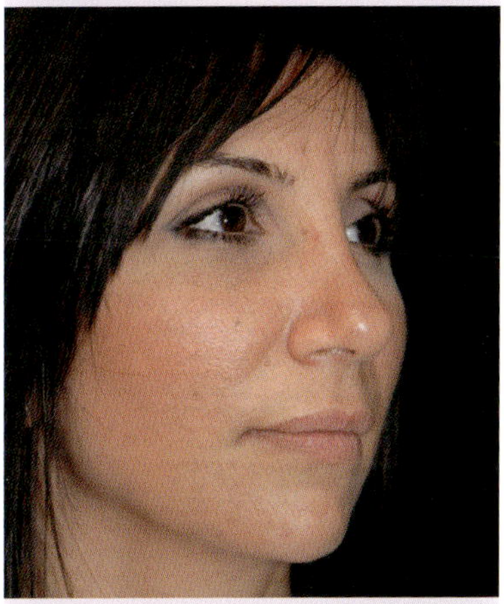

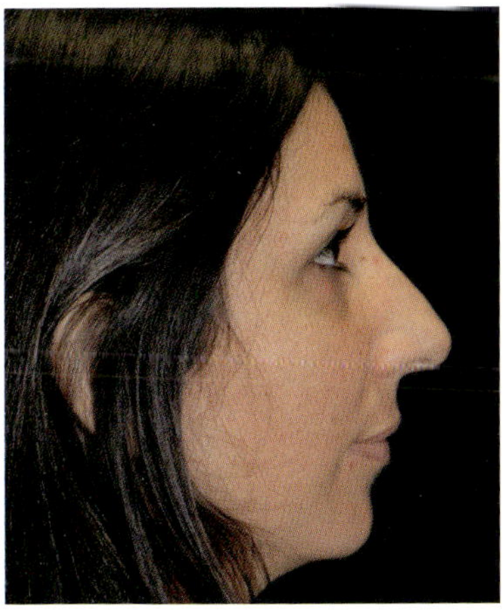

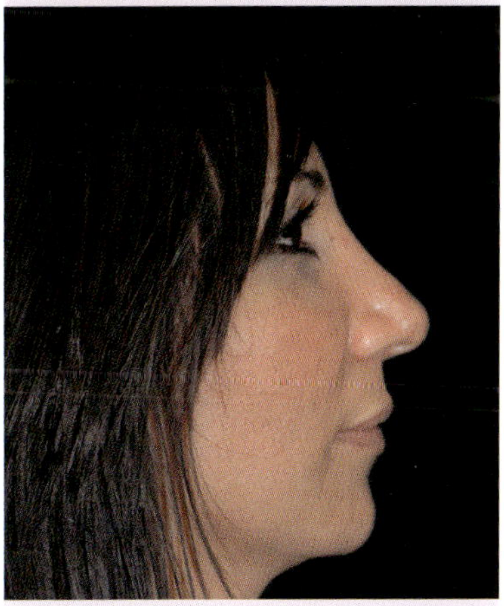

CASE 6

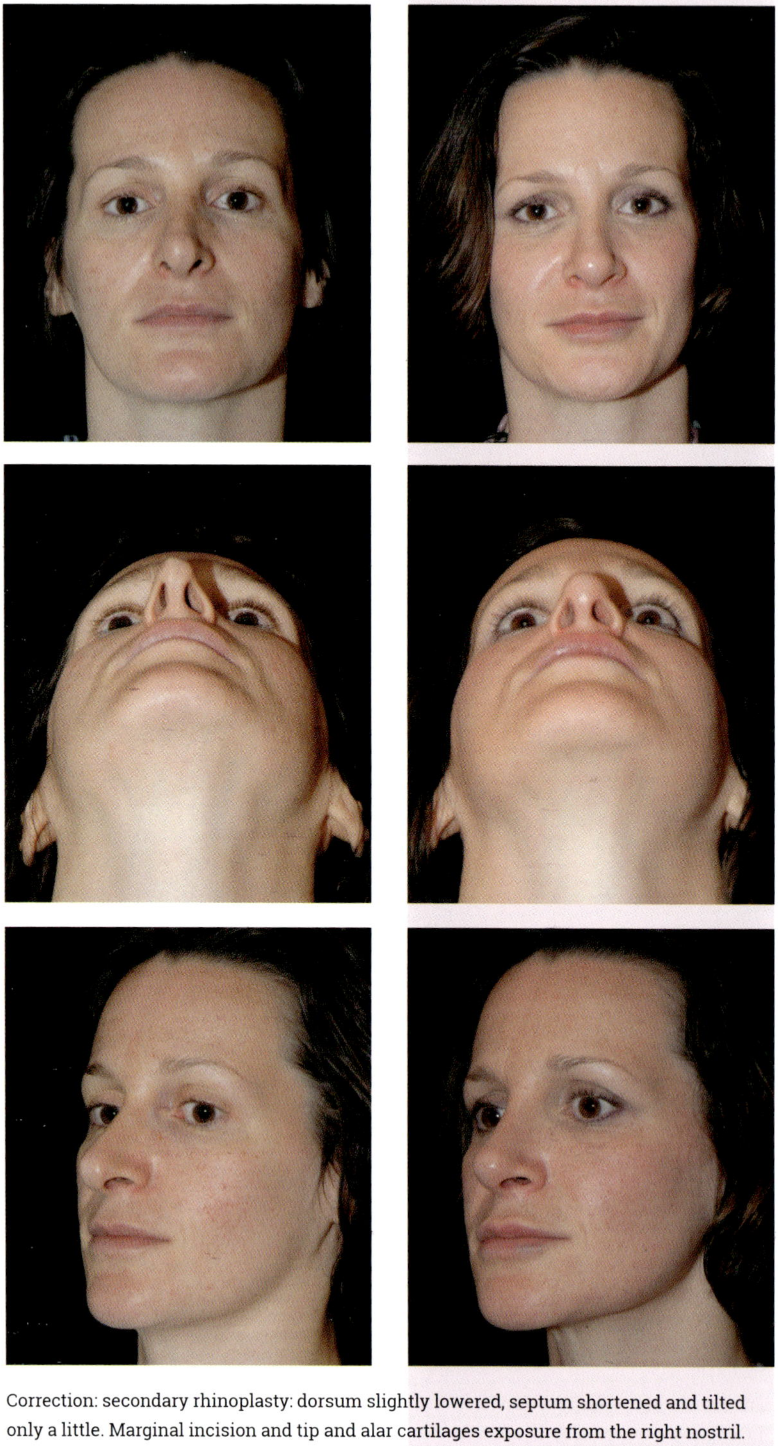

Correction: secondary rhinoplasty: dorsum slightly lowered, septum shortened and tilted only a little. Marginal incision and tip and alar cartilages exposure from the right nostril. Identification and stabilization of the Deneb point to allow symmetrization. Reduction of the projection performed by amputating the domus and opening the medial crus in order to

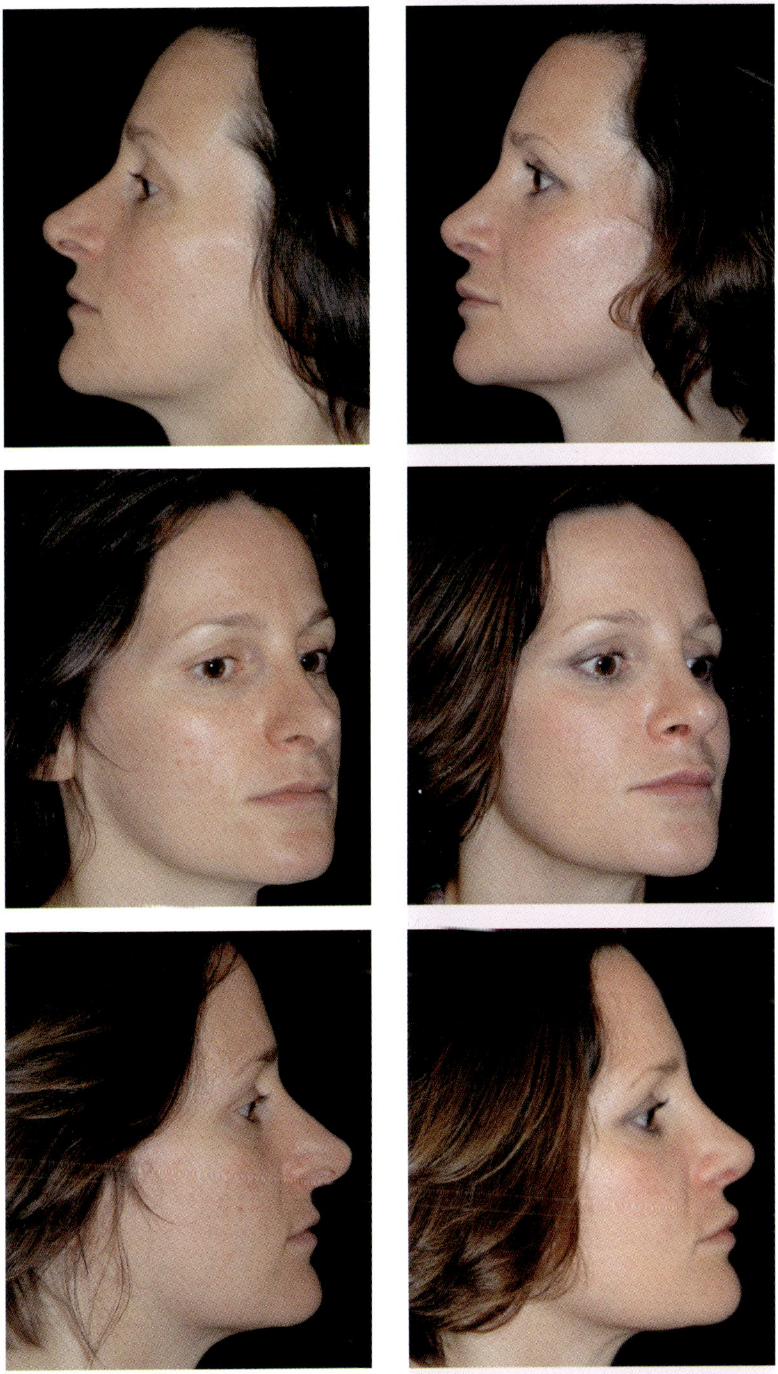

simulate Ponti's butterfly technique. The triangular cartilages are shortened maintaining the angles as indicated by Sheen. Septoplasty is performed elevating the chondromucosa and proceeding with serial incisions at the right surface to correct the anterior right deviation. Basal osteotomies.

CASE 7

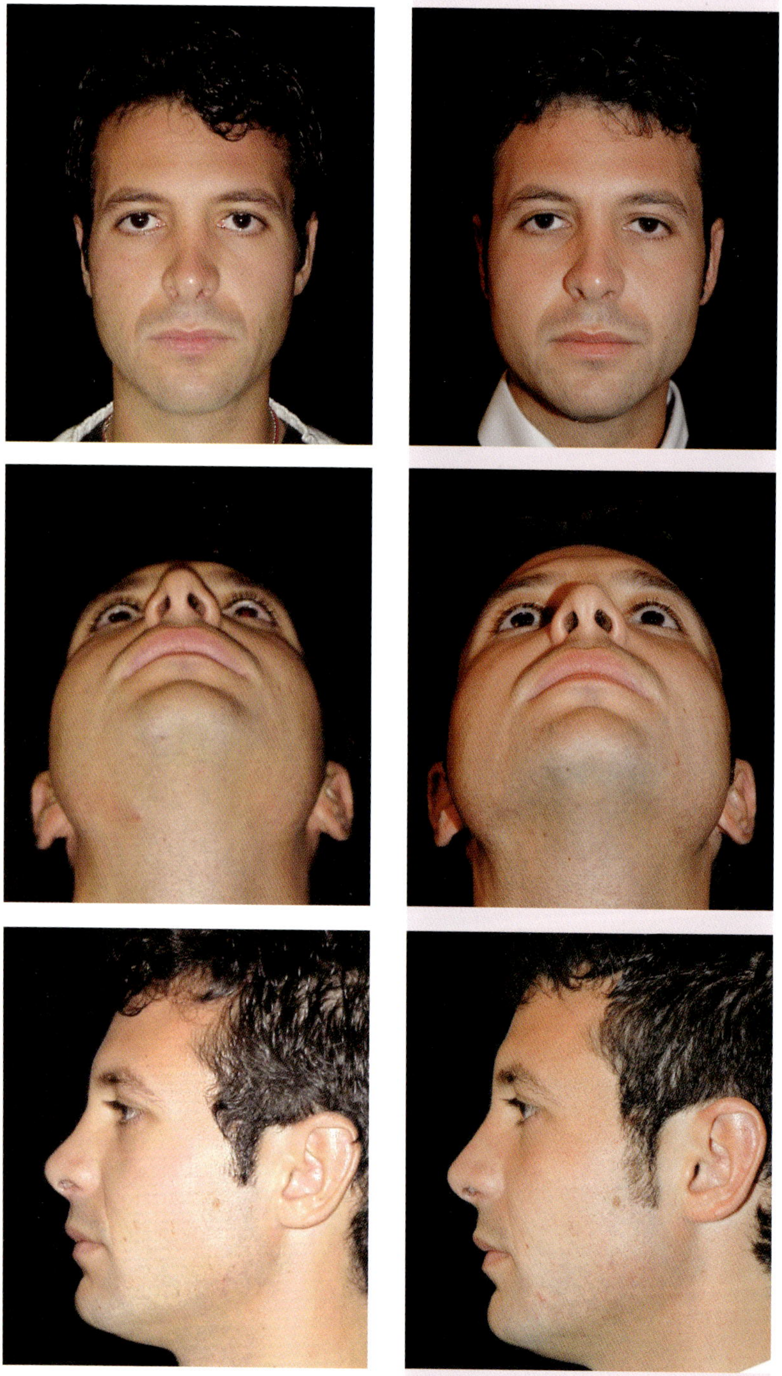

Correction: secondary rhinoplasty. Septum shortened near the anterior nasal spine. A cartilage graft is harvested from the septum and inserted along the lower edge of the lateral crus to correct the overly arched nostrils. PTFE graft placed on the dorsum.

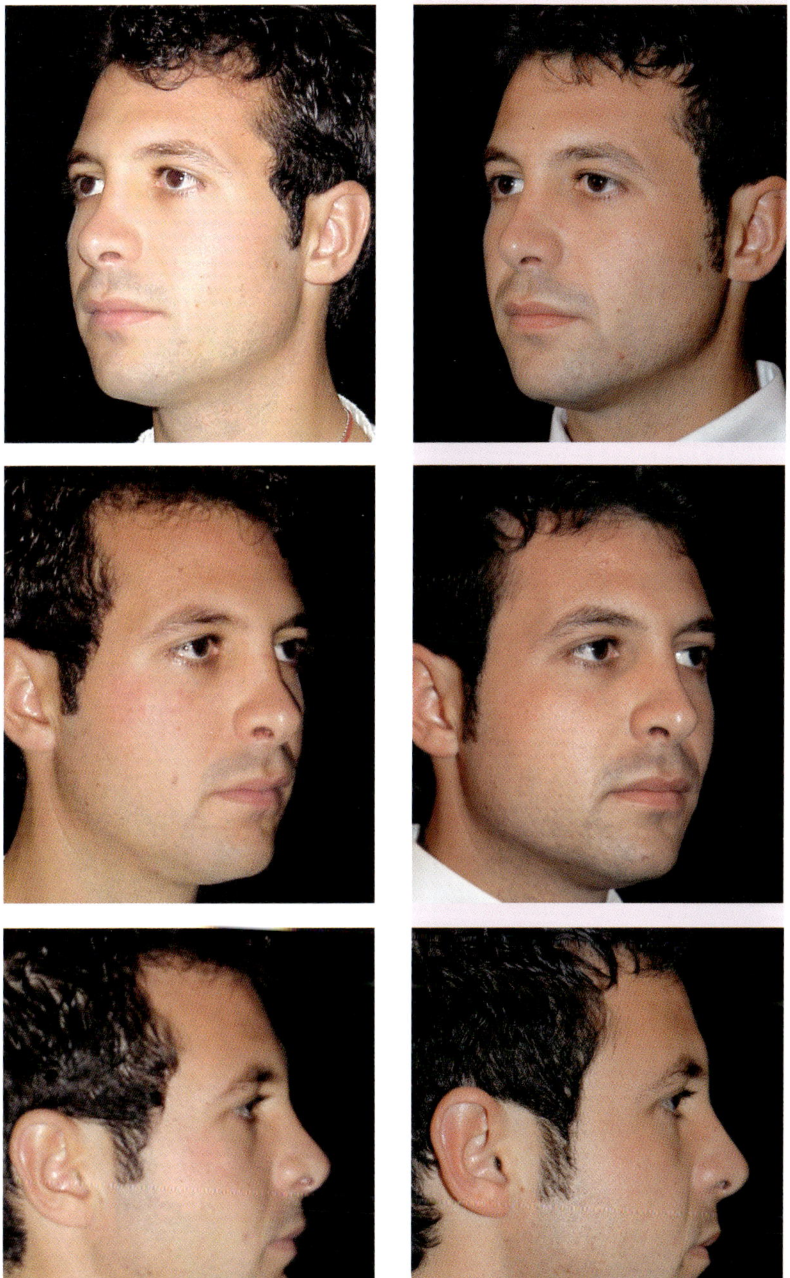

CASE 9

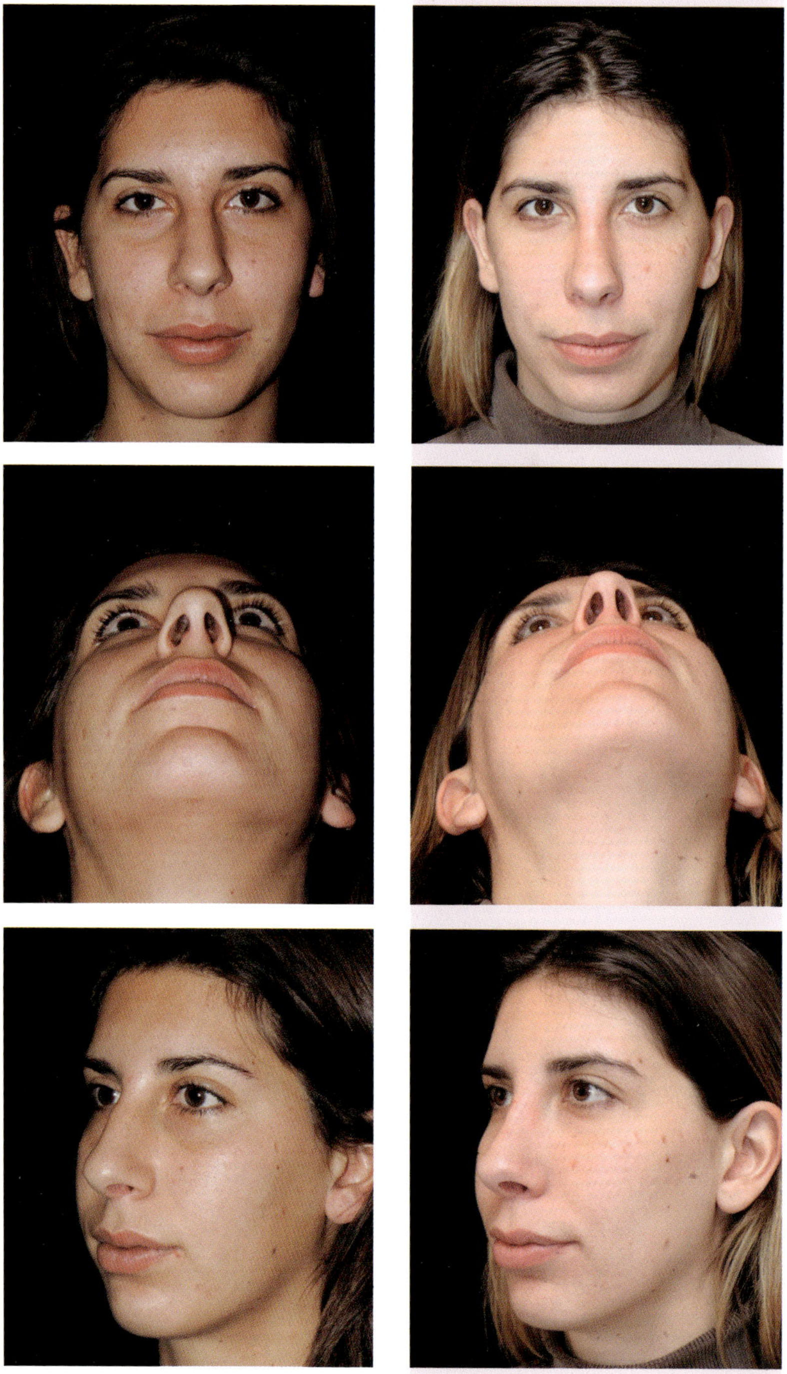

Rhinoplasty: lowered dorsum, shortened septum, reduction of the tip with hockey stick technique. The lateral crus of alar cartilages were undermined and their lateral apex reduced in order to allow a change of the relationship with the overlying skin permitting a

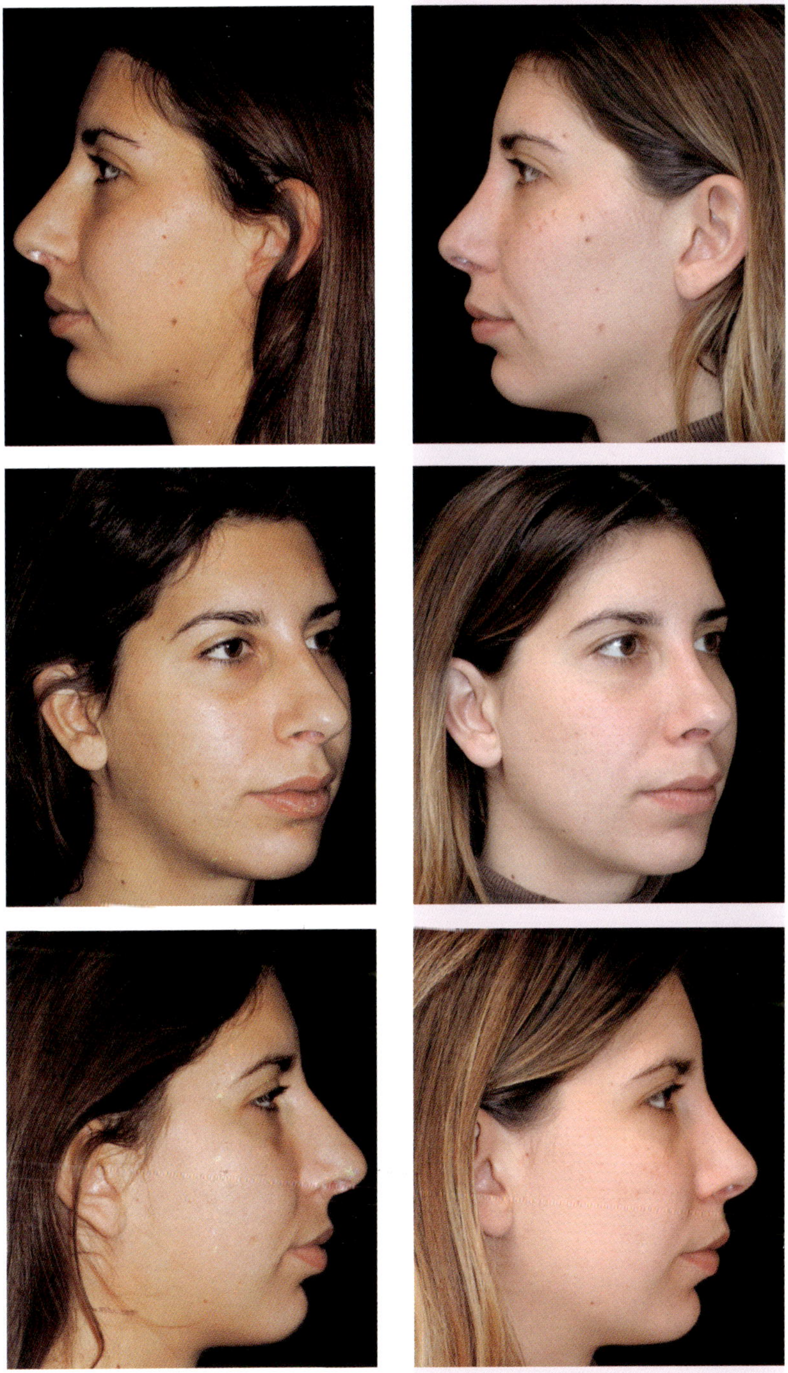

more efficient lateral sliding of the cartilages. The triangular cartilages were undermined and shortened respecting the angles as indicated by Sheen. Reduction of the nostrils. Basal osteotomies.

CASE 10

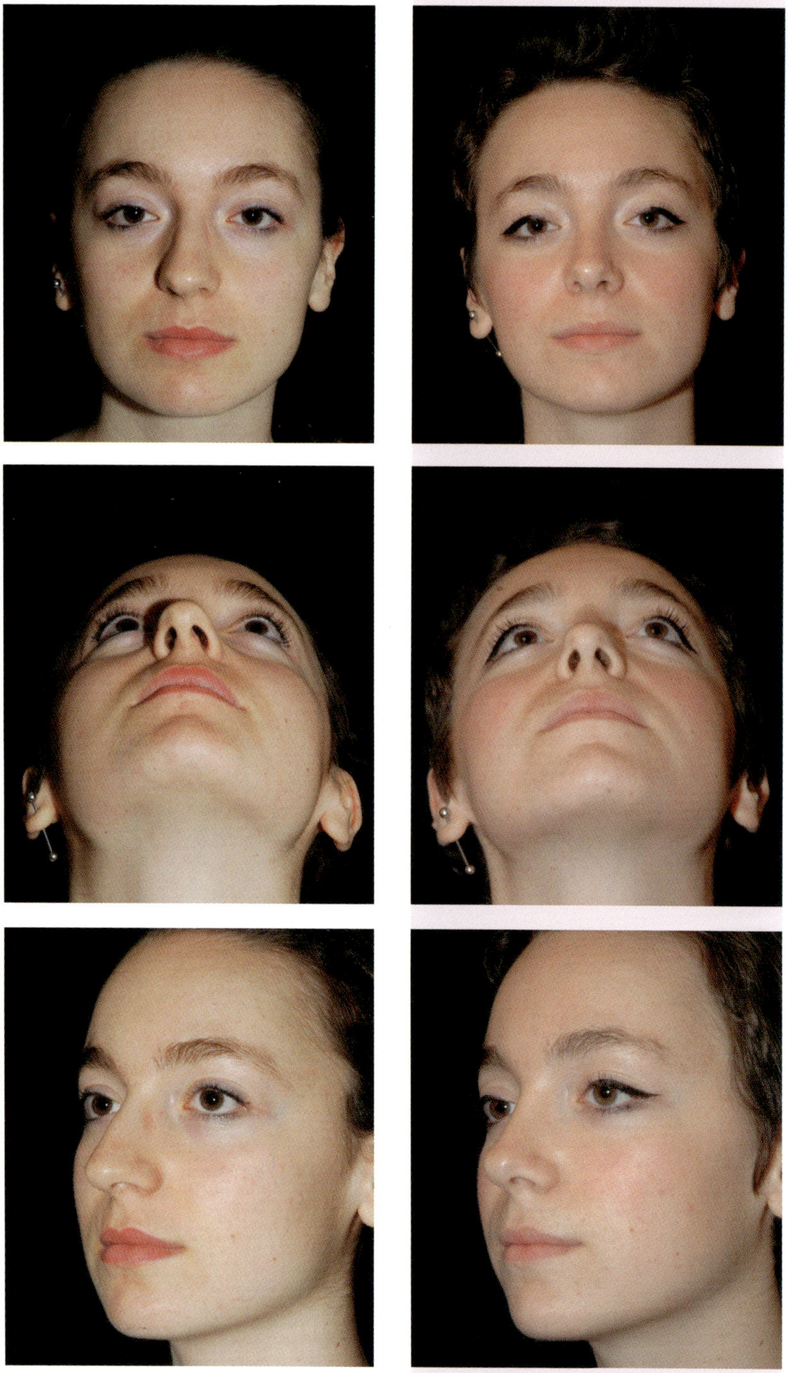

Rhinoplasty: lowered dorsum, shortened and tilted septum, reduction of the tip with hockey stick technique. Fractured nasal spine: triangular cartilages undermined and shortened according to Sheen's. Access to the septoplasty elevating bilaterally the chondromucosa

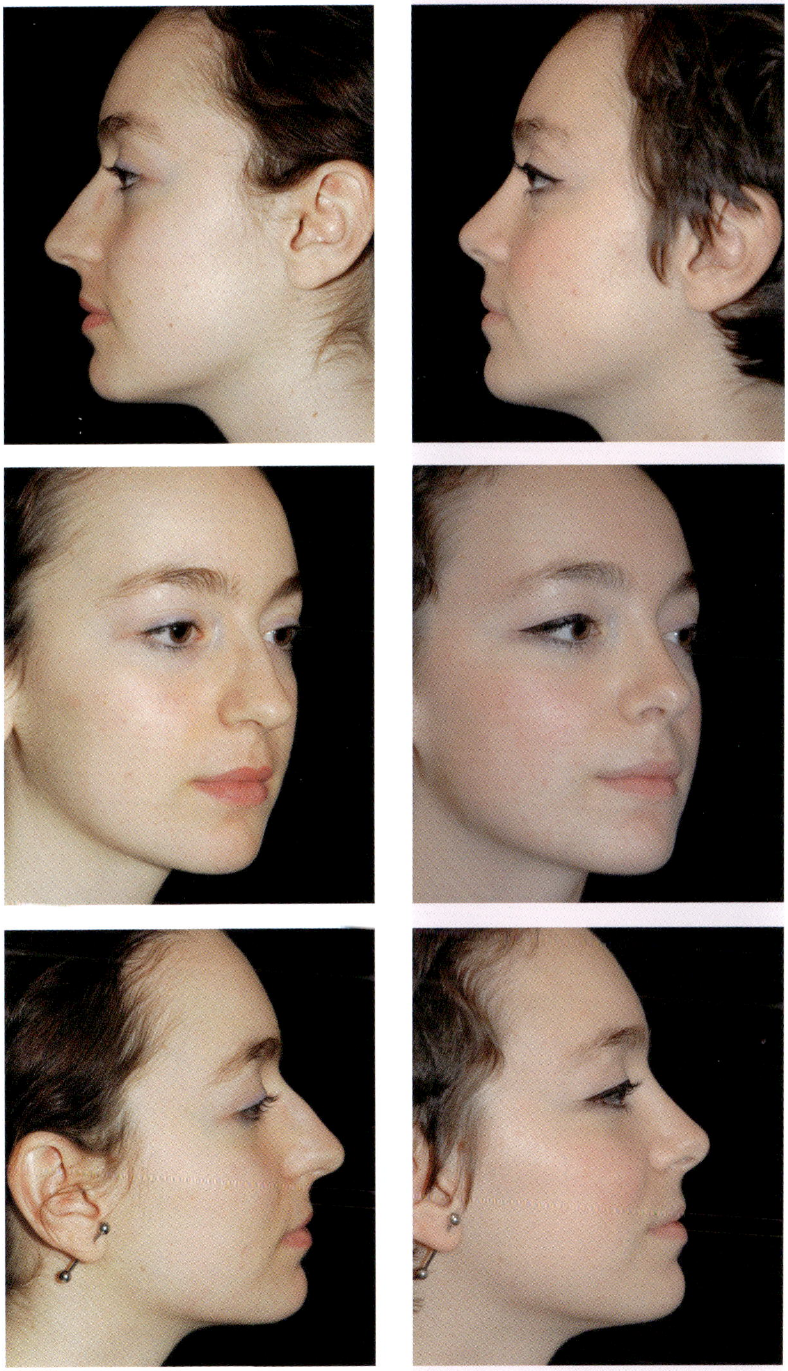

and correction of the left osteocartilagineous deviation at Cottle's area 4 according to Killian. Anteriorly to the right a Rubin morselizer was used to allow the straightening of the caudal portion of the septum. Reduction of the left nostril. Basal osteotomies.

CASE 11

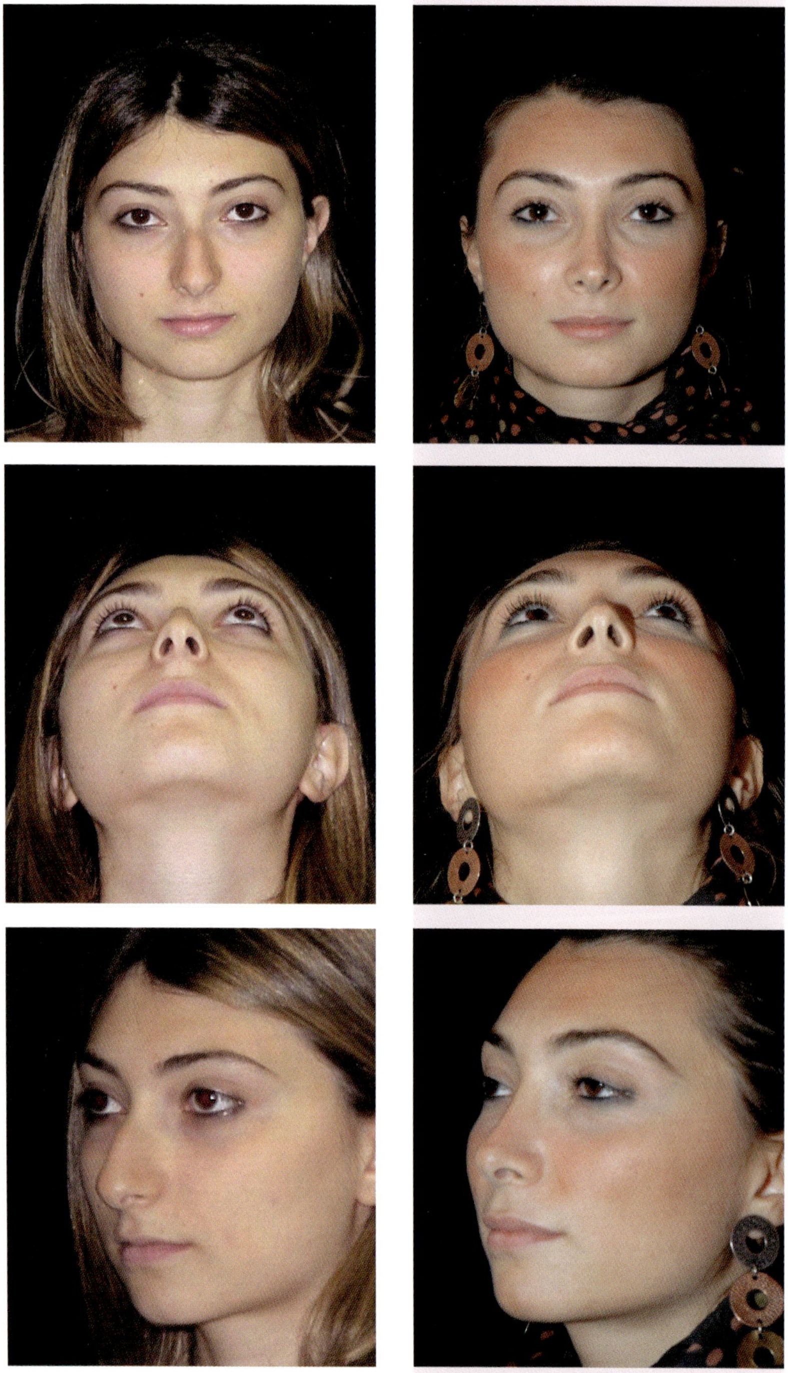

Rhinoplasty: lowered dorsum, shortened and tilted septum. Reduction of the tip with hockey stick technique. Triangular cartilages reduced according to Sheen's recommendations. Basal osteotomies.

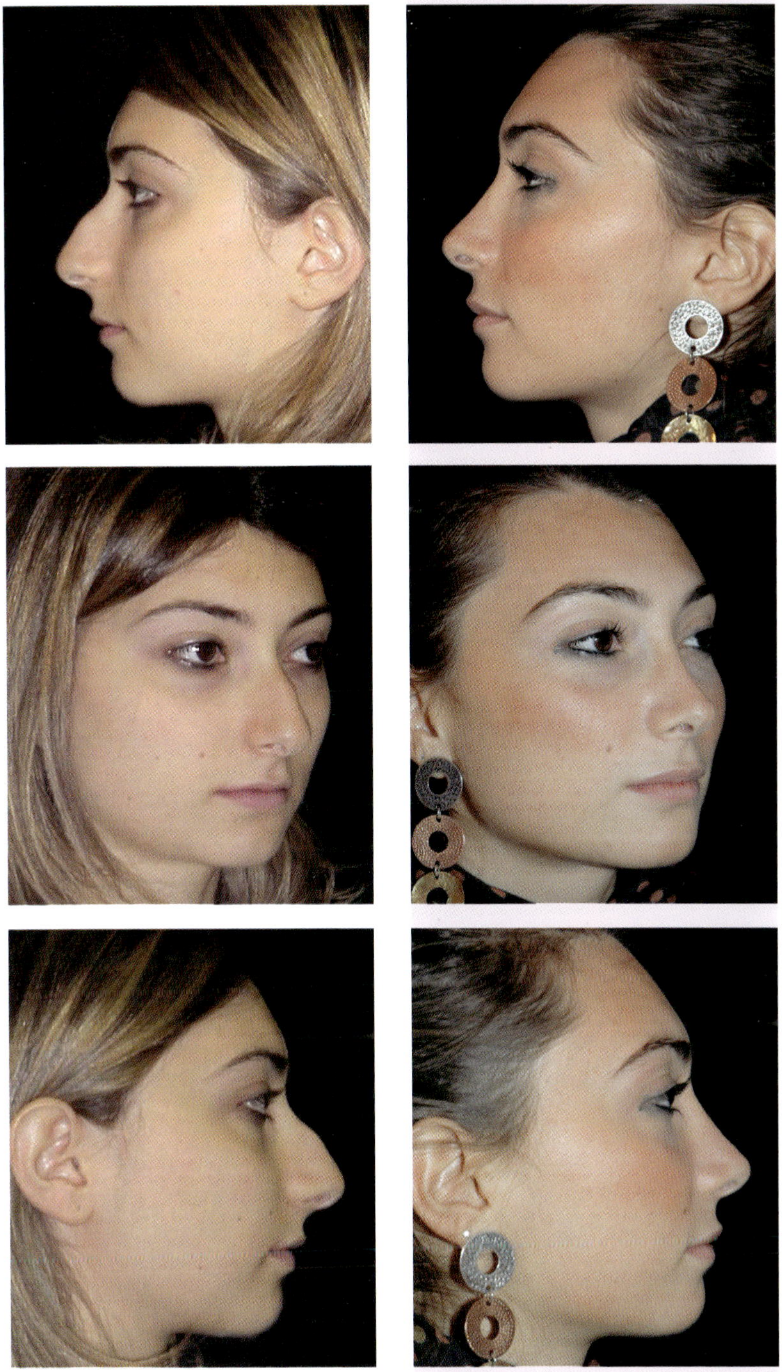

CASE 12

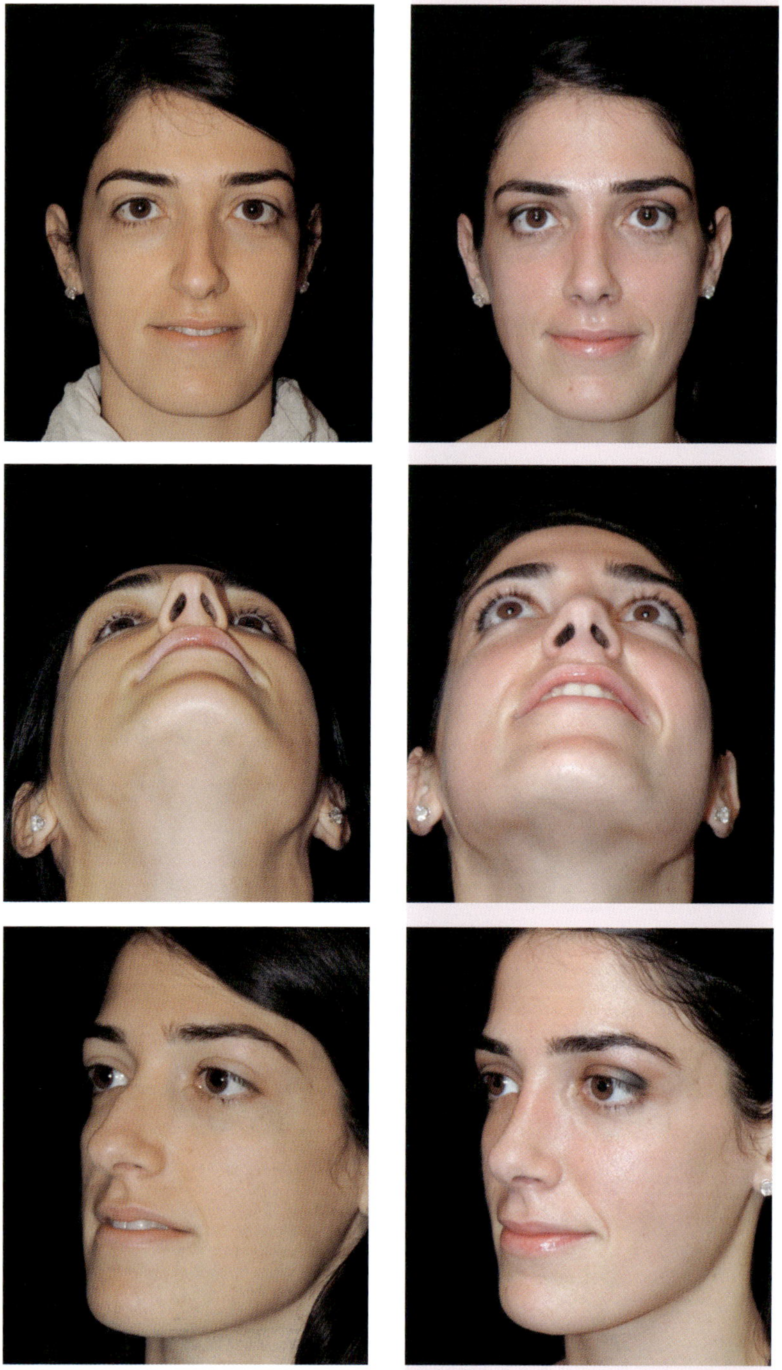

Rhinoplasty: lowered dorsum, shortened and tilted septum. Reduction of the alar cartilages with hockey stick technique. Reduction of the triangular cartilages according to Sheen's recommendations. During the surgery the apposition of cartilage graft at the level of

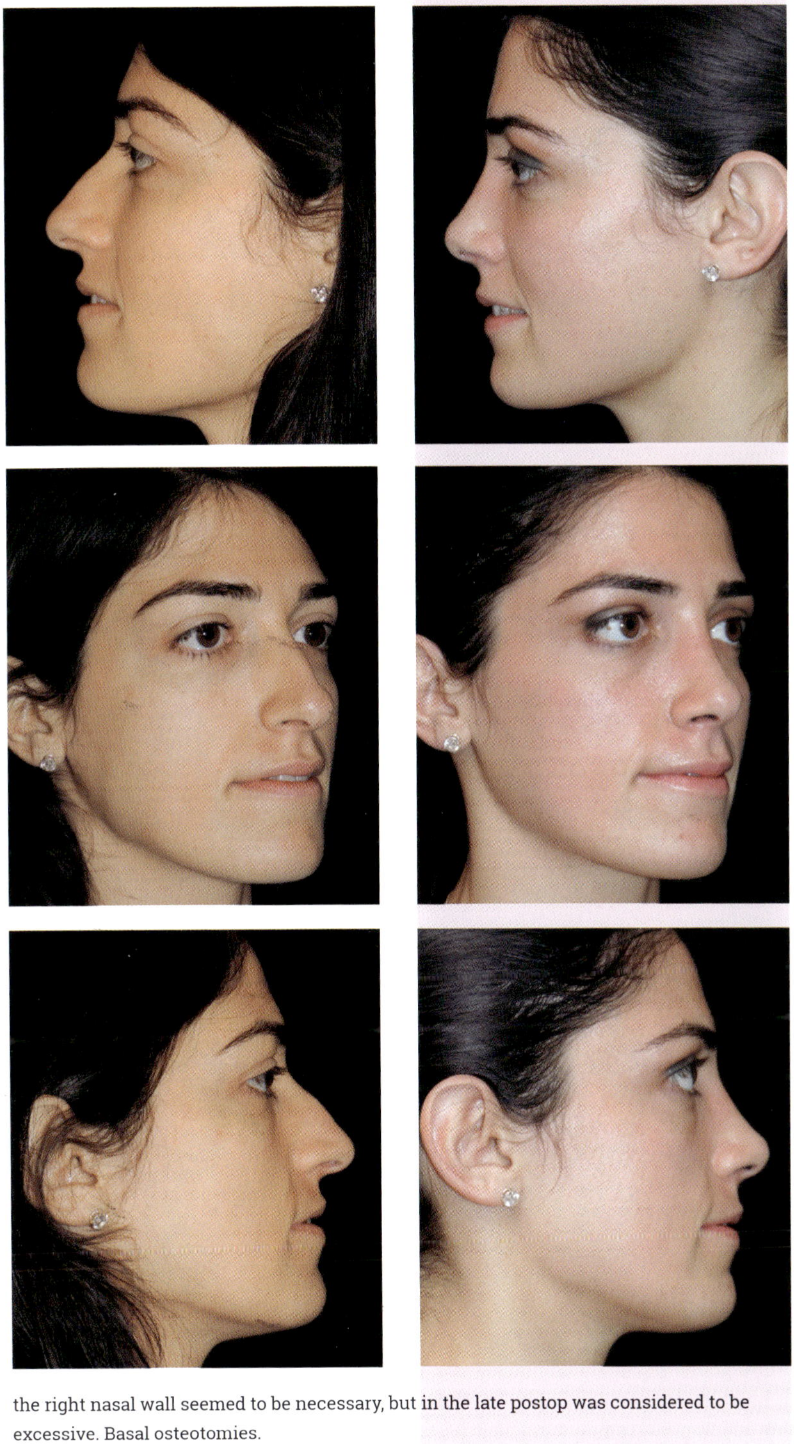

the right nasal wall seemed to be necessary, but in the late postop was considered to be excessive. Basal osteotomies.

CASE 13

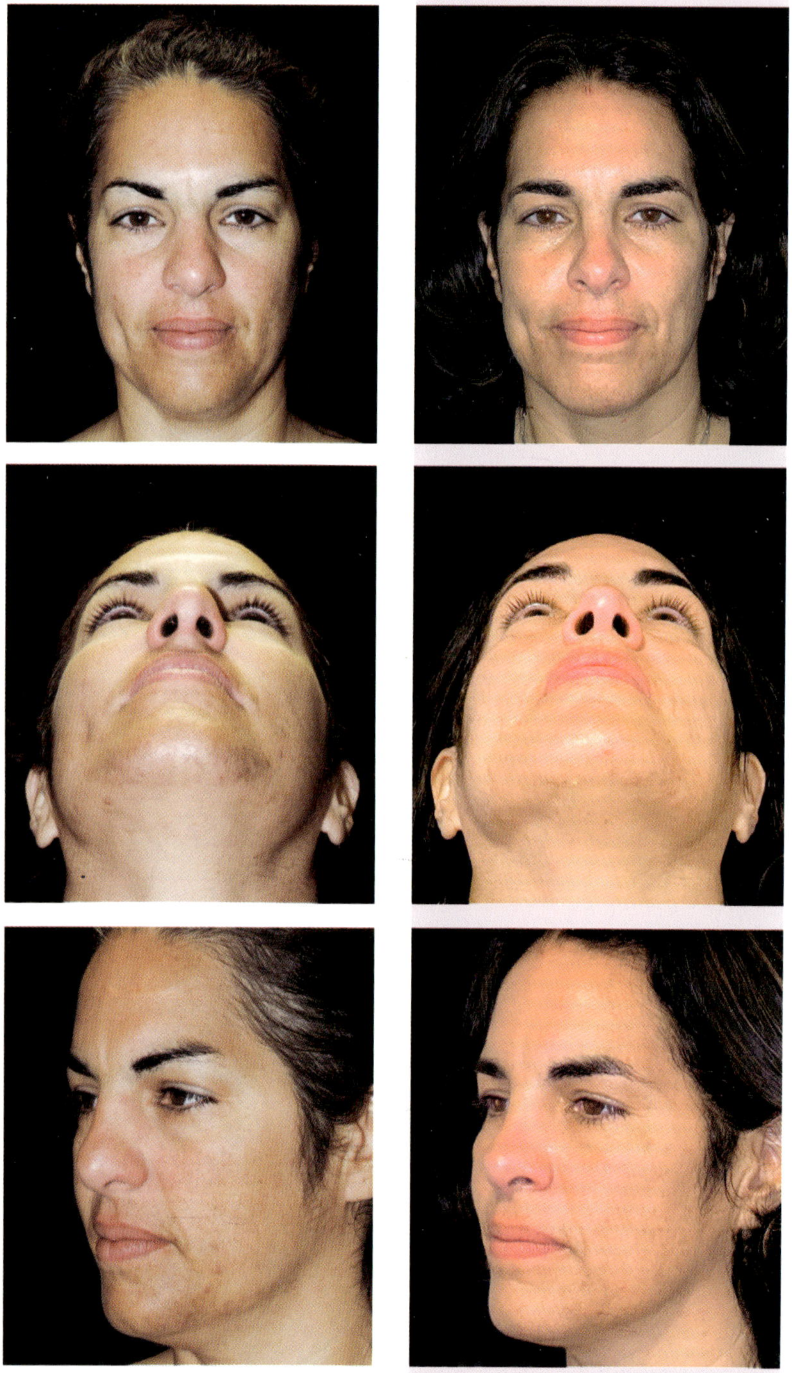

Rhinoplasty: lowered dorsum, shortened and tilted septum. Reduction of the tip with hockey stick technique. Triangular cartilages reduced according to Sheen's recommendations. Basal osteotomies.

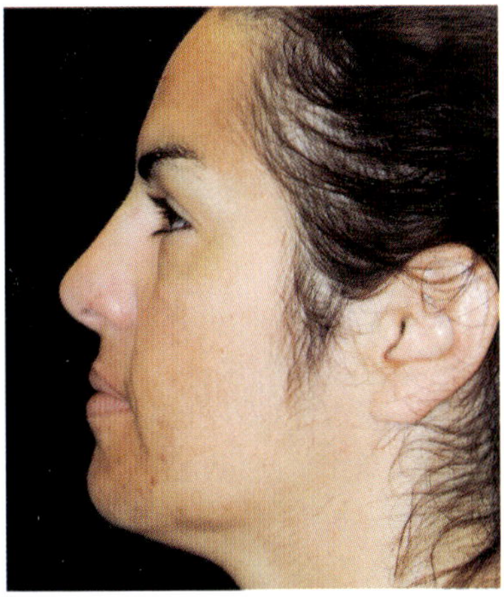

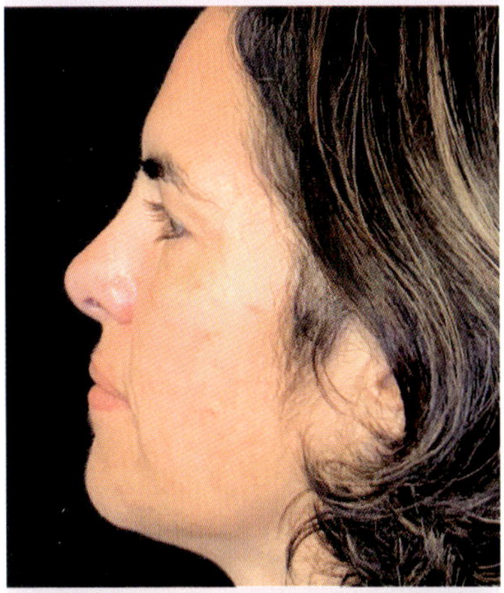

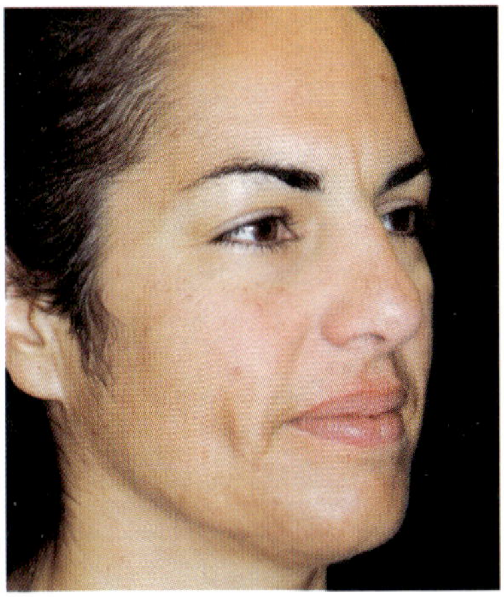

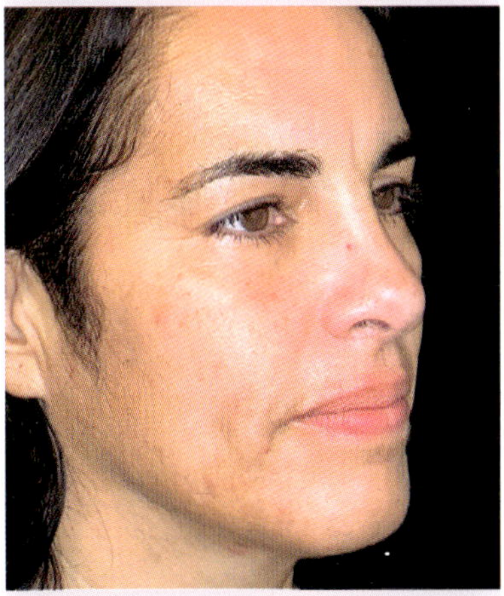

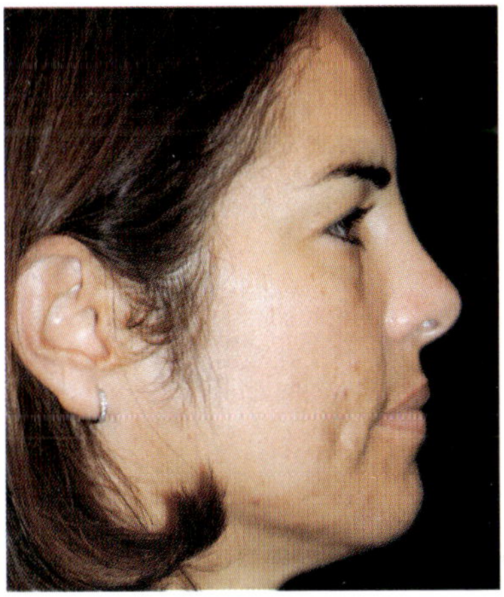

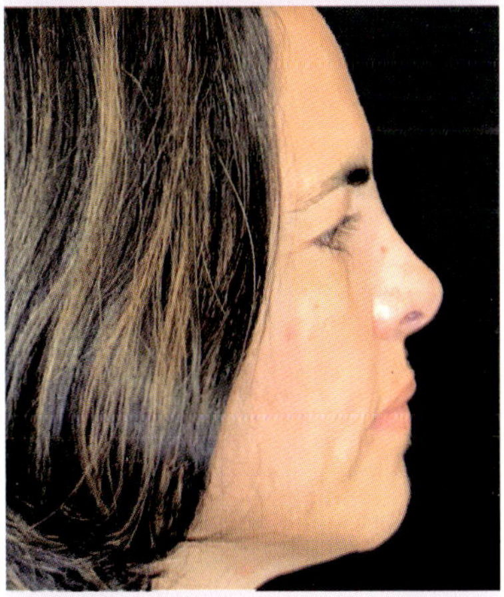

CASE 14

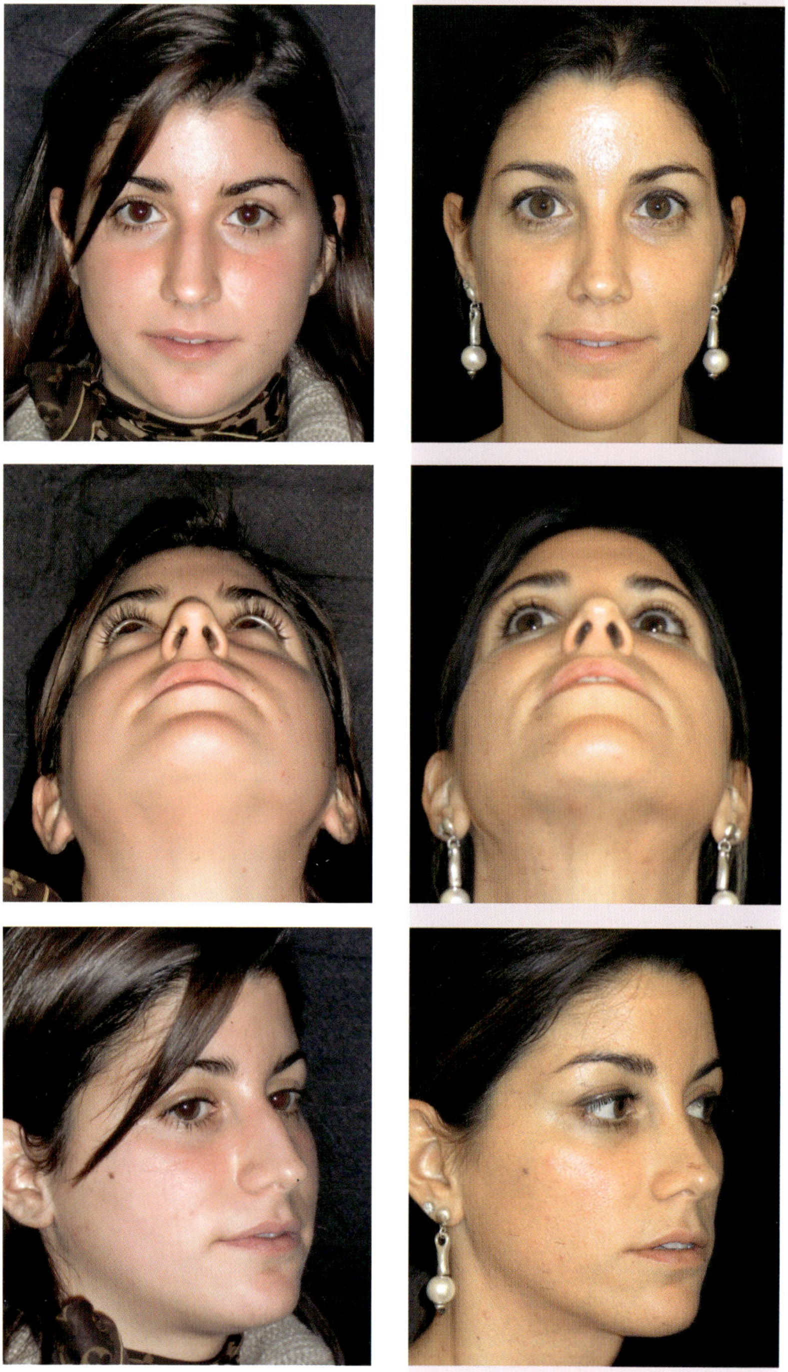

Rhinoplasty thirteen years later. Lowered dorsum, tip with hockey stick, osteotomies.

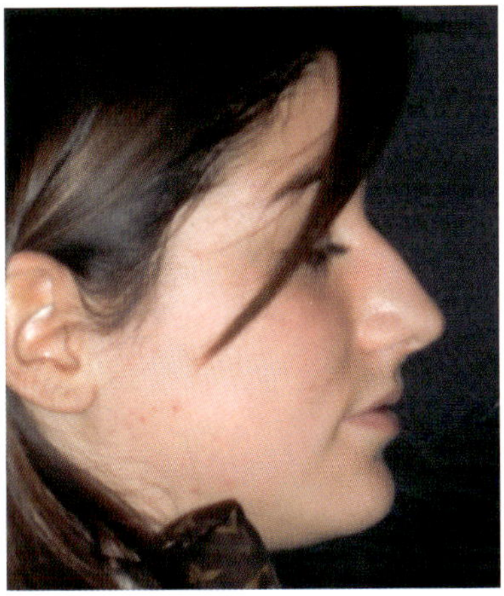
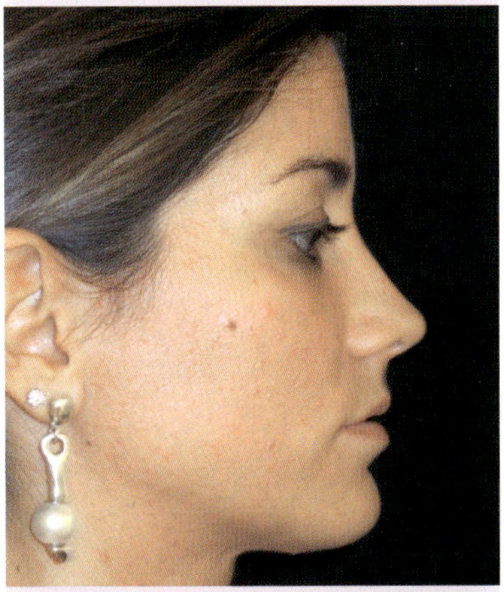
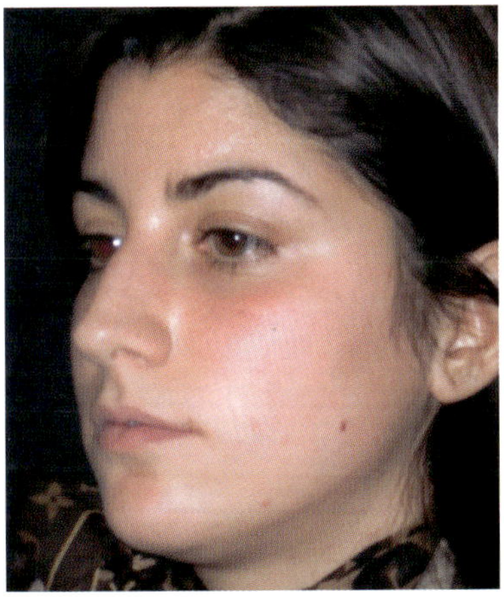
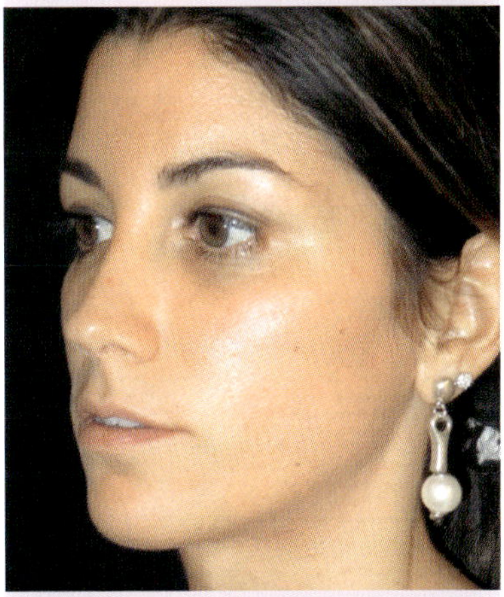
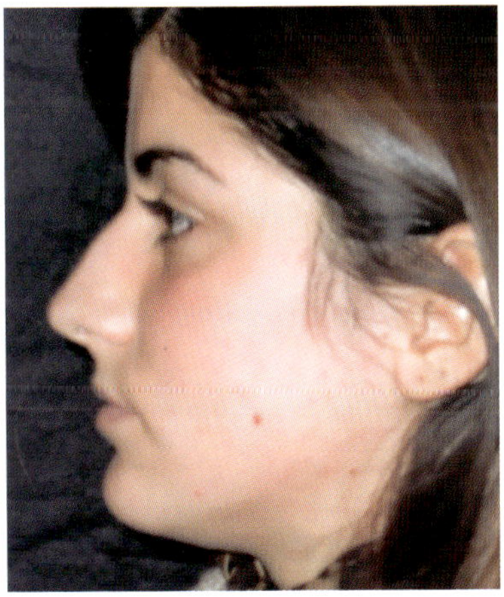
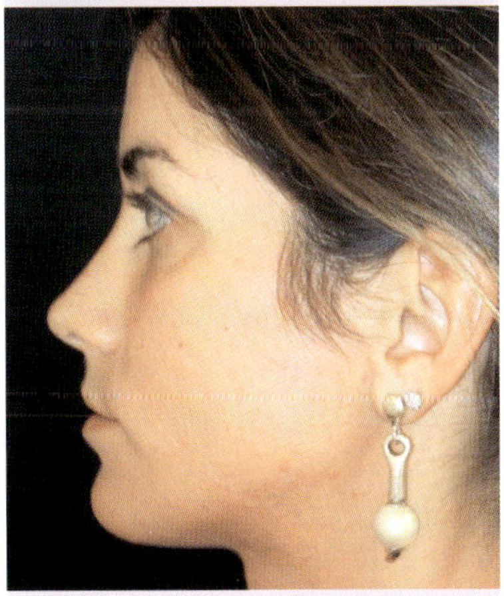

CASE 15

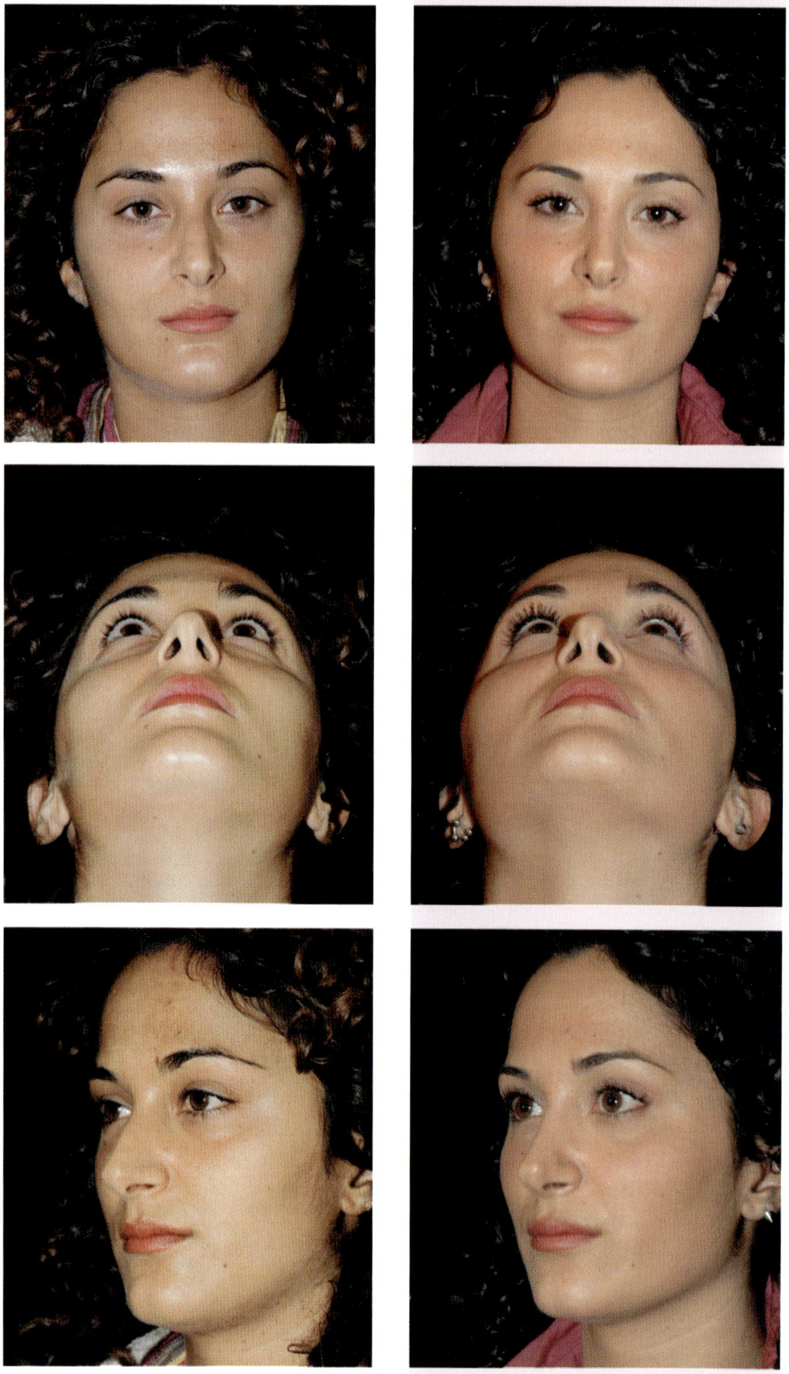

Rhinoplasty: dorsum lowered, septum shortened and tilted. Triangular cartilages reduced according to Sheen's recommendations. Tip reduction with hockey stick technique. The lateral crus of left alar cartilage was undermined and its lateral apex reduced in order to

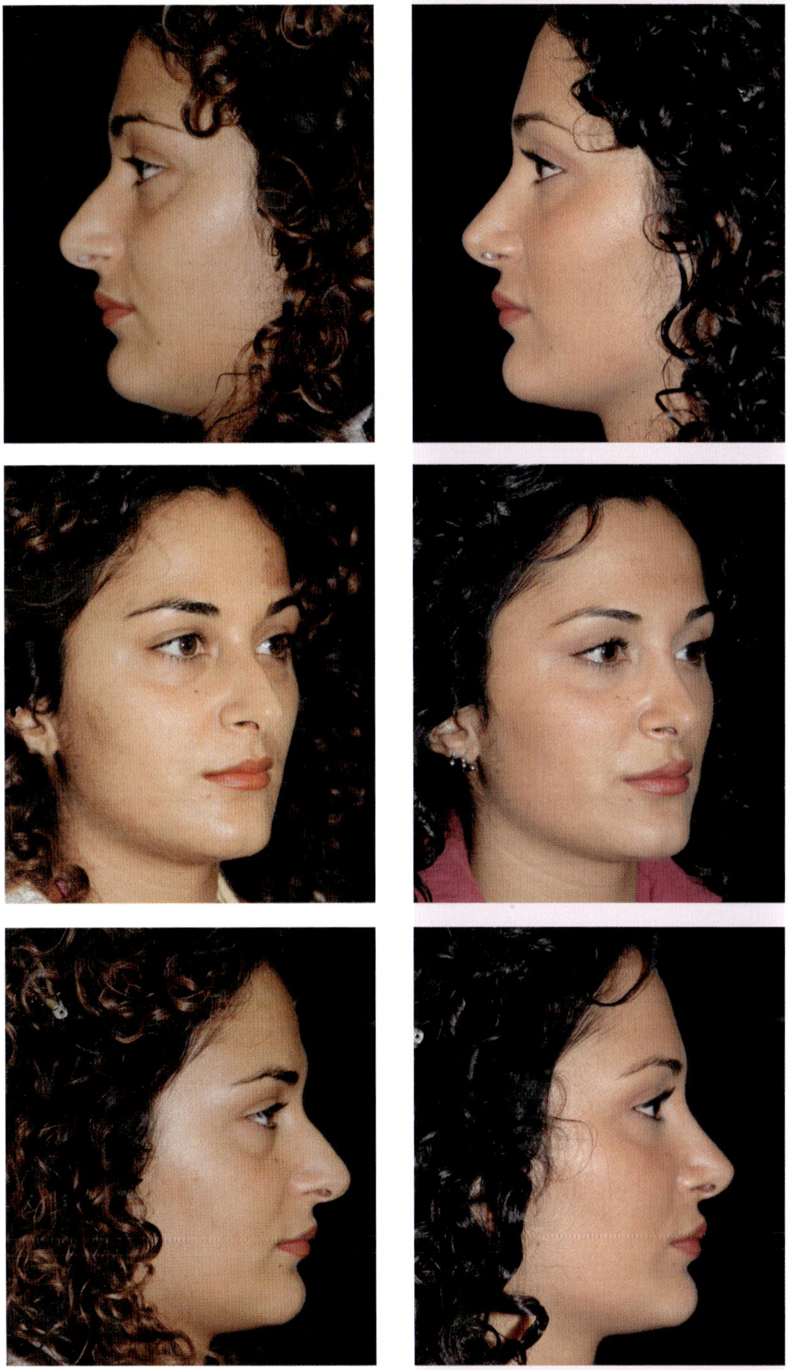

allow a change of the relationship with the overlying skin permitting a more efficient lateral sliding of the cartilages. Correction of the anterior left deviation of the septum. The anterior nasal spine was fractured to bring it to the midline. Osteotomies.